Musculoskeletal Imaging: Contemporary Perspectives

Musculoskeletal Imaging: Contemporary Perspectives

Editor: Ronnie O'Connor

AMERICAN
MEDICAL PUBLISHERS
www.americanmedicalpublishers.com

AMERICAN
MEDICAL PUBLISHERS
www.americanmedicalpublishers.com

Cataloging-in-Publication Data

Musculoskeletal imaging : contemporary perspectives / edited by Ronnie O'Connor.
p. cm.
Includes bibliographical references and index.
ISBN 978-1-63927-077-4
1. Musculoskeletal system--Imaging. 2. Musculoskeletal system--Diseases--Imaging.
3. Musculoskeletal system--Wounds and injuries--Imaging. I. O'Connor, Ronnie.
RC925.7 .M87 2022
616.707 548--dc23

American Medical Publishers,
41 Flatbush Avenue,
1st Floor, New York,
NY 11217, USA

ISBN 978-1-63927-077-4 (Hardback)

Contents

Preface

This book has been an outcome of determined endeavour from a group of educationists in the field. The primary objective was to involve a broad spectrum of professionals from diverse cultural background involved in the field for developing new researches. The book not only targets students but also scholars pursuing higher research for further enhancement of the theoretical and practical applications of the subject.

Musculoskeletal imaging is a technique of creating a visual representation of the musculoskeletal system for clinical analysis and medical intervention. It also helps in the assessment of musculoskeletal functions. Musculoskeletal imaging comprises of computed tomography scans, radiographs, magnetic resonance imaging, bone scans and musculoskeletal ultrasonography. High-resolution imaging has facilitated the evaluation of joint injuries, determines the cause of chronic pain, assesses joint replacements, image muscle disorders, and bone and soft tissue tumors. Several clinical procedures are image-guided such as certain biopsies, joint aspirations, peripheral nerve pain management, etc. This book discusses the fundamentals as well as modern approaches of musculoskeletal imaging. The various studies that are constantly contributing towards advancing technologies and evolution of musculoskeletal imaging are examined in detail. As this domain is emerging at a fast pace, this book will help the readers to better understand the contemporary perspectives in musculoskeletal imaging.

It was an honour to edit such a profound book and also a challenging task to compile and examine all the relevant data for accuracy and originality. I wish to acknowledge the efforts of the contributors for submitting such brilliant and diverse chapters in the field and for endlessly working for the completion of the book. Last, but not the least; I thank my family for being a constant source of support in all my research endeavours.

Editor

1

Manually defining regions of interest when quantifying paravertebral muscles fatty infiltration from axial magnetic resonance imaging: a proposed method for the lumbar spine with anatomical cross-reference

Rebecca J. Crawford[1,2*], Jon Cornwall[3,1], Rebecca Abbott[4] and James M. Elliott[4,5,1]

Abstract

Background: There is increasing interest in paravertebral muscle composition as a potential prognostic and diagnostic element in lumbar spine health. As a consequence, it is becoming popular to use magnetic resonance imaging (MRI) to examine muscle volume and fatty infiltration in lumbar paravertebral muscles to assess both age-related change and their clinical relevance in low back pain (LBP). A variety of imaging methods exist for both measuring key variables (fat, muscle) and for defining regions of interest, making pooled comparisons between studies difficult and rendering post-production analysis of MRIs confusing. We therefore propose and define a method as an option for use as a standardized MRI procedure for measuring lumbar paravertebral muscle composition, and to stimulate discussion towards establishing consensus for the analysis of skeletal muscle composition amongst clinician researchers.

Method: In this descriptive methodological study we explain our method by providing an examination of regional lumbar morphology, followed by a detailed description of the proposed technique. Identification of paravertebral muscles and vertebral anatomy includes axial E12 sheet-plastinates from cadaveric material, combined with a series of axial MRIs that encompass sequencing commonly used for investigations of muscle quality (fat-water DIXON, T1-, and T2-weighted) to illustrate regional morphology; these images are shown for L1 and L4 levels to highlight differences in regional morphology. The method for defining regions of interest (ROI) for multifidus (MF), and erector spinae (ES) is then described.

Results: Our method for defining ROIs for lumbar paravertebral muscles on axial MRIs is outlined and discussed in relation to existing literature. The method provides a foundation for standardising the quantification of muscle quality that particularly centres on examining fatty infiltration and composition. We provide recommendations relating to imaging parameters that should additionally inform a priori decisions when planning studies examining lumbar muscle tissues with MRI.

(Continued on next page)

* Correspondence: rebecca.crawford@zhaw.ch
[1]Institute for Health Sciences, Zurich University of Applied Sciences, Technikumstrasse 81, Postfach, CH-8401 Winterthur, Switzerland
[2]Faculty of Health Professions, Curtin University, Perth, Australia
Full list of author information is available at the end of the article

(Continued from previous page)

Conclusions: We intend this method to provide a platform towards developing and delivering meaningful comparisons between MRI data on lumbar paravertebral muscle quality.

Keywords: Lumbar spine, Paravertebral muscles, Fat infiltration, Magnetic resonance imaging, Region of interest, Manual segmentation, Multifidus, Erector spinae

Background

Magnetic resonance imaging (MRI) has been used for several decades to examine musculoskeletal morphology and pathology, providing insight into tissue composition, disease characterization, response to injury, and changes due to mechanical stress [1, 2]. Advances in MRI technology have elevated the ubiquitous analysis of skeletal muscle composition, and as a consequence, measures towards quantifying muscle fatty infiltration (MFI) have become widely reported with equivocal results.

While data for age-related, degenerative changes to lumbar bones and joints in asymptomatic people have been published [3], few studies assess age-related alterations in paravertebral muscle morphology [4–7]. Cross-sectional [8–12] and longitudinal studies [13] evaluating paravertebral muscle quality indicate a positive relationship between MFI and low back pain (LBP) (i.e. increased fat infiltration is associated with the presence and severity of LBP). It is also suggested that examining muscle quality through MFI measurement is potentially complimentary, if not more relevant, to measurement of quantity (e.g. cross sectional area and/or volume alone) in the assessment of muscle degeneration [14–17]. However, inconsistent associations are also reported [18] and confounded by normative age-related changes [5, 7, 19], degenerative features of the vertebrae or discs [9, 19, 20], and spinal curvature [21, 22].

While several MRI approaches are possible to measure the water and fat species of skeletal muscle, the contemporary standard for evaluating muscle size and structure is chemical-shift MRI, producing water- and fat-only images from dual- and/or multi-echo acquisitions [11, 23–25]. Excellent accuracy has been shown for manual segmentation based on these imaging techniques against spectroscopy [11] and histology [26], and for some common neuromusculoskeletal conditions [23, 27] including LBP [11, 28]. The chemical shift (DIXON in the Siemens environment, IDEAL [iterative least squares solution] in the General Electric environment, mDIXON (Philips), FatSep™ (Hitachi), or WFS (Toshiba)) method collects data at echo times when fat and water are in-phase and out-of-phase. The data can then be combined to generate a co-registered fat and water image, although this method is not immune to field inhomogeneities. Current methods towards improving the estimation of fat and water images have used the IDEAL method, which has been applied successfully for the liver and musculoskeletal system [29, 30]. Despite such reports and technological advances, the vast majority of population-based studies examining pathoanatomical features of the lumbar spine (e.g. including muscle, other soft-tissues such as the intervertebral disc, and the skeletal vertebral column) use conventional T1-weighted [18, 31] or T2-weighted [13, 32] MRI. While different, and potentially less accurate when compared to chemical-shift imaging [14, 29, 30, 33], the data derived from these investigations represent a resource of immeasurable value to investigators interested in the role of all spinal elements.

Despite the obvious usefulness of assessing spinal muscle quality using MRI, a robust and easily replicated platform for acquiring and assessing imaging data on muscle composition remains elusive. Currently, comparisons between studies are challenging and often not possible when investigators have used different manual, semi-automated, or automated segmentation software, programmes, or methods for defining the regions of interest for each muscle (see Table 1 for a summary of published methods). As such, the aetiological significance of MFI in spinal muscles remains unclear. Moreover, efforts to simulate and model muscle activity in both healthy and clinical populations are dependent on accuracy in defining where tissues with different tensile properties (e.g. muscle versus fatty deposits) are located, and there are no widely adopted or standardized assessment tools currently utilized for this purpose. In order to better understand the influence of MFI content on spinal health, it is imperative that common methodologies are developed and adopted in order to facilitate standardization and accurate comparison of data between studies.

We consider that standardized and easily replicated methods enabling consistent MFI quantification are urgently required to facilitate widespread adoption of an agreed technique in measuring muscle quality. While there is a general trend toward optimising automated methodologies that quantify muscle composition based on differential tissue signal intensities, even the newest, time-efficient tools require a degree of manual input in defining regions of interest (ROI) [34–36]. A standardised ROI method is arguably most important for these studies where it has been speculated that difficulties identifying morphology results in poorer repeatability

Table 1 Representative literature summary of methods in investigations describing paravertebral muscle analysis using magentic resonance imaging (MRI)

Citation	Reliability	MRI Sequence	Slice Selection	Muscles of Interest	ROI Selection	Fat Detection	Measure
Antony et al., 2016 [52]	No	T2 FRFSE	1 slice per level at IVD L3-S1	MF, ES	Semi-Automated interactive Segmentation (intelligent scissors)	Semi-Automated User set pixel intensity threshold	FCSA = (CSAFat)/(CSATotal)
Battaglia et al. 2014 [53]	2 raters ($n = 25$); Qualitative: Intra-rater weighted kappa = 0.71–0.93, Inter-rater kappa = 0.76–0.85; Quantitative: Inter-rater ICC = 0.73–0.90	T1	1 slice per level at IVD L4-5, L5-S1	MF	Qualitative: visual inspection; Quantitative ImageJ manual trace, exclude fascial boder between MF and ES	Qualitative: Goutallier Classification (0,1,2,3,4); Quantitative: pixel intensity range set by user selected fat ROI within MF	% fat = (# of fat pixels)/(total # of pixels)
Beneck et al., 2012 [12]	1 rater; intra-rater: ICC (3,1) = 0.961 for CSA	T1	All slices spanning L4, L5-S1, and S2-S3 vertebral bodies	MF, ES	Slice-o-matic manual trace	Muscle divided into 6–9 regions. Gray-scale signal threshold semi-automatically determined for each region based on user selected small region of muscle	Muscle volume = total volume – fat volume
Bhadresha et al., 2016 [19]	2 raters ($n = 20$); inter-rater ICC = 0.33–0.76, Cronbach's alpha = 0.59–0.91	T2 FSE	I slice per level at IVD L3-4, L4-5, L5-S1	MF, ES, PS	Visual inspection	18x27 (1 cm apart) grid applied to image. By visual inspection: # of grid points touching fat vs. muscle counted	Muscle to Fat Ratio= Muscle/#fat pixels
Crawford et al., 2016 [5]	No	2-point DIXON (3D fast-field echo T1) whole body	Every 3rd slice L1-L5 (with interpolation to full volume)	MF, ES	Semiautomatic segmentation with linear interpolation (Myrian Intrasense, Paris, France)	Semi-automated ROI from water to fat image	Fat signal fraction (FSF) = (Signalfat/[Signalwater + Signalfat])*100
D'Hooge et al., 2012 [10]	No	T1 FSE	1 slice per level at L3 superior endplate, L4 superior endplate, L4 inferior endplate	MF, ES, PS	ImageJ manual trace	Automated based on pixel intensity gray-scale threshold	MFI = (signal intensity of "lean muscle")/(signal intensity of user defined fat ROI)
Fortin et al., 2014 [13]	1 rater; intra-rater: ICC = 0.90 –0.96)	T2	1 slice per level at IVD L3-4 and L5-S1	MF, ES, MF + ES	ImageJ manual trace following fascial borders	User selected pixel intensity gray-scale threshold selected from 4–6 sample ROIs within visible 'lean muscle'	FCSA = (CSAFat)/(CSATotal); Proportion estimate of muscle fat content = Average signal intensity of Total ROI
Hebert et al., 2014 [18]	1 rater; intra-rater ($n = 30$) ICC (3 1) = 0.93, Bias = −0.70, 95% LOA = −8.11-6.72	T1 SE (0.2 Tesla)	1 slice per level at L4 and L5	MF	Manual trace	Custom MatLab script; threshold set from midpoint between histogram peaks for 'fat and muscle'	% IMAT = CSAFat/CSATotal (IMAT = intramuscular adipose tissue)

Table 1 Representative literature summary of methods in investigations describing paravertebral muscle analysis using magentic resonance imaging (MRI) *(Continued)*

Hu et al., 2011 [54]	3 raters ($n = 29$); intra-rater ICC (3,1) for FCSA = 0.832–0.847, for T2 SI = 0.926–0.957; inter-rater CC for FCSA = 0.858–0.894, for T2 SI = 0.891–0.923	T2 FSE	1 slice per level at IVD L3-4, L4-5, L5-S1	MF, ES	PACS workstation manual trace: lean muscle CSA Drawn avoiding visible fat; Fat% - following outer perimeter	PACS embedded ROI and gray-scale histogram software calculated from mean T2 signal intensity	Lean muscle FCSA = Manually traced Muscle CSA Fat Infiltration = T2 signal intensity
Kjaer et al., 2007 [8]	2 raters ($n = 50$); intra-rater k = 0.86; inter-rater k = 0.58	T1 SE (0.2 Tesla)	1 slice per level at IVD L3-4, L4-5, L5-S1	MF	Visual Inspection	Visual categorization: Normal 0–10%, slight 10–50%, severe > 50% fat	Fat infiltration = (0,1,2)
Paalanne et al., 2011 [28]	2 raters ($n = 35$); intra-rater ICC = 0.86–0.88, inter-rater ICC = 0.85–0.87	T1 FSPGR (In-Phase and Opposed-Phase)	1 slice at upper endplate of L4	MF, ES	neaView Radiology; manual trace	Average Signal Intensity	Relative signal loss = (IP SI – OP SI)/ (IP SI)*100%
Pezolato et al., 2012 [22]	2 raters ($n = 10$); intra-rater ICC = 0.90–0.94, inter-rater ICC = 0.86–0.83	T2 FSE	2 slices per level at upper and lower endplates of L1-L5	MF, MF + ES	ImageJ manual trace	Grayscale threshold	Fat infiltrate = TotalCSA – FCSA
Ranson et al., 2005 [55]	1 rater ($n = 6$) × 3: average intra-rater ICC = 0.97	T2	1 slice per level at lower vertebral endplate of L1-L5; upper vertebral end plate of L5-S1	MF, ES, PS, QL	ImageJ manual trace following fascial borders	Grey scale pixel intensity range for muscle, fat, and bone were determined from histogram of manual ROIs of "lean paraspinal muscle", inter-muscular fat, and vertebral body for either: method 1: global grey scale range (0–120); Method 2: slice specific grey scale range	FCSA = TotalCSA of pixels within grey-scale range for fat
Shahidi et al., 2016 [48]	No	T2	1 slice at L4 (to standardize CSA across individuals)	MF, ES	Quantitative manual trace using MatLab	Pixels identified as either fat or muscle by fitting a two term Gaussian model to the pixel intensities histogram of from segmented ROIs; identified intersection where pixel values above classified as fat and pixels below classified as muscle.	Cross Sectional Area Fat signal fraction = *n*pixels fat/*n*pixels fat + *n*pixels muscle
Valentin et al., 2015 [7]	1 rater ($n = 24$); intra-rater ICC = 0.88–0.99	T1	All slices spanning lower endplate of L5 to upper endplate of L1 (10 mm slice thickness)	MF, ES, PS, RA	Analyze Direct Manual trace	Average SI	MFI = (Muscle SI)/ (Subcutaneous Fat SI)

PS **Psoas Major,** ***MF*** **Multifidus,** ***ES*** **Erector Spinae,** ***QL*** **Quadratus Lumborum,** ***RA*** **Rectus Abdominus,** ***FCSA*** **Functional Cross Sectional Area,** ***SI*** **Signal Intensity,** ***IP*** **In-Phase (Water),** ***OP*** **Opposed-Phase (Fat),** ***FSPGR*** **Fast-Spoiled Gradient Echo,** ***ROI*** **Region of Interest**

[34]. With continued improvements and uptake of MRI technology, analyses utilizing a common method for the identification of ROI's could result in increasing insight and clinical translation within this important area of study. The purpose of this proposed method is therefore to provide an option for use as a standardized MRI procedure for measuring lumbar paravertebral muscle composition, and to stimulate discussion towards establishing consensus for the analysis of skeletal muscle composition amongst clinician researchers.

Method

Challenges for producing a region of interest of lumbar muscles: Important background for developing the proposed method

Detailed descriptions of the complex anatomy of lumbar paravertebral muscles and definitions regarding the spatial distribution of MFI on axial MRI are limited [37–40]. Published images demonstrating investigators' definition of ROI for these muscles predominantly depict the lower lumbar levels, with limited identification of separate muscles. Further, descriptions lack details towards acknowledging the complex three-dimensional structure that produces a changing spatial relationship observed across lumbar segmental levels. The lumbar paravertebral muscles typically examined in such studies include: multifidus (MF) as the largest lumbar spinotransverse muscles; erector spinae (ES) including lumbar longissimus and iliocostalis; and less frequently, psoas (including major and minor), and quadratus lumborum (see Fig. 1). This paper intentionally focuses on MF and ES as these are presumed to have the greatest clinical significance. However, other paravertebral muscles exist in the lumbar spine (e.g. the lumbar interspinales and intertransversarii, and thoracic semispinalis), yet they are generally not mentioned in descriptive investigations. This may relate to a lack of image resolution with available sequences, making it challenging to accurately delineate individual muscles from adjacent structures, and it therefore remains unclear how they should be treated when defining ROIs.

Our proposed method outlined in the results section, provides a foundational solution for the problem of how to measure muscles traversing the lumbar spine, and includes suggestions on operational characteristics for acquiring MR images. While we offer this starting point for a common methodology to facilitate accurate definition of lumbar muscle ROI, we are cognisant that the method is not a definitive end-point on 'how to'. We hope that with time and new research findings these methods will be modified, expanded, and refined.

Anatomically defining the muscles of interest

Figure 1 presents axial E-12 sheet-plastinates from cadaveric material (A&C) and schematic representations of the same (B&D) for approximately the L1 (A&B) and L4 (C&D) levels to depict the paravertebral muscles and adjacent anatomy for cross reference to the descriptive text to follow. The seminal anatomical studies we use for reference are those of Cornwall et al.[38], Macintosh et al. [39–41], and Bogduk [37].

Spinotransverse muscles

This group is located immediately lateral to the spinous processes of vertebrae throughout the length of the vertebral column (Fig. 1b and d). These muscles maintain a consistent morphology in all vertebral regions [38], where fibres in the cervical and thoracic spines originate from the spinous process of the cranial vertebra, to insert into the transverse processes of several more caudal vertebrae. In the lumbar spine, where the transverse processes have evolved to become the mammillary processes (and the costal elements - the ribs - are now the transverse processes), these muscles insert into the mammillary processes of the vertebrae caudal [42]. In the cervical and thoracic spine the longest, multisegment-spanning muscles of this group are named the semispinalis; in the lumbar spine, this entire muscle group is all termed the multifidus (MF) despite the commonality in morphology with spinotransverse muscles in the other spinal regions. The lumbar multifidus occupy the space between the mammillary processes (laterally) and spinous processes (medially), with multiple fascicles originating from each lumbar level. These fascicles pass caudally to insert into vertebrae sequentially, and due to their architecture (fascicles from each segmental level inserting into those that are adjacent via a myomyonal junction) it is extremely difficult to determine where each fascicle has originated when assessing MR images. This is because some individual epaxial muscles (broadly, those muscles which developmentally arise to form the post and paravertebral muscles [43], such as the erector spinae and spinotransverse muscles) are not encapsulated by their own, independent layer of epimysium - a factor which normally assists in identifying or delineating a skeletal muscle as an individual entity [38, 42]. The epaxial muscles are therefore different to hypaxial muscles (those muscles that developmentally include all trunk muscles that are not epaxial in origin) in regards to being able to identify each individual muscle via easily distinguishable borders, and this adds to the problems interpreting MRI of these muscles when a clear fascial boundary does not exist (e.g. different segmental levels of multifidus, or between iliocostalis and longissimus). This means interpretation of muscle quality can be problematic when looking to identify where each multifidus fascicle may be originating or inserting. Other muscles within this space include the interspinales and intertransversarii (see Fig. 1c and d insert), although these are not considered part of the spinotransverse muscle group. The

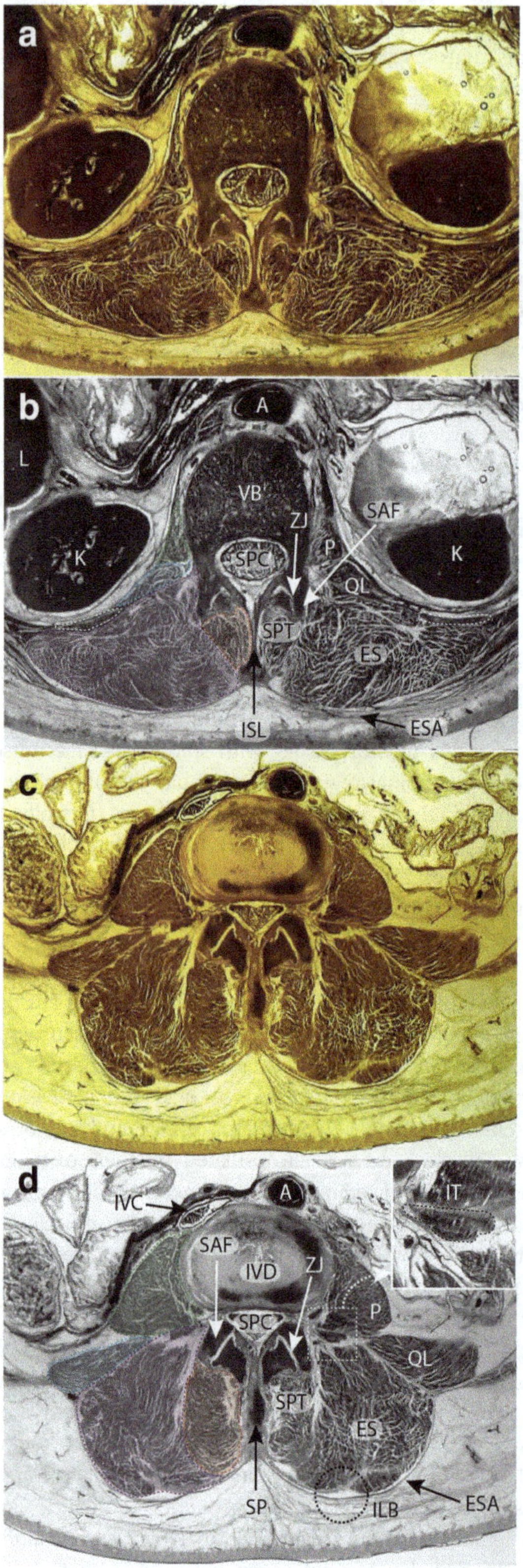

Fig. 1 Axial E12 plastinated sections (**a, c**) and schematic illustrations (**b, d**) at approximately L1 (**a, b**) and L4 (**c, d**) highlighting anatomical structures at these vertebral levels. **b, d** Dotted lines and shading, *Green* - psoas major muscle; *Blue* – quadratus lumborum muscle; *Purple* – erector spinae muscles; *Red* – spinotransverse muscles. **b** round white dotted regions (bilateral) denote 12th rib. **d** square dotted box surrounds enlarged inset; round dotted circle indicates morphological feature of interest (ILB fatty 'tent'). *Legend:* A – aorta; ES – erector spinae muscles; ESA – erector spinae aponeurosis; ILB – iliocostalis – longissimus boundary and indentation; ISL – interspinous ligament; IT – intertransversarii muscle; IVC – inferior vena cava; K – kidney; L – liver; P – psoas major muscle; QL – quadratus lumborum muscle; SAF – superior articular facet; SP – spinous process; SPC – spinal canal; SPT – spinotransverse muscle group; ZJ – zygapophysial joint

rotatores muscles, apparent in other spinal regions, do not exist in the lumbar spine [38].

Lumbar erector spinae

The lumbar erector spinae (ES) is part of a large group that extends the full length of the spine comprising longissimus and iliocostalis and occupying a lateral position compared to the spinotransverse group of muscles (see Fig. 1b and d). In anatomical terminology, the lumbar region is the location of the erector spinae muscles iliocostalis lumborum pars lumborum, and longissimus thoracis pars lumborum. It is difficult to accurately delineate between each of these two muscles on most forms of imaging due to the fact these muscles are not encapsulated with their own sheath of epimysium at their boundary, making visualisation of their anatomical border difficult to distinguish (similar to the problems identifying different segmental levels of multifidus).

Results

Defining the regions of interest from MRI

First, in discerning lumbar level from MRI, we suggest using the iliac crest tangent sign [44] by connecting a tangent between the iliac crests, which bisect either the L4 vertebra or the L4/5 intervertebral disc. This should be achieved using the coronal image with cross-reference to the sagittal and then axial images in the full imaging dataset. It should be noted that in following the method outlined, the user may need to scroll between adjacent MRI slices to visualise landmark structures to those on the level being segmented; the method is applicable to studies examining paravertebral ROIs for single or multiple slices. Second, in terms of commencement order for defining separate regions of interest, we recommend a randomised approach for the left or right side, and/or separate muscles as recent evidence has shown their influence on repeatability [34, 45]. Third, definitions for ROI for MF, and longissimus and iliocostalis lumborum (together as ES) are included, describing the medial, anterior, lateral, and posterior borders in order (cross reference to Figs. 2 (L1/2) and

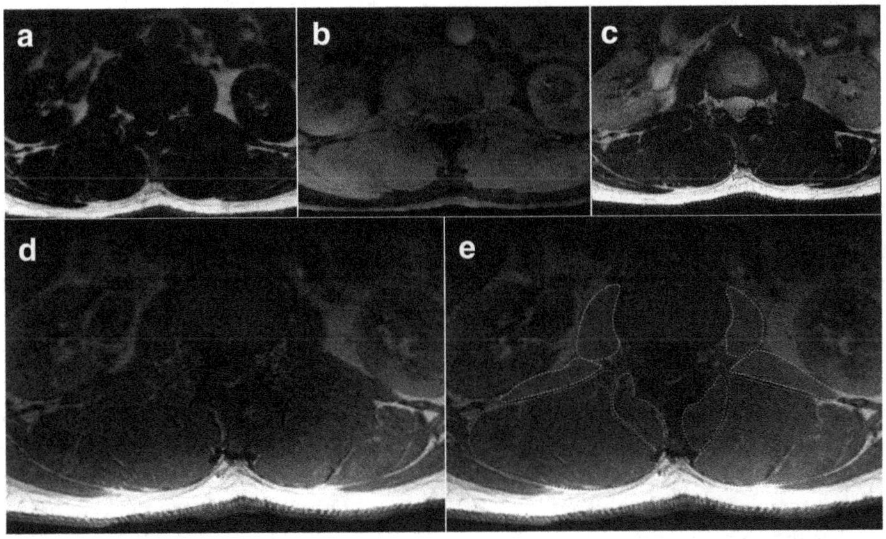

Fig. 2 Axial MRIs at the L1/2 disc level of a 47 year old male depicting fat- (**a**) and water-separated (**b**) chemical shift, and T2- (**c**) and T1-weighted (**d** and **e**, same) images. **e** Dotted lines and shading depicting the regions of interest for: *Green* - psoas muscle; *Blue* – quadratus lumborum muscle; *Purple* – erector spinae group (longissimus and iliocostalis together); and *Red* – spinotransverse muscles (predominantly multifidus)

3 (L4/5)). All muscles are present at the first lumbar level with their distal attachments described.

1. Multifidus (MF): medial border is defined by the most superficial aspect of the spinous process following the spinous process deep to where it forms the lamina; the deeper, more anterior border follows the lamina laterally to the anterior aspect of the mammillary process and zygapophyseal joint; the lateral border follows the fascial line (the epimysium of the spinotransverse group) extending from the lateral aspect of the mammillary process between MF and ES toward a small visible indentation at the subcutaneous tissue superficially; the posterior, more superficial border extends along the epimysium of MF that is clearly distinct from the thoracolumbar fascia and adjacent subcutaneous adipose tissue (Figs. 1, 2, and 3). MF is present medially at each lumbar level with increasing volume toward the lower levels of the lumbar spine, with it then

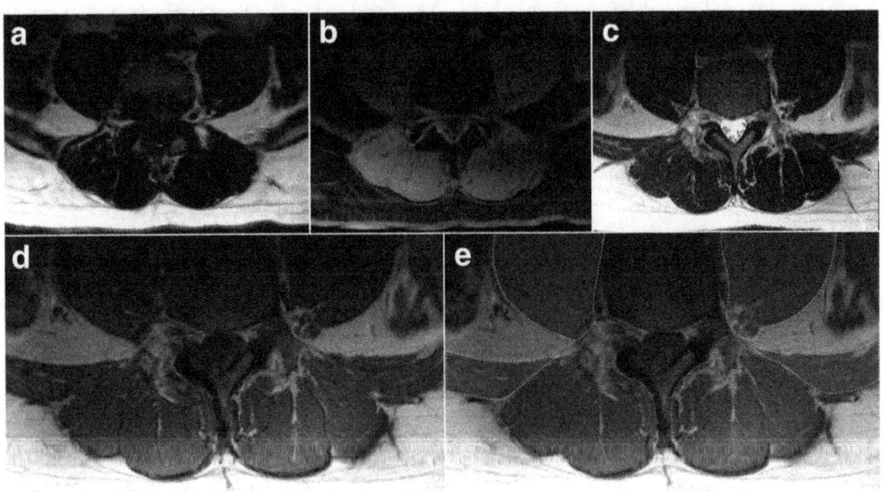

Fig. 3 Axial MRIs at the L4/5 disc level of a 47 year old male depicting fat- (**a**) and water-separated (**b**) chemical shift, and T2- (**c**) and T1-weighted (**d** and **e**; same image cropped anteriorly therein truncating psoas) images. **e** Dotted lines and shading depicting the regions of interest for: *Green* - psoas muscle (truncated at the ventral border due to limited visibility in image); *Blue* – quadratus lumborum muscle; *Purple* – erector spinae group (longissimus and iliocostalis together); and *Red* – spinotransverse muscles (predominantly multifidus)

diminishing to terminate at its distal attachments to the sacrum where it blends with the lumbosacral fascia. Further technical considerations are included below:

a. This definition is best applied at the lower lumbar levels where distinction between MF and ES is generally clearer (Fig. 1c and d); in the upper lumbar levels (only), thoracic semispinalis (ES) will be captured as part of the spinotransverse group due to its medial position. With current technology it is generally not possible to consistently or accurately delineate between semispinalis and multifidus in axial scans through the lumbar spine.
b. Fat approximating the spinous process or lamina is included within the ROI defining MF. For slices transecting the interspinous space, this fat generally overlies the spinous process but remains defined and should be included.
c. When the interspinales muscle and/or interspinous ligament are clearly distinct with a slightly irregular and darkened edge, their lateral contour can be followed rather than the spinous process in defining the medial border.
d. Should deposits of fat be visible at the mid-sagittal line and within the interspinales muscle fibres (rather than in MF), this should not be considered to be MF and therefore excluded from the ROI.

2. Erector spinae (ES): the medial border is defined by the fascial line between MF and ES and abutting the outer aspect of the mammillary process and/or zygapophyseal joint; the anterior border runs along the transverse process laterally as distinct from the quadratus lumborum muscles that lay anterolateral to it and the transverse process, following the anterior thoracolumbar; the lateral border follows the rounded contour of the fascial boundary surrounding iliocostalis; the posterior border follows the ES muscle and aponeurosis as distinct from the thoracolumbar fascia and adjacent subcutaneous adipose tissue; the lumbar intermuscular aponeurosis is included within this ROI (Figs. 1, 2, and 3). The ES longissimus and iliocostalis are present at all levels of the lumbar spine with diminishing size toward the low lumbar levels where they terminate at the posteromedial aspect of the iliac crest and toward the posterior superior iliac spine. Further technical considerations are included below:

a. If distinct, the lumbar intertransversarii that attach adjacent transverse processes should be included as part of the ES (see Fig. 1d square insert).
b. When fat is accumulated between the MF and ES (longissimus), a vertical line from the mammillary process/zygapophyseal joint where a thin fascial line is often present to follow can be used as a guide. When uncertainty exists, take the lateral border of MF.
c. When a large fat-filled 'tent' exists between longissimus and iliocostalis at the lumbar intermuscular aponeurosis posteriorly (applicable when including these together as ES), the border is defined by following the most posterior aspect of visible muscle tissue. Refer to Fig. 1d dotted circular line depicting fatty 'tent'.
d. Particularly at the low lumbar levels, the most anterior fibres of the ES (in the region of the intertransversarii) can be seen to blend with fat tissue in a striated pattern; however, a clear fascial line can direct the ROI.

MR imaging - operational parameters

There are many different variables that can influence the type and quality of image that is acquired from MR scans, and operational parameters are an important consideration in regards to determining final image output. This method for defining ROI in the lumbar paravertebral muscles has been proposed to facilitate improved comparison between studies, and we consider it important to suggest reporting a minimum set of MRI sequencing parameters. This aspect has been variably described in the literature (refer to Table 1) but in order to improve the study's relevance to a wider readership, we suggest the following reported inclusions as minimum: Field strength (e.g. 3 Tesla); sequence type (e.g. 2-point DIXON (3D fast-field echo T1) whole body); repetition time (e.g. TR 4.2 ms); echo time (e.g. TE 1.2 and 3.1 ms); flip angle (e.g. 5°); field of view (e.g. FOV 560 × 352 mm); acquired voxel dimensions (e.g. 2.0 × 2.0 × 4.0 mm); reconstructed voxel dimensions (e.g. 1.0 × 1.0 × 2.0 mm); bandwidth (e.g. 120 Hz/Px), acquisition time (e.g. TA 5 min 22 s) and slice thickness (e.g. 4.0 mm).

Discussion

This paper has proposed a foundational directive (method) for defining lumbar paravertebral ROI's for studies quantifying MFI from MRI images in the axial plane. We present this method with the aim of standardizing and homogenizing the definition of ROIs for research teams, utilizing several different visual representations of vertebral morphology including E-12 sheet-plastinated anatomical sections, schematic representations of spinal structures, fat- and water-based chemical-shift MRIs, and images demonstrating demarcated ROI as per the described method.

Anatomical boundaries for ROIs can be difficult to define and are a point for discussion. Specifically, whether

ROIs should include what might be considered extra-muscular fat. To rationalise our approach, we consider that if fat is occupying space within the epimysia of either ES or SPT, it is potentially compromising the functional integrity of that muscle tissue and should be included in the ROI. For example, fat that is occupying space that approximates bony tissue (spinous processes, laminae, zygapophyseal joint, and transverse processes) where the epimysium abuts, is included in the ROI. We base this decision in part on the findings for the lumbar spine of He et al. [46] who have shown this definition to have superior clinical relevance to the alternative non-inclusive definition. In addition, our wider group has recently shown improved repeatability for defining MF over ES, which we speculate is related to ease of definition based on MF approximating these bony landmarks [34]. Further, research has shown improved inter- and intra-rater reliability when following the spinous process and/or lamina in the cervical spine, while retaining the ability to discriminate between clinical groups [47].

Including fat that approximates the muscle at non-bony borders, particularly posteriorly where the definition between the thoracolumbar fascia can be variable, we err on the side of non-inclusivity. Our overarching rationale for this is that we intend to capture tissues that are or were, muscular, and not tissues that were unlikely to have a muscular origin. There is clear distinction of the rounded epimysium that encapsulates iliocostalis, longissimus, and the SPT, with small fascial 'tents' in the posterior border between each; these 'tents' are typically fat-filled (see Fig. 1d insert). The vast majority of investigators have employed this ROI definition (see Table 1), which allows for comparisons between studies. In using a different approach, Shahidi et al. [48] recently describe their posterior border for MF and ES as following the margin of the thoracolumbar fascia. However, their definition and representative figure indicate that this ROI includes a significant volume of fat extraneous (posterior and lateral) to the epimysium of the lumbar ES and SPT muscles. We contend that this space does not contain any muscle tissue, and therefore should not be included in measurement that seeks to provide comment on the functional capacity or quality of contractile elements such as the spinal muscles. We appreciate there may be strong value in recording the quantity and spatial distribution of this fatty deposition in terms of clinical relevance and potential to impede adjacent muscle function. However, we would suggest this fat be captured as a separate ROI rather than considered with any measure of muscle quality involving the paravertebral muscles.

Rater experience of anatomy, particularly cadaveric or three-dimensional, could influence the definition of lumbar paravertebral musculature on axial MRI images (e.g. greater experience results in less error). However, larger numbers of raters with varying levels of anatomical and post-production MRI experience would be required before deriving definitive conclusions on the influence of experience in quantifying MFI. Two studies examining the influence of rater experience on quantifying MFI in lumbar paravertebral muscles have indicated comparably high repeatability between novice and experienced raters given adequate training and practise of the novice rater [34, 45].

Challenges for the consistent and accurate quantification of MFI exist. These include, but are not limited to, a wide-variety of available whole-body human MRI scanners worldwide and the potential for varying results across field strengths (e.g. 1.5 Tesla to 3 Tesla). Accordingly, the question of how best to optimise the analysis of lumbar paravertebral muscle composition is a consideration that warrants comment. It is reasonable to assume that the higher the magnetic field (e.g. 3 Tesla versus 1.5 Tesla) the better the signal-to-noise and contrast-to-noise, but this is overly simplistic. While the quantification of muscle fat with MRI (and the Dixon sequence) is not without some complexities, we feel such discussion is beyond the scope of this paper. However, based on the available literature [49], discussions with experts in the field, experiential, and empirical evidence [26, 50], the authors opine that 1.5 Tesla and above is suitable when using the proposed MFI quantification method.

While methods employing a single MR slice are time efficient in determining fat proportion within an ROI, typically based on cross sectional area (mm^2), the MR slice has a thickness [14, 15]. Accordingly, volumetric measures are more appropriate and have shown to be more meaningful functionally [47, 51]. We therefore recommend a multi-slice approach that derives fat content based on a three-dimensional volume across L1-L5 (or the levels of interest). It is acknowledged that acquiring such data is time-consuming, even using semi-automated or automated programmes. By way of potential compromise toward a time-efficient capture of lumbar paravertebral MFI on the basis of volume, Crawford et al. [5] have shown that the fat content at L4 best represents that of the entire lumbar region in healthy participants. Measuring multiple slices at this level alone may present an effective option in busy clinical radiology environments, although further data are required to support the validity and reliability of the technique. Research efforts should strive to comprehensively include the entire lumbar spine toward a stronger body of evidence regarding age-aggregated lumbar paravertebral muscle composition, which should be undertaken for healthy volunteers, and in asymptomatic and symptomatic disease cohorts.

Conclusion

We present a foundational method for defining the ROIs of the lumbar paravertebral muscles MF and ES from axial MRIs. This includes a detailed and step-by-step description of the proposed technique to facilitate accurate reproduction of the method. This method has been proposed to provide a platform for standardizing measurement of lumbar paravertebral muscle ROI, with the aim of allowing accurate and reliable comparison of muscle quality between studies in (and beyond) this field.

Abbreviations

ES: Erector Spinae; FCSA: Functional Cross Sectional Area; FI: Fatty infiltration; FSPGR: Fast-spoiled gradient echo; IP: In-phase (water); L1,4: Lumbar levels L1 and L4; LBP: Low back pain; MF: Multifidus; MRI: Magnetic resonance imaging; OP: Opposed-phase (Fat); PS: Psoas major; QL: Quadratus lumborum; RA: Rectus abdominis; ROI: Region of interest; SI: Signal intensity; SPT: Spinotransverse muscles

Acknowledgements

Not applicable.

Funding

No funding was received.

Authors' contributions

RJC and JME conceived the study, while RJC, JC, RA, and JME each made substantial contributions to its design. RJC, JC, RA, and JME have been involved in drafting the manuscript or revising it critically for important intellectual content and each given final approval of the version to be published. RJC, JC, RA, and JME agree to be accountable for all aspects of the work in ensuring that questions related to the accuracy or integrity of any part of the work are appropriately investigated and resolved.

Competing interests

Authors RJC, JC, and RA have no disclosures to declare. In unrelated activities, JME is principle investigator on NIH grant [HD079076-01A1; 09/2014-05/2019; cervical spine study] and 35% investor/owner in a medical consulting start-up, Pain ID, LLC.

Consent for publication

Approval to use images of the E-plastinated sections was granted by Department of Anatomy, University of Otago. All MRIs were derived from the same informed and consenting adult subject.

Author details

[1]Institute for Health Sciences, Zurich University of Applied Sciences, Technikumstrasse 81, Postfach, CH-8401 Winterthur, Switzerland. [2]Faculty of Health Professions, Curtin University, Perth, Australia. [3]Graduate School of Nursing, Midwifery and Health, Victoria University of Wellington, Wellington, New Zealand. [4]Department of Physical Therapy and Human Movement Sciences, Feinberg School of Medicine, Northwestern University, Chicago, USA. [5]School of Health and Rehabilitation Sciences, University of Queensland, Brisbane, Australia.

References

1. D'Aprile P, Tarantino A, Jinkins JR, Brindicci D. The value of fat saturation sequences and contrast medium administration in MRI of degenerative disease of the posterior/perispinal elements of the lumbosacral spine. Eur Radiol. 2007;17(2):523–31.
2. Kumar Y, Hayashi D. Role of magnetic resonance imaging in acute spinal trauma: a pictorial review. BMC MusculoskeletDdisord. 2016;17(1):310.
3. Brinjikji W, Luetmer PH, Comstock B, Bresnahan BW, Chen LE, Deyo RA, Halabi S, Turner JA, Avins AL, James K, et al. Systematic literature review of imaging features of spinal degeneration in asymptomatic populations. Am J Neuroradiol. 2015;36(4):811–6.
4. Amabile C, Moal B, Chtara OA, Pillet H, Raya JG, Iannessi A, Skalli W, Lafage V, Bronsard N. Estimation of spinopelvic muscles' volumes in young asymptomatic subjects: a quantitative analysis. Surg Radiol Anat. 2016 Sep 16 [Epub ahead of print] doi:10.1007/s00276-016-1742-6.
5. Crawford R, Filli L, Elliott J, Nanz D, Fischer M, Marcon M, Ulbrich E. Age- and level-dependence of fatty infiltration in lumbar paravertebral muscles of healthy volunteers. Am J Neuroradiol. 2016;37(4):742–8.
6. Crawford R, Volken T, Valentin S, Melloh M, Elliott J. Rate of lumbar paravertebral muscle fat infiltration versus spinal degeneration in asymptomatic populations: An age- aggregated cross-sectional simulation study. BMC Scol & Spinal Disord. 2016;11:21–9.
7. Valentin S, Licka T, Elliott J. Age and side-related morphometric MRI evaluation of trunk muscles in people without back pain. Man Ther. 2015;20(1):90–5.
8. Kjaer P, Bendix T, Sorensen JS, Korsholm L, Leboeuf-Yde C. Are MRI-defined fat infiltrations in the multifidus muscles associated with low back pain? BMC Med. 2007;5:2.
9. Teichtahl AJ, Urquhart DM, Wang Y, Wluka AE, Wijethilake P, O'Sullivan R, Cicuttini FM. Fat infiltration of paraspinal muscles is associated with low back pain, disability, and structural abnormalities in community-based adults. The Spine J. 2015;15(7):1593–601.
10. D'Hooge R, Cagnie B, Crombez G, Vanderstraeten G, Dolphens M, Danneels L. Increased intramuscular fatty infiltration without differences in lumbar muscle cross-sectional area during remission of unilateral recurrent low back pain. Man Ther. 2012;17(6):584–8.
11. Fischer MA, Nanz D, Shimakawa A, Schirmer T, Guggenberger R, Chhabra A, Carrino JA, Andreisek G. Quantification of muscle fat in patients with low back pain: comparison of multi-echo MR imaging with single-voxel MR spectroscopy. Radiol. 2013;266(2):555–63.
12. Beneck GJ, Kulig K. Multifidus atrophy is localized and bilateral in active persons with chronic unilateral low back pain. Arch PhysMed & Rehab. 2012;93(2):300–6.
13. Fortin M, Videman T, Gibbons LE, Battie MC. Paraspinal muscle morphology and composition: a 15-yr longitudinal magnetic resonance imaging study. Med & Sci in Sports & Ex. 2014;46(5):893–901.
14. Elliott JM, Kerry R, Flynn T, Parrish TB. Content not quantity is a better measure of muscle degeneration in whiplash. Man Ther. 2013;18(6):578–82.
15. Elliott JM, Pedler AR, Jull GA, Van Wyk L, Galloway GG, O'Leary SP. Differential changes in muscle composition exist in traumatic and nontraumatic neck pain. Spine. 2014;39(1):39–47.
16. Hodges PW, James G, Blomster L, Hall L, Schmid A, Shu C, Little C, Melrose J. Multifidus muscle changes after back injury are characterized by structural remodeling of muscle, adipose and connective tissue, but not muscle atrophy: molecular and morphological evidence. Spine. 2015;40(14):1057–71.
17. Kumar D, Karampinos DC, MacLeod TD, Lin W, Nardo L, Li X, Link TM, Majumdar S, Souza RB. Quadriceps intramuscular fat fraction rather than muscle size is associated with knee osteoarthritis. Osteoarthritis & Cartilage. 2014;22(2):226–34.
18. Hebert JJ, Kjaer P, Fritz JM, Walker BF. The relationship of lumbar multifidus muscle morphology to previous, current, and future low back pain: a 9-year population-based prospective cohort study. Spine. 2014;39(17):1417–25.
19. Bhadresha A, Lawrence OJ, McCarthy MJ. A comparison of magnetic resonance imaging muscle Fat content in the lumbar paraspinal muscles with patient-reported outcome measures in patients with lumbar degenerative disk disease and focal disk prolapse. Global Spine J. 2016;6(4):401–10.
20. Kalichman L, Hodges P, Li L, Guermazi A, Hunter DJ. Changes in paraspinal muscles and their association with low back pain and spinal degeneration: CT study. Eur Spine J. 2010;19(7):1136–44.
21. Meakin JR, Fulford J, Seymour R, Welsman JR, Knapp KM. The relationship between sagittal curvature and extensor muscle volume in the lumbar spine. J Anatomy. 2013;222(6):608–14.
22. Pezolato A, de Vasconcelos EE, Defino HL, Nogueira-Barbosa MH. Fat infiltration in the lumbar multifidus and erector spinae muscles in subjects with sway-back posture. Eur Spine J. 2012;21(11):2158–64.

23. Elliott JM, Courtney DM, Rademaker A, Pinto D, Sterling MM, Parrish TB. The rapid and progressive degeneration of the cervical multifidus in whiplash: a MRI study of fatty infiltration. Spine. 2015;40(12):E694–700.
24. Reeder SB, Hu HH, Sirlin CB. Proton density fat-fraction: a standardized MR-based biomarker of tissue fat concentration. JMRI. 2012;36(5):1011–4.
25. Samagh SP, Kramer EJ, Melkus G, Laron D, Bodendorfer BM, Natsuhara K, Kim HT, Liu X, Feeley BT. MRI quantification of fatty infiltration and muscle atrophy in a mouse model of rotator cuff tears. J Ortho Research. 2013; 31(3):421–6.
26. Smith AC, Parrish TB, Abbott R, Hoggarth MA, Mendoza K, Chen YF, Elliott JM. Muscle-fat MRI: 1.5 Tesla and 3.0 Tesla versus histology. Muscle & Nerve. 2014;50(2):170–6.
27. Gaeta M, Scribano E, Mileto A, Mazziotti S, Rodolico C, Toscano A, Settineri N, Ascenti G, Blandino A. Muscle fat fraction in neuromuscular disorders: dual-echo dual-flip-angle spoiled gradient-recalled MR imaging technique for quantification–a feasibility study. Radiol. 2011;259(2):487–94.
28. Paalanne N, Niinimaki J, Karppinen J, Taimela S, Mutanen P, Takatalo J, Korpelainen R, Tervonen O. Assessment of association between low back pain and paraspinal muscle atrophy using opposed-phase magnetic resonance imaging: a population-based study among young adults. Spine. 2011;36(23):1961–8.
29. Reeder SB, Pineda AR, Wen Z, Shimakawa A, Yu H, Brittain JH, Gold GE, Beaulieu CH, Pelc NJ. Iterative decomposition of water and fat with echo asymmetry and least-squares estimation (IDEAL): application with fast spin-echo imaging. Mag Res in Med. 2005;54(3):636–44.
30. Reeder SB, Wen Z, Yu H, Pineda AR, Gold GE, Markl M, Pelc NJ. Multicoil Dixon chemical species separation with an iterative least-squares estimation method. Mag Res in Med. 2004;51(1):35–45.
31. Maatta J, Karppinen J, Luk KD, Cheung KM, Samartzis D. Phenotype profiling of Modic changes of the lumbar spine and its association with other MRI phenotypes: a large-scale, population-based study. The Spine J. 2015;15(9):1933–42.
32. Maatta JH, Wadge S, MacGregor A, Karppinen J, Williams FM. ISSLS prize winner: vertebral endplate (modic) change is an independent risk factor for episodes of severe and disabling Low back pain. Spine. 2015;40(15):1187–93.
33. Elliott JM, Walton DM, Rademaker A, Parrish TB. Quantification of cervical spine muscle fat: a comparison between T1-weighted and multi-echo gradient echo imaging using a variable projection algorithm (VARPRO). BMC Med Imaging. 2013;13:30.
34. Mhuiris AN, Volken T, Elliott JM, Hoggarth M, Samartzis D, Crawford RJ. Reliability of quantifying the spatial distribution of fatty infiltration in lumbar paravertebral muscles using a new segmentation method for T1-weighted MRI. BMC Musculoskelet Disord. 2016;17(1):234–40.
35. Putzier M, Hartwig T, Hoff EK, Streitparth F, Strube P. Minimally invasive TLIF leads to increased muscle sparing of the multifidus muscle but not the longissimus muscle compared with conventional PLIF-a prospective randomized clinical trial. The Spine J. 2016;16(7):811–9.
36. Valenzuela W, Ferguson SJ, Ignasiak D, Diserens G, Vermathen P, Boesch C, Reyes M. Correction tool for active shape model based lumbar muscle segmentation. PloS one. 2015;2015:3033–6.
37. Bogduk N. A reappraisal of the anatomy of the human lumbar erector spinae. J Anatomy. 1980;131(Pt 3):525–40.
38. Cornwall J, Stringer MD, Duxson M. Functional morphology of the thoracolumbar transversospinal muscles. Spine. 2011;36(16):E1053–1061.
39. Macintosh JE, Bogduk N. Volvo award in basic science. The morphology of the lumbar erector spinae. Spine 1987. 1987;12(7):658–68.
40. Macintosh JE, Valencia F, Bogduk N, Munro RR. The morphology of the human lumbar multifidus. Clin Biomech. 1986;1(4):196–204.
41. Macintosh JE, Bogduk N. The attachments of the lumbar erector spinae. Spine. 1991;16(7):783–92.
42. Standring SE: Gray's Anatomy, 40th edn. London: Churchill Livingstone; 2009, 1576 pages; ISBN: 9780443066849.
43. Deries M, Schweitzer R, Duxson MJ. Developmental fate of the mammalian myotome. Developmental Dynamics. 2010;239(11):2898–910.
44. Farshad-Amacker NA, Aichmair A, Herzog RJ, Farshad M. Merits of different anatomical landmarks for correct numbering of the lumbar vertebrae in lumbosacral transitional anomalies. Eur Spine J. 2015;24(3):600–8.
45. Valentin S, Yeates TD, Licka T, Elliott J. Inter-rater reliability of trunk muscle morphometric analysis. J Back Musculoskelet Rehab. 2015;28(1):181–90.
46. He J, Nakajima T, Espinoza Orias A, An H, Inoue N: Characterizing lumbar multifidus fatty infiltration with MRI: Is there a correct region of interest? Paper 0290 in: Orthopaedic Research Society Conference. Orlando, USA; 2016.
47. Abbott R, Pedler A, Sterling M, Hides J, Murphey T, Hoggarth M, Elliott J. The geography of fatty infiltrates within the cervical multifidus and semispinalis cervicis in individuals with chronic whiplash-associated disorders. J Orthop & Sports Phys Ther. 2015;45(4):8.
48. Shahidi B, Parra CL, Berry DB, Hubbard JC, Gombatto S, Zlomislic V, Allen RT, Hughes-Austin J, Garfin S, Ward SR. Contribution of lumbar spine pathology and age to paraspinal muscle size and fatty infiltration. Spine. 2016 Aug 11 [Epub ahead of print] DOI: 10.1097/BRS.0000000000001848.
49. Friedman SD, Poliachik SL, Carter GT. Muscle-fat magnetic resonance imaging: applications. Muscle & Nerve. 2014;50(2):157–8.
50. Andersson T, Romu T, Karlsson A, Noren B, Forsgren MF, Smedby O, Kechagias S, Almer S, Lundberg P, Borga M, et al. Consistent intensity inhomogeneity correction in water-fat MRI. JMRI. 2015;42(2):468–76.
51. Boom HP, van Spronsen PH, van Ginkel FC, van Schijndel RA, Castelijns JA, Tuinzing DB. A comparison of human jaw muscle cross-sectional area and volume in long- and short-face subjects, using MRI. Archives Oral Biol. 2008; 53(3):273–81.
52. Antony J, McGuinness K, Welch N, Coyle J, Franklyn-Miller A, O'Connor NE, Moran K. An interactive segmentation tool for quantifying fat in lumbar muscles using axial lumbar-spine MRI. IRBM. 2016;37(1):11–22.
53. Battaglia PJ, Maeda Y, Welk A, Hough B, Kettner N. Reliability of the Goutallier classification in quantifying muscle fatty degeneration in the lumbar multifidus using magnetic resonance imaging. Journal of Manipulative and Physiological Therapeutics. 2014;37(3):190–7.
54. Hu ZJ, He J, Zhao FD, Fang XQ, Zhou LN, Fan SW. An assessment of the intra- and inter-reliability of the lumbar paraspinal muscle parameters using CT scan and magnetic resonance imaging. Spine. 2011;36(13):E868–874.
55. Ranson CA, Burnett AF, Kerslake R, Batt ME, O'Sullivan PB. An investigation into the use of MR imaging to determine the functional cross sectional area of lumbar paraspinal muscles. European Spine Journal. 2006;15(6):764–73.

2

Early detection of osteoarthritis in rabbits using MRI with a double-contrast agent

Okihiro Onishi[1], Kazuya Ikoma[1*], Masamitsu Kido[1], Yukichi Kabuto[1], Keiichiro Ueshima[1], Ken-ichi Matsuda[2], Masaki Tanaka[2] and Toshikazu Kubo[1]

Abstract

Background: Articular cartilage degeneration has been evaluated by magnetic resonance imaging (MRI). However, this method has several problems, including its time-consuming nature and the requirement of a high magnetic field or specialized hardware. The purpose of this study was to sequentially assess early degenerative changes in rabbit knee articular cartilage using MRI with a new double-contrast agent.

Methods: We induced osteoarthritis (OA) in the right knee of rabbits by anterior cruciate ligament transection and partial medial meniscectomy. Proton density-weighted images and T_2-calculated images were obtained before and after contrast agent injection into the knee. The signal intensity ratio (SIR) values on the proton density-weighted images were calculated by dividing the signal intensity of the articular cartilage by that of joint fluid. Six rabbits were examined using MRI at 2 (designated 2-w OA) and 4 weeks (4-w OA) after the operation. Histological examination was performed 4 weeks after the operation. One rabbit was histologically examined 2 weeks after the operation. The control consisted of six rabbits that were not subjected to the operation. The SIR values, T_2 values and the thicknesses of the cartilage of the 2-w OA, 4-w OA and the control before and after contrast agent injection were analyzed. The Mankin score and OARSI (Osteoarthritis Research Society International) score were used for the histological evaluation.

Results: Significant differences in the SIR and T_2 values of the medial and lateral condyles of the femur were found between the control and the 4-w OA only after contrast agent injection. No significant differences were found in the SIR and T_2 values before contrast agent injection between the control, the 2-w OA and 4-w OA. The thickness of the articular cartilage revealed no significant differences. In the histological assessment, the Mankin score and OARSI score sequentially increased from the control to the 4-w OA.

Conclusion: We evaluated the SIR and T_2 values of the knees in a rabbit OA model and a control model using a new double-contrast agent. MRI with this agent enabled OA detection earlier than using conventional MRI.

Keywords: Contrast agent, Rabbit model, Osteoarthritis

Background

Osteoarthritis (OA) leads to degeneration and wear of the articular cartilage, sclerosis of the subchondral bone, and synovitis, causing joint pain, limitation of joint movement, and muscular atrophy [1]. Many older individuals suffer from OA, which reduces their quality of life and increases the mortality rate [2, 3]. The progression of OA requires painkillers and surgery, such as prosthetic arthroplasty, osteotomy, and arthroscopic operations. Early diagnosis and treatment of OA would not only prevent the development of more severe OA in many patients but would also decrease social costs, including medical expenses and human resources.

Exercise therapy, orthosis, and oral administration of non-steroid anti-inflammatory drugs, opioids, and acetaminophen are used to treat early-stage OA, and the effects of these agents are being examined. However, a method for early detection of articular cartilage degeneration has not been established [4]. The Kellgren and Lawrence scale is clinically used to

* Correspondence: kazuya@koto.kpu-m.ac.jp
[1]Department of Orthopaedics, Graduate School of Medical Science, Kyoto Prefectural University of Medicine, 602-8566 465, Kajiicho, Kamigyo-ku Kyoto-shi, Kyoto, Japan
Full list of author information is available at the end of the article

evaluate the grade of knee OA [5]; however, this scale evaluates the grade of OA based on articular cartilage wear and is therefore not applicable for evaluating early-stage OA, in which the articular cartilage thickness has not decreased [6]. Computed tomography exposes patients to high radiation doses and is therefore not an ideal choice for evaluating OA [7, 8].

Recently, the use of magnetic resonance imaging (MRI) has been evaluated to determine the quality of articular cartilage. OA reduces proteoglycan (PG) and collagen content in articular cartilage and increases the content of water molecules. Qualitative evaluations of articular cartilage using MRI can be divided into two types. One type mainly detects hydration and reductions in collagen density in articular cartilage, whereas the other type mainly detects decreases in PG in articular cartilage. The former includes T_2 mapping and diffusion-weighted imaging, whereas the latter includes delayed gadolinium-enhanced MRI (dGEMRIC), $T_{1\rho}$ mapping, glycosaminoglycan chemical exchange saturation transfer (gag CEST), and ^{23}Na MRI [9–11]. Recht et al. reported that T_2-weighted images showed articular cartilage of the human knee, although thin-layered cartilage, such as that in the hip joint and ankle joint, is difficult to depict clearly [12]. It is difficult to use $T_{1\rho}$-calculated images because their acquisition requires a long period of time, and the reference values cannot be set because $T_{1\rho}$ values vary with the magnetic field of the MRI device [13]. dGEMRIC is used to detect degenerative changes in articular cartilage; however, problems with this technique include a long acquisition time and restrictions for use in patients with renal impairment [14, 15]. Gag CEST requires an MRI device with a high magnetic field [16–18]. ^{23}Na MRI requires specialized hardware; therefore, it is difficult to obtain these images in many facilities [19].

Manganese ions shorten T_2 relaxation times and have been used as components of contrast agents in MRI studies examining the brain and digestive organs [20–22]. In a previous study, the selective visualization of articular cartilage using MRI with a new double-contrast agent containing manganese ions as a positive contrast agent and ferrous and copper ions as negative contrast agents revealed thin-layered structures that were difficult to visualize using conventional methods [23]. Accordingly, rabbit knee cartilage was successfully and vividly delineated ex vivo in that study. As articular cartilage degenerates, its T_2 relaxation time of articular cartilage becomes longer. We hypothesized that selective visualization of articular cartilage using MRI could be used to detect early degenerative changes in articular cartilage. The purpose of this study was to sequentially assess degenerative changes in rabbit knee articular cartilage using MRI with a new double-contrast agent and compare the results with observations obtained using histological methods.

Methods

Animals

This study was conducted in compliance with the guidelines in the Guide for the Care and Use of Laboratory Animals published by the National Institutes of Health and was approved by the Ethics Committee on Animal Experimentation of our institution. Thirteen male Japanese white rabbits (13 to 15-week-old; weighing 3.0 to 3.2 kg; Shimizu Laboratory Supplies Co., Ltd. Kyoto, Japan) were housed in separate cages at the Animal Center of our institution's animal facility. The rabbits were anesthetized by the inhalation of isoflurane at a rate of 2.5 L/min. OA was induced in the right knee joint by anterior cruciate ligament transection and a partial medial meniscectomy, and the left knee remained intact. Seven rabbits underwent the operation. Six rabbits were examined using MRI at 2 (designated 2-w OA) and 4 weeks (4-w OA) after the operation. Histological examination was performed 4 weeks after the operation. One rabbit was histologically examined 2 weeks after the operation. The control consisted of six rabbits that were not subjected to the operation.

MRI protocol

MRI was performed on a large-bore gradient coil (inside diameter, 210 mm) MRI unit for animals (Varian MRI System 7.04 Tesla; Agilent Technologies, Palo Alto, CA) using a transmitter/receiver surface coil (4 × 3-cm diameter). The rabbits were placed in a supine position, and the knee joint was placed in 90° flexion under the surface coil on the cradle. Each rabbit was anesthetized by the inhalation of isoflurane at a rate of 1.5 L/min while performing MRI. Sagittal images through the medial and lateral condyle of the right femur in a supine position of the 2-w OA and 4-w OA rabbits and the control rabbits were obtained at 2 and 4 weeks postoperatively. MR images were obtained before and 5 min after contrast agent injection (1.0 mL) into the knee joints. A microelement preparation of a high-caloric infusion preparation (Mineric® Nipro Pharma Corp., Osaka, Japan) was used as the contrast agent [23]. Mineric® contains 0.5 mmol/L $MnCl_2$, 2.5 mmol/L $CuSO_4$, and 17.5 mmol/L $FeCl_3$. To evaluate the efficacy of the contrast agent in vivo, proton density-weighted images were obtained before and 5 min after contrast agent injection (Fig. 1). The parameters were as follows: spin-echo sequence; TR, 2000 ms; TE,

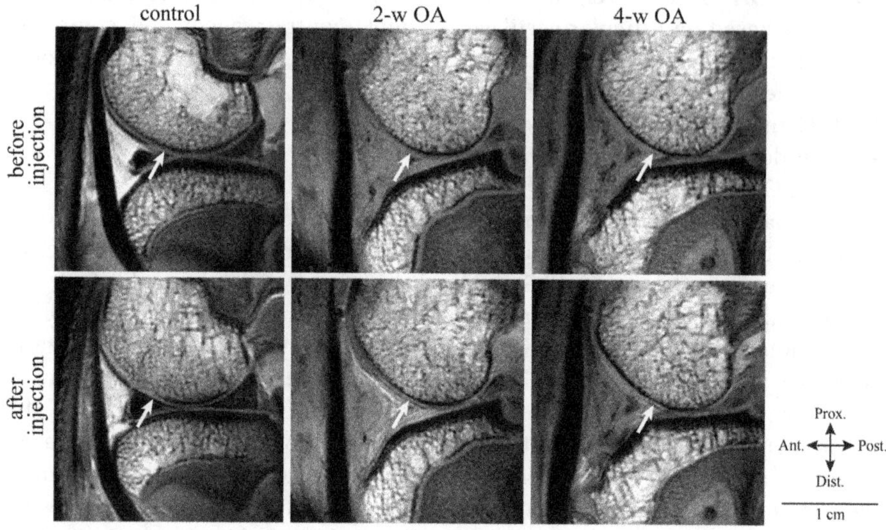

Fig. 1 MR images from the present study. Representative proton density-weighted images are shown. The top row shows MR images of the control, the 2-w OA and 4-w OA before contrast agent injection, and the bottom row after contrast agent injection. The arrows indicate the surface of the cartilage in the control, 2-w OA and 4-w OA. Scale bar, 1 cm. Ant. = anterior, Post. = posterior, Prox. = proximal, and Dist. = distal

11.55 ms; flip angle, 20 degrees; 10 sagittal slices; slice thickness, 1 mm; matrix, 512 × 512 after zero-filling; acquisition time = 8 min 36 s. The signal intensity of the articular cartilage and joint fluid were measured, and the signal intensity ratio (SIR), which was obtained by dividing the signal intensity of the articular cartilage by that of joint fluid, was calculated.

T_2-calculated images were obtained from fast spin-echo images with 8 TEs. The parameters were as follows: TR, 2000 ms; 8 TEs, 11.55–92.4 ms; echo train length, 2; echo spacing, 11.55; field of view, 40 × 40 mm; 10 sagittal slices; slice thickness, 1 mm; matrix, 256 × 256; acquisition time = 34 min 12 s. Regions of interest (ROI) were selected that corresponded to the weight-bearing areas in the medial and lateral condyle of the femur and the fluid near the area on the sagittal slices. The sagittal slices were obtained perpendicular to the line through the medial and lateral condyle of the femur on the axial slice and parallel to the bone axis of the tibia on the coronal slice. The proton density-weighted images were then referenced when the ROI was set. The MRI findings were reviewed by two orthopedic surgeons.

The thickness of the articular cartilage was measured in proton density-weighted images after contrast agent injection as a conventional assessment of osteoarthritis.

The SIR and T_2 values of 6 knees of each group were compared.

Statistical analysis

The SIR values and T_2 values of the articular cartilage of the medial and lateral condyles of the femur before and after injection of the agent were compared between the control and the 2-w OA, as well as between the control and the 4-w OA by the Mann-Whitney U test. They were compared between the 2-w OA and the 4-w OA by the Wilcoxon signed-rank test. A significant difference was defined as a Bonferroni-corrected P-value less than 0.017. The thickness of the articular cartilage of the medial and lateral condyle after injection of the agent was compared between the control and the 2-w OA, as well as between the control and the 4-w OA by the Mann-Whitney U test, and was compared between the 2-w OA and the 4-w OA by the Wilcoxon signed-rank test. A significant difference was defined as a Bonferroni-corrected P-value less than 0.017. We assessed variations in the SIR and T_2 values before injection to after injection by the Wilcoxon signed-rank test. A significant difference was defined as a P-value less than 0.05. SPSS ver. 22 (IBM Corp., Armonk, NY, USA) was used for the analysis.

Histology

One rabbit from the 2-w OA, the four evaluable rabbits from the 4-w OA and one rabbit from the control were assessed. The rabbits were sacrificed by the inhalation of isoflurane at a rate of 2.5 L/min and the intravenous injection of 4.0 mL of pentobarbital sodium (Somnopentyl®, Kyoritsuseiyaku Corp., Tokyo, Japan); each rabbit's knee joint was then dissected. The knee joint was preserved in 10% neutral-buffered formalin solution and decalcified in 10% ethylenediaminetetraacetic acid solution. The tissues were embedded in paraffin and cut at the location in the same manner as the MR images were selected. The tissues were stained with hematoxylin and

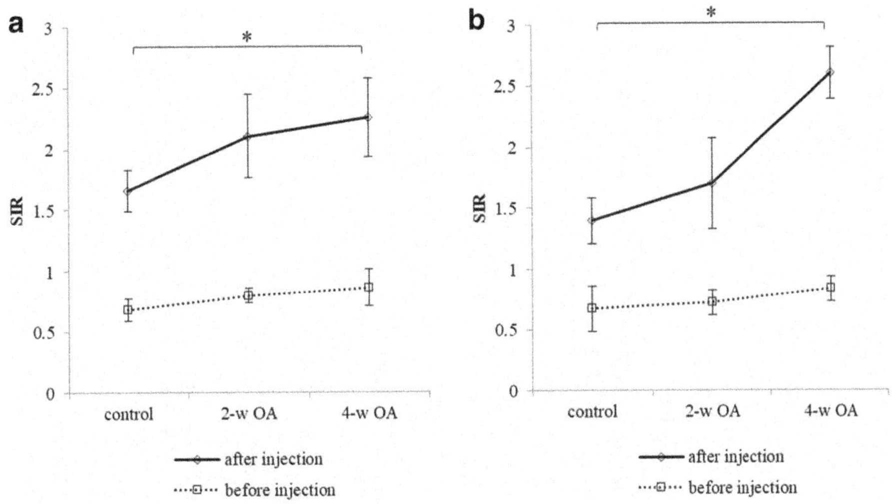

Fig. 2 SIR values in proton density-weighted images. The SIR values of the medial condyle of the femur before and after contrast agent injection (**a**) and those of the lateral condyle of the femur before and contrast agent injection (**b**) are shown. * indicates $P < 0.017$, which was defined as a significant change

eosin (H&E) and Safranin O according to the previous study [23]. Histological evaluation of OA was performed using the Mankin score and OARSI (Osteoarthritis Research Society International) score of articular cartilage changes in three slices per rabbit [24, 25]. The averages of the scores of the 2-w OA, 4-w OA and the control were treated as the overall scores of the groups.

Results

Comparison of SIRs

Significant differences were observed in the SIR values of the medial condyle ($P = 0.004$) and the lateral condyle ($P = 0.002$) only after contrast agent injection between the control and the 4-w OA (Fig. 2). On the contrary, no significant differences were noted in the SIR values of the medial and lateral condyles of the femur before contrast agent injection between the control, 2-w OA, and 4-w OA (Fig. 2). The SIR values after contrast agent injection were significantly greater than those before contrast agent injection (Table 1).

Comparison of T_2 values

Significant differences in the SIR values of the medial condyle ($P = 0.009$) and the lateral condyle ($P = 0.002$)

Table 1 The comparison of the SIR values before and after contrast agent injection

	Before injection SIR (SI of cartilage (× 10^4) / SI of fluid (× 10^4))	After injection SIR (SI of cartilage (× 10^4) / SI of fluid (× 10^4))	*P*-value
(a)			
Control	0.683 ± 0.092 (0.921 ± 0.171 / 1.360 ± 0.268)	1.660 ± 0.169 (1.102 ± 0.188 / 0.680 ± 0.193)	0.028
2-w OA	0.797 ± 0.061 (1.125 ± 0.200 / 1.416 ± 0.247)	2.106 ± 0.344 (1.176 ± 0.306 / 0.573 ± 0.179)	0.028
4-w OA	0.863 ± 0.150 (1.167 ± 0.088 / 1.377 ± 0.179)	2.258 ± 0.322 (1.437 ± 0.324 / 0.641 ± 0.150)	0.028
(b)			
Control	0.674 ± 0.186 (1.016 ± 0.219 / 1.546 ± 0.270)	1.396 ± 0.187 (1.200 ± 0.251 / 0.865 ± 0.167)	0.028
2-w OA	0.723 ± 0.104 (1.059 ± 0.234 / 1.464 ± 0.261)	1.700 ± 0.374 (1.236 ± 0.376 / 0.729 ± 0.158)	0.028
4-w OA	0.835 ± 0.104 (1.196 ± 0.216 / 1.438 ± 0.229)	2.605 ± 0.212 (1.363 ± 0.350 / 0.525 ± 0.141)	0.028

(a) medial condyle, (b) lateral condyle

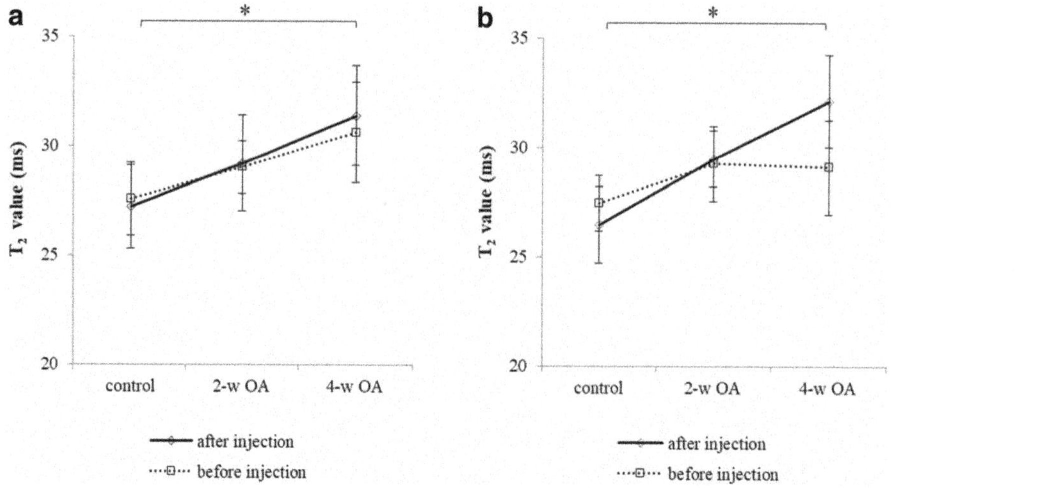

Fig. 3 T_2 values of articular cartilage. The T_2 values of the medial condyle of the femur before and after contrast agent injection (**a**) and those of the lateral condyle of the femur before and contrast agent injection (**b**) are shown. * indicates $P < 0.017$, which was defined as a significant change

were observed only after contrast agent injection between the control and 4-w OA (Fig. 3). On the contrary, no significant differences were noted in the T_2 values of the medial and lateral condyles of the femur before contrast agent injection between the control, 2-w OA and 4-w OA (Fig. 3). The T_2 values of the lateral condyle in the 4-w OA were significantly greater after contrast agent injection than those prior to injection (Table 2).

Comparison of the thickness of the articular cartilage on MRI

No significant differences were noted in the thickness of the articular cartilage of the medial and lateral condyles of the femur between the control, 2-w OA and 4-w OA (Fig. 4).

Comparison of histological findings

We examined the four evaluable rabbits from the 4-w OA, one rabbit from the 2-w OA and one rabbit from the control. The loss of Safranin O staining and the erosion of the cartilage in the 4-w OA increased compared with the 2-w and control (Fig. 5). For H&E staining, the control exhibited normal findings, and the 2-w OA and 4-w OA exhibited decreased chondral cells (Fig. 6). The Mankin score and the OARSI score were used for the histological evaluation of OA (Table 3). The scores sequentially increased from the control to the 4-w OA.

Discussion

Assessment of this study

In this study, histological findings revealed substantial changes at 4 weeks after surgery and minimal changes at 2 weeks after surgery. The SIR values of the 2-w OA, 4-w OA and the control after the agent injection were significantly greater than those before the injection. This indicated that selective visualization of the articular cartilage using MRI with this contrast agent could provide a strong contrast between the articular cartilage and joint fluid. This feature allowed the delineation of thin structures, such as rabbit articular cartilage.

The 4-w OA exhibited no significant differences in the thickness of the articular cartilage. The SIR and T_2 values were significantly different between the control and the 4-w OA only after contrast agent injection. Therefore, MRI with contrast agent enabled us to detect articular cartilage degeneration before we could detect it using conventional MRI.

Table 2 T_2 Values before and after contrast agent injection

Medial condyle	Before injection	After injection	*P*-value	Lateral condyle	Before injection	After injection	*P*-value
Control	27.6 ± 1.67	27.2 ± 1.92	0.753	Control	27.4 ± 1.25	26.5 ± 1.73	0.116
2-w OA	29.0 ± 1.20	29.2 ± 2.18	0.753	2-w OA	29.3 ± 1.73	29.5 ± 1.29	0.600
4-w OA	30.6 ± 2.29	31.4 ± 2.27	0.249	4-w OA	29.1 ± 2.16	32.1 ± 2.09	0.028

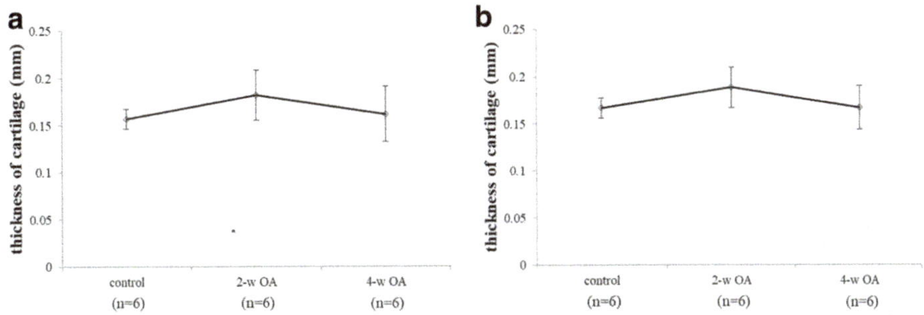

Fig. 4 The thickness of articular cartilage in proton density-weighted images. The thickness of the articular cartilage of the medial condyle (**a**) and that of the lateral condyle (**b**) are shown

These findings were consistent with the histological findings.

In histological assessment, the lateral condyle indicated more progressive degeneration in articular cartilage. This might relate to the result that the T_2 values of the lateral condyle in the 4-w OA were significantly greater after contrast agent injection than before the injection.

Other studies on articular cartilage

$T_{1\rho}$-calculated images, T_2-calculated images, dGEMRIC, gag CEST, and ^{23}Na MRI have been investigated as MRI methods that can potentially be used to evaluate degenerative changes in articular cartilage [9–11]. Li X et al. reported increased $T_{1\rho}$ and T_2 relaxation times of patellofemoral joint articular cartilage in OA patients compared to those in normal individuals [9]. Rakhra KS et al. measured the $T_{1\rho}$ relaxation time of hip articular cartilage of femoroacetabular impingement patients and normal control individuals [26]. The values were increased in middle and deep layers in the femoroacetabular impingement patients compared to those in the control patients, indicating cartilage changes. Despite these results, the histological evaluation of OA has been difficult to perform in humans. Wei et al. measured the T_2 relaxation time of an OA model generated by immobilization of the rabbit knee, which exhibited increased values 2 weeks after immobilization and reduced Safranin O staining and PG content [27]. Evaluation by histology and by MRI findings requires an animal model, such as a rabbit. However, the articular cartilage of experimental animals such as rabbits is thinner than that of humans, and the articular cartilage of the femorotibial joint is too thin for clear delineation. The researchers performed qualitative MRI of the articular cartilage of animals [9–11, 26]; however, few studies have delineated the articular cartilage vividly and evaluated it qualitatively [12]. Therefore, methods have not been established to detect earlier stages of OA.

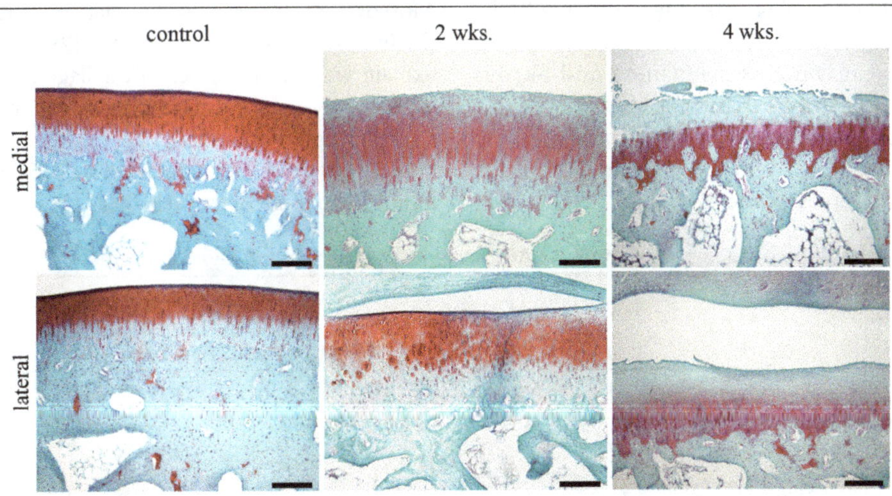

Fig. 5 Articular cartilage of the rabbit knee with Safranin O staining. Histological images with Safranin O staining of the medial and lateral condyle of the femur are shown. The top row shows the images of the medial condyle of the control, the 2-w OA and 4-w OA, and the bottom row of the lateral condyle. Scale bar, 200 μm

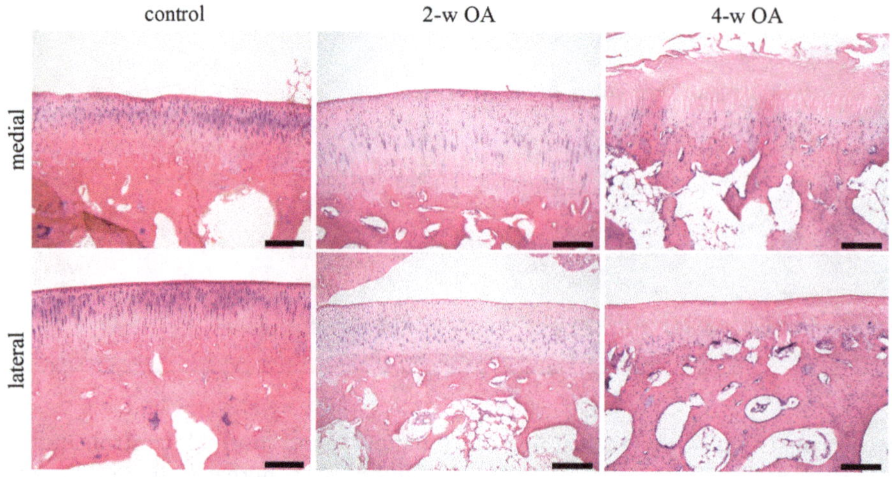

Fig. 6 Articular cartilage of the rabbit knee with H&E staining. Histological images with H&E staining of the medial and lateral condyle of the femur are shown. The top row shows the images of the medial condyle of the control, the 2-w OA and 4-w OA, and the bottom row of the lateral condyle. Scale bar, 200 μm

Characteristics of MRI with the double-contrast agent

Special conditions are needed to clearly visualize thin structures, such as articular cartilage. Wesbey et al. used oral iron solutions to enhance the signal of the gastrointestinal tract of rats and humans during MRI [26]. This method could vividly delineate the gastrointestinal tract because the signal intensity of the cavity was decreased. Similarly, in the present study, the double-contrast agent increased the signal intensity of the articular cartilage and reduced the signal intensity of the joint fluid, which enabled more vivid delineation of the articular cartilage than that achieved by conventional imaging. The SIR values were increased in more progressive OA. This method was effective not only for visualizing articular cartilage but also for detecting OA before articular cartilage degeneration could be detected via conventional MRI.

The contrast agent contains manganese and ferrous ions, which shorten T_1 and T_2 relaxation times [20–22, 28]. $FeCl_3$ is colloidal; therefore, it cannot infiltrate into the normal cartilage and remains in the joint fluid. The ferrous ions decreased the T_2 values of the joint fluid, which decreased the signal intensity of the joint fluid, resulting in an increased SIR [23]. The agent contains 0.5 mmol/L $MnCl_2$ and 2.5 mmol/L $CuSO_4$. The previous study showed that the copper ions have T_1 shortening effect, though the manganese ions dominated the effect of these ions [23].

Articular cartilage consists of a matrix, including PGs and type II collagen, which has a low T_2 value, and free water, which has a high T_2 value [29]. The irregularity and the fissure of degenerative cartilage allowed more manganese ions to enter the cartilage. The T_2 relaxation time of the matrix with manganese ions was reduced, possibly to less than 11.55 ms, which was the TE of the T_2-calculated images; therefore, the signal of the matrix was small enough to be negligible. Moreover, an increase in the relative water content caused the increase in T_2 relaxation time [29]. These reasons may explain why the T_2 values of cartilage in the 4-w OA were significantly greater than those in the control after contrast agent injection. To explain our results more completely, the mechanism should be ascertained using a multi-exponential analysis of T_2 times [30].

Table 3 Histological evaluation using Mankin score and OARSI score for the 2-w OA and 4-w OA Models

3 slices per rabbit		Mankin score					OARSI score				
		Structure	Cells	Safranin-O staining	Tidemark	Total	Safranin-O staining	Structure	Chondrocyte density	Cluster formation	Total
control (*n* = 1)	medial	0.0 ± 0.0	0.0 ± 0.0	0.0 ± 0.0	0.0 ± 0.0	0.0 ± 0.0	0.0 ± 0.0	0.0 ± 0.0	0.0 ± 0.0	0.0 ± 0.0	0.0 ± 0.0
	lateral	0.0 ± 0.0	0.0 ± 0.0	0.0 ± 0.0	0.0 ± 0.0	0.0 ± 0.0	0.0 ± 0.0	0.0 ± 0.0	0.0 ± 0.0	0.0 ± 0.0	0.0 ± 0.0
2-w OA (*n* = 1)	medial	0.0 ± 0.0	2.0 ± 0.0	1.0 ± 0.0	0.0 ± 0.0	3.0 ± 0.0	1.0 ± 0.0	0.0 ± 0.0	1.0 ± 0.0	1.0 ± 0.0	3.0 ± 0.0
	lateral	0.3 ± 0.6	2.0 ± 0.0	1.7 ± 0.6	0.0 ± 0.0	4.0 ± 1.0	2.3 ± 1.2	1.0 ± 1.7	2.0 ± 0.0	2.3 ± 1.2	7.7 ± 1.5
4-w OA (*n* = 4)	medial	3.0 ± 0.6	3.0 ± 0.0	2.6 ± 0.5	0.1 ± 0.3	8.7 ± 0.8	5.1 ± 1.0	4.9 ± 0.8	4.0 ± 0.0	1.0 ± 0.7	15.0 ± 1.5
	lateral	3.0 ± 0.9	3.0 ± 0.0	2.8 ± 0.4	0.1 ± 0.3	8.9 ± 1.1	5.5 ± 0.8	5.2 ± 0.3	4.0 ± 0.0	1.8 ± 0.6	16.4 ± 1.7

The significant difference in the SIR values between the control and the 4-w OA was thought to be caused by the increased signal intensity of cartilage. The increase in T_2 values of degenerative cartilage contributed to the increased signal intensity of cartilage. Additionally, T_1 relaxation time of free water in cartilage was 3 s. Manganese ions shortened T_1 relaxation time of water, which strengthened the signal intensity of cartilage in the MR images, with a TR of 2000 ms.

Limitations

This study had several limitations, one of which is toxicity. Specifically, neurotoxicity has been noted when manganese ions are used in contrast agents [31]. However, abnormal functions and respiratory rates were not observed in this study. Toxicity should be assessed in future studies via cell culture in vitro and animal experiments. The contrast agent contains ferrous ions as negative contrast agents; therefore, low levels of manganese ions were required to obtain sufficient contrast. Inflammatory findings were not observed in this study, which may indicate the safety of this procedure. Another limitation of the study was that only one rabbit from the control group and one from the 2-w OA were assessed histologically.

Conclusions

We evaluated T_2 values and SIR values of the knees in a rabbit OA model and in a control model using a new contrast agent. The OA model had significantly higher values for these parameters than the control model after intra-articular injection of contrast agent. MRI with the double-contrast agent enabled us to detect OA earlier than using conventional MRI.

Abbreviations

dGEMRIC: Delayed gadolinium-enhanced MRI; gag CEST: Glycosaminoglycan chemical exchange saturation transfer; H&E: Hematoxylin and eosin; MRI: Magnetic resonance imaging; OA: Osteoarthritis; OARSI: Osteoarthritis Research Society International; PG: Proteoglycan; ROI: Regions of interest; SIR: Signal intensity ratio

Acknowledgements

We would like to thank Dr. Masahiro Umeda and Dr. Maki Asada for advice on writing the text, and Dr. Masataka Minami for help with making figures.

Funding

This work was supported by JSPS (Japan Society for the Promotion of Science) KAKENHI, Grant Number 26462311.

Authors' contributions

OO, KI, MK, and KU designed the study. OO mainly performed the procedures. KI organized this study. KI and OO contributed substantially to the writing of the paper. OO and MK obtained the MRI data. YK performed the operations with OO. TK supervised the MRI experiment. OO and KM performed the histological assessments. MT supervised the histological assessments. All authors have read and approved the manuscript.

Consent for publication

Not applicable.

Competing interests

The authors declare that they have no competing interests.

Author details

[1]Department of Orthopaedics, Graduate School of Medical Science, Kyoto Prefectural University of Medicine, 602-8566 465, Kajiicho, Kamigyo-ku Kyoto-shi, Kyoto, Japan. [2]Department of Anatomy and Neurobiology, Graduate School of Medical Science, Kyoto Prefectural University of Medicine, Kyoto, Japan.

References

1. Guccione AA, Felson DT, Anderson JJ, Anthony JM, Zhang Y, Wilson PW, et al. The effects of specific medical conditions on the functional limitations of elders in the Framingham study. Am J Public Health. 1994;84(3):351–8.
2. Montero A, Mulero JF, Tornero C, Guitart J, Serrano M. Pain, disability and health-related quality of life in osteoarthritis-joint matters: an observational, multi-specialty trans-national follow-up study. Clin Rheumatol. 2016;35(9):2293–305.
3. Cerhan JR, Wallace RB, el-Khoury GY, Moore TE, Long CR. Decreased survival with increasing prevalence of full-body, radiographically defined osteoarthritis in women. Am J Epidemiol. 1995;141(3):225–34.
4. Madry H, Kon E, Condello V, Peretti GM, Steinwachs M, Seil R, et al. Early osteoarthritis of the knee. Knee Surg Sports Traumatol Arthrosc. 2016;24(6):1753–62.
5. Kellgren JH, Lawrence JS. Rheumatism in miners. II. X-ray study. Br J Ind Med. 1952;9(3):197–207.
6. Felson DT, Niu J, Guermazi A, Sack B, Aliabadi P. Defining radiographic incidence and progression of knee osteoarthritis: suggested modifications of the Kellgren and Lawrence scale. Ann Rheum Dis. 2011;70(11):1884–6.
7. Intema F, Thomas TP, Anderson DD, Elkins JM, Brown TD, Amendola A, et al. Subchondral bone remodeling is related to clinical improvement after joint distraction in the treatment of ankle osteoarthritis. Osteoarthr Cartilage OARS, Osteoarthr Res Soc. 2011;19(6):668–75.
8. Bijlsma JW, Berenbaum F, Lafeber FP. Osteoarthritis: an update with relevance for clinical practice. Lancet (London, England). 2011;377(9783):2115–26.
9. Li X, Pai A, Blumenkrantz G, Carballido-Gamio J, Link T, Ma B, et al. Spatial distribution and relationship of T1rho and T2 relaxation times in knee cartilage with osteoarthritis. Magn Reson Med. 2009;61(6):1310–8.
10. Borthakur A, Shapiro EM, Beers J, Kudchodkar S, Kneeland JB, Reddy R. Sensitivity of MRI to proteoglycan depletion in cartilage: comparison of sodium and proton MRI. Osteoarthr Cartilage OARS Osteoarthr Res Soc. 2000;8(4):288–93.
11. Raya JG, Arnoldi AP, Weber DL, Filidoro L, Dietrich O, Adam-Neumair S, et al. Ultra-high field diffusion tensor imaging of articular cartilage correlated with histology and scanning electron microscopy. Magma (New York, NY). 2011;24(4):247–58.
12. Recht MP, Goodwin DW, Winalski CS, White LM. MRI of articular cartilage: revisiting current status and future directions. AJR Am J Roentgenol. 2005;185(4):899–914.
13. Ling W, Regatte RR, Navon G, Jerschow A. Assessment of glycosaminoglycan concentration in vivo by chemical exchange-dependent saturation transfer (gagCEST). Proc Natl Acad Sci U S A. 2008;105(7):2266–70.
14. Gray ML, Burstein D, Kim YJ, Maroudas A. 2007 Elizabeth Winston Lanier award winner. Magnetic resonance imaging of cartilage glycosaminoglycan: basic principles, imaging technique, and clinical applications. J Orthop Res. 2008;26(3):281–91.

15. McAlindon TE, Nuite M, Krishnan N, Ruthazer R, Price LL, Burstein D, et al. Change in knee osteoarthritis cartilage detected by delayed gadolinium enhanced magnetic resonance imaging following treatment with collagen hydrolysate: a pilot randomized controlled trial. Osteoarthr Cartil OARS Osteoarthr Res Soc. 2011;19(4):399–405.
16. Ward KM, Aletras AH, Balaban RS. A new class of contrast agents for MRI based on proton chemical exchange dependent saturation transfer (CEST). J Magnetic Resonance (San Diego, Calif : 1997). 2000;143(1):79–87.
17. Rehnitz C, Kupfer J, Streich NA, Burkholder I, Schmitt B, Lauer L, et al. Comparison of biochemical cartilage imaging techniques at 3 T MRI. Osteoarthr Cartilage OARS Osteoarthr Res Soc. 2014;22(10):1732–42.
18. Felson DT, Hodgson R. Identifying and treating preclinical and early osteoarthritis. Rheum Dis Clin N Am. 2014;40(4):699–710.
19. Wheaton AJ, Borthakur A, Shapiro EM, Regatte RR, Akella SV, Kneeland JB, et al. Proteoglycan loss in human knee cartilage: quantitation with sodium MR imaging–feasibility study. Radiology. 2004;231(3):900–5.
20. Kuo YT, Herlihy AH, So PW, Bhakoo KK, Bell JD. In vivo measurements of T1 relaxation times in mouse brain associated with different modes of systemic administration of manganese chloride. J Magn Reson Imaging. 2005;21(4):334–9.
21. Sheppard D, Allan L, Martin P, McLeay T, Milne W, Houston JG. Contrast-enhanced magnetic resonance cholangiography using mangafodipir compared with standard T2W MRC sequences: a pictorial essay. J Magn Reson Imaging. 2004;20(2):256–63.
22. Geraldes CF, Sherry AD, Brown RD 3rd, Koenig SH. Magnetic field dependence of solvent proton relaxation rates induced by Gd3+ and Mn2+ complexes of various polyaza macrocyclic ligands: implications for NMR imaging. Magn Reson Med. 1986;3(2):242–50.
23. Kido M, Ikoma K, Hara Y, Matsuda K, Kawata M, Umeda M, et al. Selective visualization of rabbit knee cartilage using MR imaging with a double-contrast agent. J Magn Reson Imaging. 2014;39(5):1186–90.
24. Mankin HJ, Dorfman H, Lippiello L, Zarins A. Biochemical and metabolic abnormalities in articular cartilage from osteo-arthritic human hips. II. Correlation of morphology with biochemical and metabolic data. J Bone Joint Surg Am. 1971;53(3):523–37.
25. Laverty S, Girard CA, Williams JM, Hunziker EB, Pritzker KP. The OARSI histopathology initiative - recommendations for histological assessments of osteoarthritis in the rabbit. Osteoarthr Cartilage OARS Osteoarthr Res Soc. 2010;18(Suppl 3):S53–65.
26. Rakhra KS, Lattanzio PJ, Cardenas-Blanco A, Cameron IG, Beaule PE. Can T1-rho MRI detect acetabular cartilage degeneration in femoroacetabular impingement? A pilot study. J Bone Joint Surg Br Volume. 2012;94(9):1187–92.
27. Wei B, Mao F, Guo Y, Yao Q, Tang C, Xu Y, et al. Using 7.0T MRI T2 mapping to detect early changes of the cartilage matrix caused by immobilization in a rabbit model of immobilization-induced osteoarthritis. Magn Reson Imaging. 2015;33(8):1000–6.
28. Mitchell DG, Alam F. Mangafodipir trisodium: effects on T2- and T1-weighted MR cholangiography. J Magn Reson Imaging. 1999;9(2):366–8.
29. Dunn TC, Lu Y, Jin H, Ries MD, Majumdar S. T2 relaxation time of cartilage at MR imaging: comparison with severity of knee osteoarthritis. Radiology. 2004;232(2):592–8.
30. Lattanzio PJ, Marshall KW, Damyanovich AZ, Peemoeller H. Macromolecule and water magnetization exchange modeling in articular cartilage. Magn Reson Med. 2000;44(6):840–51.
31. Takeda A. Manganese action in brain function. Brain research. Brain Res Rev. 2003;41(1):79–87.

3

Systematic review of quantitative imaging biomarkers for neck and shoulder musculoskeletal disorders

Judith E. Gold[1,5*], David M. Hallman[1], Fredrik Hellström[1], Martin Björklund[1,2], Albert G. Crenshaw[1], Svend Erik Mathiassen[1], Mary F. Barbe[3] and Sayed Ali[4]

Abstract

Background: This study systematically summarizes quantitative imaging biomarker research in non-traumatic neck and shoulder musculoskeletal disorders (MSDs). There were two research questions: 1) Are there quantitative imaging biomarkers associated with the presence of neck and shoulder MSDs?, 2) Are there quantitative imaging biomarkers associated with the severity of neck and shoulder MSDs?

Methods: PubMed and SCOPUS were used for the literature search. One hundred and twenty-five studies met primary inclusion criteria. Data were extracted from 49 sufficient quality studies.

Results: Most of the 125 studies were cross-sectional and utilized convenience samples of patients as both cases and controls. Only half controlled for potential confounders via exclusion or in the analysis. Approximately one-third reported response rates. In sufficient quality articles, 82% demonstrated at least one statistically significant association between the MSD(s) and biomarker(s) studied. The literature synthesis suggested that neck muscle size may be decreased in neck pain, and trapezius myalgia and neck/shoulder pain may be associated with reduced vascularity in the trapezius and reduced trapezius oxygen saturation at rest and in response to upper extremity tasks. Reduced vascularity in the supraspinatus tendon may also be a feature in rotator cuff tears. Five of eight studies showed an association between a quantitative imaging marker and MSD severity.

Conclusions: Although research on quantitative imaging biomarkers is still in a nascent stage, some MSD biomarkers were identified. There are limitations in the articles examined, including possible selection bias and inattention to potentially confounding factors. Recommendations for future studies are provided.

Keywords: MRI, MSD, Near-infrared spectroscopy, Pain, Ultrasound

Background

Soft tissue neck and shoulder musculoskeletal disorders (MSDs), namely, disorders of the muscles, tendons, ligaments, nerves, or blood vessels, are prevalent worldwide [1–4], are a common cause of work absence and disability [5], and impose a sizeable societal economic burden [1, 3, 4, 6–11].

Most options for screening, surveillance and diagnosis of proximal upper extremity MSDs depend on symptoms. Improved diagnostic and screening methods, especially objective techniques, are needed [12, 13]. A biomarker has been defined as "a characteristic that is objectively measured and evaluated as an indicator of normal biologic processes, pathogenic processes, or pharmacologic responses to a therapeutic intervention"[14]. Quantitative medical imaging techniques are increasingly used in clinical practice and MSD research, and enable detection of potential MSD biomarkers, including functional and morphological changes. The Quantitative Imaging Biomarkers Alliance and the Terminology Working Group define a quantitative imaging biomarker as "an objective characteristic derived from an in vivo image measured on a ratio or interval scale as an indicator of normal biological

* Correspondence: JudithEGold@gmail.com
[1]Centre for Musculoskeletal Research, Department of Occupational and Public Health Sciences, University of Gävle, Gävle, Sweden
[5]Gold Standard Research Consulting, 830 Montgomery Ave, Bryn Mawr, PA, USA
Full list of author information is available at the end of the article

processes, pathogenic processes or a response to a therapeutic intervention" [15]. Valid and reliable biomarkers could improve diagnosis and screening methods [16] and provide objective means to evaluate medical treatments and workplace interventions. Use of such biomarkers may also elucidate MSD pathomechanisms.

Three biomarkers classes are conventionally described: exposure, effect (disease), and susceptibility [17]. Herein, we have reviewed biomarkers of effect, defined as "any change that is qualitatively or quantitatively predictive of health impairment or potential impairment..." [17]. Through measurement of biomarkers of effect, pathophysiological processes may be illuminated and used to stage MSD severity, such as early biomarkers that precede disease diagnosis versus late biomarkers in already diagnosed subjects.

Previous biomarker reviews

Prior reviews on this topic include a pioneering paper highlighting the potential for MSD biomarkers to detect subclinical disease and monitor MSD severity [18], and a later MSD review article [19] focused on biochemical markers. Neither paper mentioned medical imaging. Our recent systematic review also focused on biochemical biomarkers in MSDs [20]. To our knowledge, there have been no published reviews of quantitative imaging biomarkers in neck and shoulder MSDs.

The purpose of this systematic review was to conduct a comprehensive assessment of quantitative imaging biomarkers in neck and shoulder MSDs. We aimed to answer the following two research questions:

1. Are there quantitative imaging biomarkers associated with the presence of neck and shoulder MSDs?
2. Are there quantitative imaging biomarkers associated with the severity of neck and shoulder MSDs?

Methods

Review team and process overview. Our review team consisted of eight researchers with expertise in musculoskeletal radiology and in epidemiologic, intervention and experimental studies, including studies on pathomechanisms within the field of work-related MSD research. The review process was as follows: 1) research questions were formulated; 2) principal concepts of the review were defined; 3) a search strategy and terms were developed (Additional file 1); 4) PubMed and Scopus databases were searched, with results pooled with articles identified from the authors' files; 5) identified papers were screened based on pre-defined criteria (Additional files 1, 2 and 3) using a two-step procedure of primary (title and abstract) and secondary (quality) screens; 6) summary tables were created from sufficient quality papers; and 7) evidence was synthesized with respect to the two research questions. A consensus process was used throughout the review process. See Gold et al. for further details [20].

Neck and shoulder MSDs were defined as clinical diagnoses or musculoskeletal symptoms in the neck and shoulder region. These included both specific and non-specific conditions related to muscles, tendons, nerves, blood vessels or ligaments [21]. The scope of this review encompassed MSDs that occur in a work-related context [22].

Quantitative imaging biomarker was defined as an objective characteristic derived from an in vivo image or from an in vivo signal captured in response to electromagnetic radiation to detect morphology or function, measured on a ratio or interval scale as an indicator of normal biological or pathogenic processes [15]. We have focused on minimally invasive/non-invasive methods. Potential quantitative imaging biomarkers could be derived through MRI, ultrasound, far infrared thermography, near infrared spectroscopy (NIRS), laser Doppler flowmetry, and other modalities. Thus, for example, muscle oxygenation as measured through NIRS was included in this review. Because plain radiographs (x-rays) are best utilized in evaluating bone abnormalities and have poor contrast resolution, this imaging modality is not routinely indicated in soft tissue evaluation [23–26]. Thus, studies using only plain radiography were excluded from this review.

Severity was operationalized as encompassing longitudinal and cross-sectional differences in symptoms.

Inclusion criteria. The current review was limited to studies on adults (age > 18 years) with non-traumatic neck and shoulder MSDs, published between June 4, 1988 and October 14, 2016 and written in English language. Potential biomarkers were examined for the following specific MSDs, as categorized by Boocock, et al. [21]: rotator cuff syndrome/shoulder tendonitis, shoulder capsulitis and thoracic outlet syndrome. Other specific MSDs included are listed in Boocock, et al. [21] Table 2, although status post-whiplash, cervico-brachial fibromyalgia, and joint-related conditions were excluded. Upper extremity non-specific regional pain, namely, "neck pain", "shoulder pain", and "neck/shoulder pain", was also included. We included articles that met our inclusion criteria, even if some parts of the study were consistent with the exclusion criteria; however, only results in compliance with our criteria were included.

Exclusion criteria are summarized in Additional file 2.

Literature search

The search was first conducted in PubMed and combined with articles identified from the authors' files. Articles were screened for quality. If met, a second search for papers that cited the sufficient quality articles was conducted using Scopus. Additional file 1 provides an overview of the search strategy, while Fig. 1 illustrates the overall search strategy and selection procedure. PubMed search terms included both MESH terms and key words selected for two categories: neck and shoulder MSDs, and biomarkers. Search terms within each category were combined using the "OR" operator, while search terms between categories were combined using "AND". A systematic procedure was carried out for selection of appropriate MESH terms and key words, where each search term was entered by a step-wise procedure. Fifteen articles were identified by the review team and used for refining the search and testing its sensitivity. See Additional file 4 for the search string.

A total of 4002 articles were examined by members of the review team. The final PubMed search resulted in 3999 articles; three additional papers were added from the team members' personal files. Primary and secondary screens were implemented (see below and Additional files 1, 2 and 3). The Scopus search identified recently published articles in PubMed that still lacked assigned MESH terms. Since a PubMed search may miss relevant studies in other databases, the Scopus search reduced this potential search strategy bias. To assure clarity and limit reviewer bias, pilot testing of evaluation criteria was conducted at each stage of the review process.

Primary screen-selection of articles

The primary screen was conducted by two independent reviewers assessing each title and abstract for eligibility based on inclusion and exclusion criteria (Additional file 2), after importing all records from PubMed into systematic review software (EPPI-reviewer4 v4.3.4, EPPI-Centre, Social Science Research Unit, Institute of Education, University of London, UK). The full text was read if necessary. A "yes" answer on any question in Additional file 2 resulted in article exclusion. Results were compared between reviewers, and consensus agreement was reached in all cases (with input from a third person in case of disagreement between reviewers). The same procedure was repeated for articles from personal files and articles found in Scopus.

Secondary screen-quality assessment and data extraction

All articles passing the primary screen were scored for quality by five review team members. The articles were randomly allocated to five different clusters; each reviewer was assigned randomly to two of these clusters. In the quality screen, each article was assessed by two independent reviewers, scores were compared, and a consensus agreement was reached after discussing disagreements (using a third reviewer as needed). Additional file 3 lists questions used for the quality assessment. These questions were derived from reporting guidelines and checklists for quality assessment in health-related research studies [27–31]. Seventeen items were included in the scoring system, with each item scored as either "yes" (1 point), "unknown or not applicable" (0) or "no" (0). Scores were summed for each paper (range: 0–17). Articles scoring at or above 70% of the maximum (12/17) were labeled as "sufficient quality" and were included for data extraction. Articles scoring "no" on question 15 were excluded from data extraction. These included papers with less than appropriate statistical analysis methods, such as multiple comparisons without adjustment, and modeling without accounting for repeated measures. Data extraction items are listed in Additional file 5.

Research synthesis

Ulitizing a best evidence synthesis approach, we evaluated the number of sufficient quality articles in order to

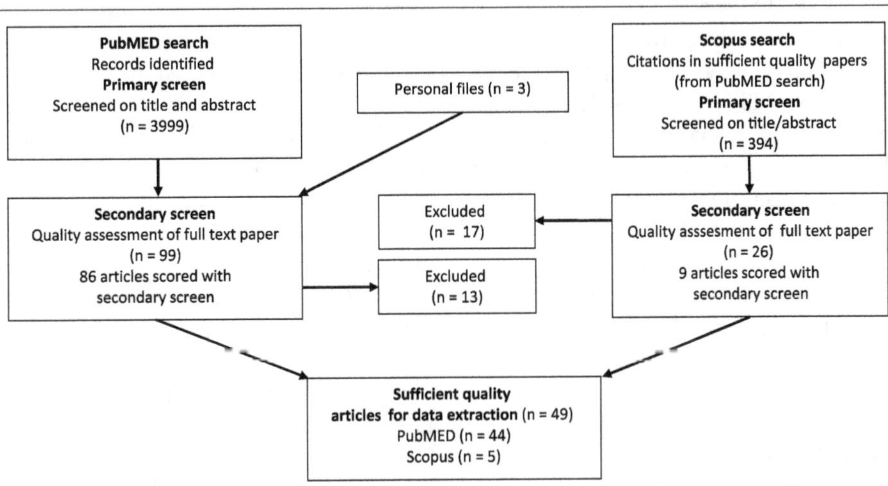

Fig. 1 Flowchart of literature search

identify a particular biomarker or class of biomarkers in their potential association with MSD(s) [32]. Considering the biomarker heterogeneity, it was not possible to conduct a meta-analysis. However, it was possible to group results according to the MSD, and then by physiological process or morphology, e.g., hemodynamic and/or oxygenation indicators or muscle dimensions, within diagnoses or symptom designations. An association between a biomarker and an MSD in three or more sufficient quality studies (and at most one sufficient quality study with a null finding) was regarded as evidence that an indicator could serve as a MSD quantitative imaging biomarker. We did not design our review to present different levels of evidence.

Results

Of the 3999 articles identified through the PubMed (primary) search (Fig. 1), and the three papers added from authors' files, 99 met secondary screening criteria. Ten papers were excluded after reading the entire article, and three eliminated due to inadequate statistical methods, leaving 86 articles to be scored in the secondary (quality) screen. Forty-four of these met the sufficient quality criteria score. The Scopus database search of these 44 sufficient quality papers yielded 394 citations of which 26 were determined to be non-duplicates and relevant through title and abstract review. Seventeen were eliminated at the secondary screening stage after reading the entire article. Nine articles were scored during the secondary screen, although one was eliminated from data extraction for less than appropriate statistical methods. Of the remaining Scopus identified articles, five scored at ≥12. These five were added to the 44 PubMed identified and similarly scored articles. Thus, 49 studies were regarded to be of sufficient quality for data extraction.

Secondary screen-quality assessment overview

Additional file 6 shows quality scores of all papers that had undergone secondary screening (n = 96; 86 from PubMed and 9 from Scopus). The majority had clearly defined aims, biomarkers, MSDs, and results. All but two unique studies (one longitudinal cohort represented by [33–35] and the other by [36]) had a cross-sectional design, and most utilized convenience samplings of patients, for both cases and referents. Just over half of the studies controlled for confounding factors through exclusion to a particular age or gender, or through a statistical adjustment in the analysis. Thirty-four studies (37%) explicitly stated that those analyzing biomarkers were blinded to case status.

Data extraction from sufficient quality studies

Additional file 7 gives a descriptive overview of the included studies. The bulk of sufficient quality studies examined neck pain, rotator cuff tears, and trapezius myalgia and other neck/shoulder pain conditions. No sufficient quality studies examined thoracic outlet syndrome. Approximately three-quarters (19/25) of the shoulder disorder studies were conducted in populations with at least one analysis group having an average age of ≥50 years. In contrast, the mean age by analysis groups in the neck pain studies ranged from 22 to 34 years, while the mean age in neck/shoulder studies ranged from 23 to 48 years.

Are there quantitative imaging biomarkers associated with the presence of neck and shoulder MSDs?

The majority of studies demonstrated an association between at least one biomarker and the MSD(s) examined (Table 1). Only 9/49 (18%) studies reported insignificant findings throughout [37–45].

Neck pain (10 studies)

Ten studies examined neck pain [37, 38, 46–53]. Decreased muscle dimensions were observed in cases in the cervical multifidus during rest [47]. In Rahnama et al. [52], no difference in multifidus muscle thickness was observed during baseline, but there was a smaller increase in cases than in controls in muscle thickness from baseline values during isometric maximum voluntary contraction (MVC). An increased muscle shape ratio (ratio between lateral and anterior-posterior dimensions) was seen in the multifidus of cases [47]. Reduced muscle dimensions were also observed in the longus colli [48, 49], and in the semispinalis capitis on cases' painful side [50]. Dorsal neck muscle thickness change from rest to MVC was different in neck pain cases than in controls, with a tendency toward increased semispinalis capitis thickness in controls, and increased semispinalis cervicis thickness in cases [53]. There was no difference in subcutaneous tissue thickness above the sternocleidomastoid or anterior scalene muscles [38].

Greater serratus anterior muscle activity, measured using fMRI, was observed at thoracic vertebral level 6 in cases [51]. However, less longus colli recruitment, measured by muscle thickness, was found at the greatest flexion angle during incremental nodding [49]. Elliott et al. [46] detected less fat infiltration in neck extensors in neck pain vs. whiplash patients. No difference in trapezius skin temperature, or temperature asymmetry between the left and right trapezii was observed in neck pain vs. controls [37].

Rotator cuff tear (11 studies)

Eleven studies investigated rotator cuff tears [33–36, 39, 54–59]. Decreased supraspinatus vascularity or blood flow was observed in two studies [55, 58], and reduced supraspinatus functional capillary density in another [54]. In

Table 1 Are there quantitative imaging biomarkers associated with the presence of neck and shoulder MSDs?

MSD Classification and diagnosis	Author(s)	Major results (case-control comparison)	Conclusion
Neck disorders and symptoms			
Neck pain	Dibai Filho (2012) [37]	Skin temperature Skin temperature (L & R trapezius), difference btwn sides (thermal asymmetry), NS.	No
Neck pain	Elliott (2008) [46]	Fat index indicating fatty infiltration (relative fat) Fat index: cases < controls, $p < 0.001$ in all muscles.	Yes ↓ fat index in cases in all neck extensor muscles (see Additional file 7).
Neck pain	Falla (2004) [38]	Subcutaneous tissue thickness over SCM, AS SCM subcutaneous tissue thickness (L & R): NS cases vs. controls AS subcutaneous tissue thickness (L & R): NS cases vs. controls	No
Neck pain	Fernández-de-las-Peñas (2008) [47]	Multifidus CSA, muscle shape ratio CSA: ANOVA, group ($p < 0.001$) & cervical level ($p < 0.001$) effects. No interactions. Cases < controls at C3, C4, C5 ($p < 0.001$) & at C6 ($p < 0.01$). Muscle shape ratio: ANOVA, group ($p < 0.001$) & cervical level ($p < 0.001$) effects. Significant interactions btwn group & level ($p = 0.01$). Cases > controls at C3 ($p < 0.001$) & C6 ($p < 0.01$).	Yes ↓ multifidus CSA in cases at C3, C4, C5, C6 ↑ muscle shape ratio in cases at C3, C6
Neck pain	Javanshir (2011) [48]	Lco CSA, anterior-posterior dimension (APD), lateral dimension (LD), and shape ratio (LD/APD) Lco CSA: cases < controls, $p < 0.001$. Lco APD: cases < controls, $p < 0.01$. Lco LD, shape ratio, NS cases vs. controls.	Yes ↓ Lco CSA in cases ↓ Lco APD in cases
Neck pain	Karimi (2016) [53]	Dorsal neck muscle thickness change w. 50% & 100% shoulder MVC in 6 directions Dorsal neck muscle thickness: During MVC: significant interaction of group x muscle, $p = 0.008$. NS, cases vs. controls group x direction; group x force.	Yes Dorsal neck muscle thickness group x muscle effect
Neck pain	Jesus-Moraleida (2011) [49]	Lco thickness, SCM thickness, change of thickness during test/thickness during rest = proportion of muscle recruitment Lco thickness increase throughout all CCFT phases: cases < controls ($p < 0.001$). SCM thickness increase throughout all CCFT phases: NS, cases vs. controls. Lco recruitment: cases < controls, phase 4 ($p = 0.02$), phase 5 ($p = 0.004$), NS other phases. SCM recruitment: NS, cases vs. controls.	Yes ↓ Lco thickness increase throughout all CCFT phases in cases ↓ Lco recruitment, phases 4 & 5
Neck pain	Park (2013) [50]	Mean difference in the bilateral semispinalis capitis muscle thickness Mean difference in the bilateral semispinalis capitis thickness: cases > controls, $p < 0.05$. Within cases mean difference in the bilateral semispinalis capitis thickness: painful side < asymptomatic side, $p < 0.05$.	Yes ↑ mean difference in the bilateral semispinalis capitis thickness in cases ↓ mean difference in the bilateral semispinalis capitis thickness in painful side
Neck pain	Rahnama (2015) [52]	Multifidus muscle thickness change w. shoulder MVC in 6 directions Multifidus muscle thickness: baseline: NS, cases vs. controls; During MVC: significant interaction of group x force, controls > cases ($p = 0.03$). NS, cases vs. controls group x direction; 3- & 4-way interactions involving group.	Yes ↓ multifidus muscle thickness increase in cases during isometric MVC

Table 1 Are there quantitative imaging biomarkers associated with the presence of neck and shoulder MSDs? *(Continued)*

Neck pain	Sheard (2012) [51]	Differences in water relaxation values (T2 relaxation) quantified from scans before and after exercise were calculated (T2 shift) as a measure of SA muscle activity T2 shift: significant effect for level ($p = .03$) and significant group × level interaction ($p = .04$) but no significant main effect for group ($p = .59$). Post hoc T2 shift: cases > controls at the T6 level ($P = .02$) only.	Yes ↑ T2 shift at T6 in cases
Shoulder disorders and symptoms			
Degenerative rotator cuff lesion	Biberthaler (2003) [54]	Mean functional capillary density, mean capillary diameterMean functional capillary density: lesion < control tissue ($p < 0.05$). Mean capillary diameter: NS, lesion vs. control tissue ($p > 0.05$).	Yes ↓ mean functional capillary density in lesion tissue
Rotator cuff tear (full thickness)	Chang (2014) [56]	Biceps long tendon (BLT) width, thickness, flattening ratio (width/thickness), cross-sectional area, echogenicity ratio BLT width, echogenicity ratio: NS, cases vs. controls BLT thickness: cases > controls, $p < 0.01$. BLT flattening ratio: cases < controls, $p < 0.01$. BLT cross-sectional area: cases > controls, $p < 0.01$.	Yes ↑ BLT thickness in cases ↓ BLT flattening ratio in cases ↑ BLT cross-sectional area in cases
Rotator cuff tear	Choo (2014) [57]	Rotator cable thickness, width Rotator cable thickness: difference among 4 groups (see shoulder tendinosis - Choo), $p < 0.001$; post-hoc analysis – full-thickness tear > normal, $p < 0.001$. Rotator cable width: difference among 4 groups (see shoulder tendinosis - Choo), $p < 0.001$; post-hoc analysis – full-thickness tear > normal, $p < 0.001$; partial-thickness tear > normal[a].	Yes ↑ rotator cable thickness in full-thickness tears ↑ rotator cable width in full-thickness tears Perhaps ↑ rotator cable width in partial-thickness tears
Rotator cuff tear	Funakoshi (2010) [55]	Vascularity in 4 ROIs: articular & bursal sides of supraspinatus tendon, medial & lateral sides of bursa Non-injected side: cases (RCT) < controls, $p < 0.0001$, in articular & bursal side of the supraspinatus tendon. Injected side: cases (contralateral to RCT) < controls, $p < 0.0001$, in articular & bursal side of the supraspinatus tendon. Cases vs. controls, NS, in medial and lateral side of bursa.	Perhaps ↓ vascularity in articular & bursal sides of supraspinatus in non-injected (rotator cuff tear) side in cases, but may be attributed to age. ↓ vascularity in articular & bursal sides of supraspinatus in injected (rotator cuff intact) side in cases, but may be attributed to age.
Rotator cuff tear	Hirano (2006) [39]	Full vs. partial rotator cuff tear, rotator cuff tear length, amount of subacrominal-subdeltoid bursal fluid Proportion of full & partial tears, NS. Proportion in categorical size of tears, NS. amount of subacrominal-subdeltoid bursal fluid, NS .	No
Rotator cuff tear	Karthikeyan (2015) [58]	Total blood flow in 4 supraspinatus zones, in anteromedial zone, in posteromedial zone Total blood flow in 4 supraspinatus zones: cases (including shoulder impingement – see below) < controls, $p = 0.001$. Anteromedial supraspinatus zone: full-thickness tears < controls, $p = 0.02$; partial-thickness tears vs. controls, NS. Posteromedial supraspinatus zone: full-thickness tears < controls, $p = 0.04$; partial-thickness tears vs. controls, NS.	Yes ↓ supraspinatus blood flow in cases ↓ anteromedial supraspinatus blood flow in full-thickness tears ↓ posteromedial supraspinatus blood flow in full-thickness tears

Table 1 Are there quantitative imaging biomarkers associated with the presence of neck and shoulder MSDs? *(Continued)*

Rotator cuff tear (full-thickness)	Keener (2015) [35]	Baseline rotator cuff tear width; Width enlargement (defined as ≥ 5 mm compared with that at baseline) percentage Baseline rotator cuff tear width: rotator cuff tear with anterior supraspinatus cable disruption > rotator cuff tear with anterior supraspinatus cable intact, $p < 0.0001$. Width enlargement percentage: NS, rotator cuff tear with anterior supraspinatus cable disruption vs. rotator cuff tear with anterior supraspinatus cable intact .	Yes ↑ baseline rotator cuff tear width with anterior supraspinatus cable disruption.
Rotator cuff tear	Mall (2010) [33]	Rotator cuff tear length, tear width, tear area, rate of substantial tear progression (transformation of a partial-thickness tear into a full-thickness tear or a size increase of > 5 mm in either the width or the length of a full thickness tear compared with that at the time of enrollment) Time of enrollment: full-thickness tear width: symptomatic > asymptomatic, $p = 0.02$; tear length, tear area, NS. Change between visit 1 & visit 2 (see paper for definitions): Shoulder remained asymptomatic: NS, tear length, width, area. Shoulder became symptomatic: tear length: visit 2 > visit 1, $p = 0.008$. tear width: visit 2 > visit 1, $p = 0.01$ tear area: visit 2 > visit 1, $p = 0.006$. Rate of substantial tear progression: symptomatic > asymptomatic, $p < 0.01$	Yes ↑ full-thickness tear width at enrollment in those who later became symptomatic in asymptomatic shoulder. ↑ tear length, width, & area at visit 2 vs. at visit 1 in those who became symptomatic in asymptomatic shoulder. ↑ rate substantial tear progression in in those who became symptomatic in asymptomatic shoulder.
Rotator cuff tear	Moosmayer (2013) [36]	Rotator cuff tear size in anteroposterior plane, in mediolateral plane, tear size increase in anteroposterior plane, in mediolateral plane. Rotator cuff tear size in anteroposterior plane: baseline: NS, symptomatic vs. asymptomatic; 3-year follow-up: symptomatic > asymptomatic, $p = 0.02$ Rotator cuff tear size in mediolateral plane: baseline: NS, symptomatic vs. asymptomatic; 3-year follow-up: NS, symptomatic vs. asymptomatic. Tear size increase in anteroposterior plane: NS, symptomatic vs. asymptomatic. Tear size increase in mediolateral plane: NS, symptomatic vs. asymptomatic.	Yes ↑ rotator cuff tear size in anteroposterior plane at follow-up in tears that became symptomatic
Rotator cuff tear (partial & full) or rotator cuff disease	Keener (2015) [34]	Rotator cuff tear enlargement (see paper for definition) Tear enlargement in 49%; median time to enlargement = 2.8 yrs. tear enlargement: assoc. w. final tear type, $p < 0.05$: full vs. control, HR = 4.17; partial vs. control, HR = 2.73; full vs. partial, HR = 1.53 (all $p < 0.05$, no CI given). New shoulder pain in 46%; median time to pain = 2.6 yrs. shoulder pain assoc. w. final tear type, $p < 0.05$. Assoc. w. tear enlargement, HR = 1.66, $p < 0.05$. 63% became painful before or at tear enlargement; 22% became painful later.	Yes ↑ risk tear enlargement in full-tears vs. controls, in partial tears vs controls, in full-tears vs. partial tears. ↑ risk new shoulder pain w. tear enlargement.

Table 1 Are there quantitative imaging biomarkers associated with the presence of neck and shoulder MSDs? *(Continued)*

Rotator cuff tear	Terabayashi (2014) [59]	Difference in blood flow peak systolic velocity (PSV), resistance index (RI) between sides Difference between sides in PSV in BA: NS, in any group. Difference between sides in PSV in AHCA: affected > unaffected side in rotator cuff tear with night pain, $p < 0.001$. NS, other groups. Difference between sides in RI in BA: NS, in any group. Difference between sides in RI in AHCA: affected < unaffected side in rotator cuff tear with night pain, $p < 0.01$.	Yes ↑ PSV in AHCA in affected vs unaffected side in rotator cuff tear with night pain. ↓ RI in AHCA in affected vs unaffected side in rotator cuff tear with night pain.
Supraspinatus tendinopathy	Arend (2014) [63]	Maximal supraspinatus tendon thickness (MSTT) MSTT: cases > controls, $p < 0.05$	Yes ↑ MSTT in cases
Rotator cuff tendinitis	Cay (2012) [60]	Subacromial distance, humeral head diameter, Glenoid APD, glenoid articular surface diameter Sagittal subacromial distance: cases < controls, $p < 0.001$ humeral head diameter, glenoid APD, axial glenoid/humerus, and axial glenoid minus humerus, NS in cases vs controls. coronal diameter of humerus: cases < controls, $p = 0.02$. coronal glenoid/humerus, coronal glenoid minus humerus: NS in cases vs controls.	Yes ↓ sagittal subacromial distance in cases ↓ coronal diameter of humerus in cases
Rotator cuff tendinosis	Choo (2014) [57]	Rotator cable thickness, width Rotator cable thickness: difference among 4 groups (see rotator cuff tear - Choo), $p < 0.001$; post-hoc analysis – NS, tendinosis vs controls. Rotator cable width: difference among 4 groups (see rotator cuff tear - Choo), $p < 0.001$; post-hoc analysis – tendinosis > normal, $p < 0.05$[a].	Perhaps ↑ rotator cable width in tendinosis
Rotator cuff tendinitis	Rechardt (2010) [61]	Carotid artery intima-media thickness Carotid artery imtima-media thickness: NS, in males and females.	No
Shoulder tendinopathy	Joensen (2009) [62]	Supraspinatus tendon thickness Tendon thickness: symptomatic side > asymptomatic side, $p < 0.01$.	Yes ↑ tendon thickness in symptomatic side
Frozen shoulder (Adhesive capsulitis)	Li (2011) [64]	CHL thickness CHL thickness: cases > controls, $p < 0.001$.	Yes ↑ CHL thickness in cases
Frozen shoulder (Adhesive capsulitis)	Michelin (2013) [67]	Joint capsule thickness Joint capsule thickness: cases > controls, $p < 0.0001$	Yes ↑ joint capsule thickness in cases
Frozen shoulder (Adhesive capsulitis)	Song (2011) [65]	Joint capsule thickness in the axillary recess, enhancing portion of the axillary recess thickness, rotator interval thickness Axillary recess: Joint capsule thickness: cases > controls, $p < 0.001$. Axillary recess enhancing portion thickness: cases > controls, $p < 0.001$. Rotator interval Enhancing portion thickness cases > controls, $p < 0.001$.	Yes ↑ axillary recess joint capsule thickness in cases ↑ Axillary recess enhancing portion thickness in cases ↑ Rotator interval Enhancing portion thickness in cases
Frozen shoulder (Adhesive capsulitis	Zhao (2012) [66]	CHL thickness, articular capsule thickness CHL thickness: cases > controls, $p < 0.001$. articular capsule thickness: cases > controls, $p < 0.05$.	Yes ↑ CHL thickness in cases ↑ articular capsule thickness in cases
Shoulder impingement syndrome	Daghir (2011) [71]	Subacromial-subdeltoid bursal thickness Greatest thickness in any view: NS cases vs. controls. Thickness in shortaxis supraspinatus view: cases > controls, $p = 0.0009$. Thickness in long-axis supraspinatus view: NS cases vs. controls.Thickness in long-axis subscapularis view: NS cases vs. controls.	Yes ↑ subacromial-subdeltoid bursal thickness in cases on shortaxis supraspinatus view

Table 1 Are there quantitative imaging biomarkers associated with the presence of neck and shoulder MSDs? *(Continued)*

Shoulder impingement syndrome	Hébert (2003) [68]	AHD Cases vs. contralateral control: Flexion: main effect of group, $p < 0.01$, and no interaction with position. Post hoc comparisons: cases < controls at 70, 90, 110 & 130 degrees, $p < 0.01$. Abduction: main effect of group, $p < 0.01$, no interaction with position. Post hoc comparisons: cases < controls at 80, 90, $p < 0.05$ and 110 degrees, $p < 0.01$. Cases vs. contralateral control vs. asymptomatic controls: Flexion - main effect of group, $p < 0.0001$, (position effect, $p < 0.0001$) interaction with position, $p = 0.01$. Post hoc comparisons: cases < asymptomatic controls at 90 & 110 degrees, $p < 0.01$. NS contralateral control vs asymptomatic controls, all positions. Abduction - main effect of group, $p = 0.052$. Post hoc comparisons: cases < asymptomatic controls at 90 & 110 degrees, $p < 0.01$. NS contralateral control vs asymptomatic controls, all positions.	Yes ↓ AHD in cases at 70, 90, 110, 130 degrees flexion vs. contralateral control ↓ AHD in cases at 80, 90, 110 degrees abduction vs. contralateral control ↓ AHD in cases at 90, 110 degrees flexion vs. asymptomatic controls ↓ AHD in cases at in 90, 110 degrees abduction vs. asymptomatic controls
Shoulder impingement syndrome	Karthikeyan (2015) [58]	Total blood flow in 4 supraspinatus zones, in anteromedial zone, in posteromedial zone Total blood flow in 4 supraspinatus zones: cases (including rotator cuff tears – see above) < controls, $p = 0.001$. Anteromedial supraspinatus zone: shoulder impingement < controls, $p = 0.01$. Posteromedial supraspinatus zone: shoulder impingement < controls, $p = 0.03$.	Yes ↓ supraspinatus blood flow in cases ↓ anteromedial supraspinatus blood flow in cases ↓ posteromedial supraspinatus blood flow in cases
Shoulder impingement syndrome	Leong (2012) [69]	AHD, supraspinatus tendon thickness AHD: NS group effect, $p = 0.08$ Supraspinatus tendon thickness: group effect, $p = 0.002$, post-hoc analysis: control volleyball players > controls, $p < 0.001$; cases > controls: $p = 0.02$; NS, control volleyball players vs. cases.	Yes ↑ supraspinatus tendon thickness in cases vs non-volleyball player controls
Shoulder impingement syndrome	Park (2007) [70]	Difference in mean skin temperature btwn sh sides in 5 ROIs Difference in mean skin temperature btwn sh sides anteromedial ROI: cases > controls, $p = 0.004$. anterolateral: cases > controls, $p = 0.001$. posteromedial: cases > controls, $p = 0.013$. posterolateral: cases > controls, $p = 0.030$. lateral: cases > controls, $p = 0.039$.	Yes ↑ difference in mean skin temperature btwn sides in all 5 ROIs in cases
Shoulder pain w. rotator cuff disease (multiple diagnoses)	Kalra (2010) [40]	AHD No group effects at rest ($p = 0.43$) or 45 degrees abduction ($p = 0.84$). No interaction between group and posture.	No
Shoulder pain	O'Sullivan (2012) [41]	Trapezius muscle thickness % change in thickness during contraction vs. rest: NS btwn cases & controls in any of the 4 trapezius regions, at 90 degrees or 120 degrees abduction. Muscle thickness difference between sides at rest or during contractions in cases: NS in any of the 4 trapezius regions, at 0, 90, or 120 degrees abduction.	No

Table 1 Are there quantitative imaging biomarkers associated with the presence of neck and shoulder MSDs? *(Continued)*

Shoulder pain	Rechardt (2010) [61]	Carotid artery intima-media thickness Carotid imtima-media thickness, NS in males and females. For each standard deviation increase in carotid IMT, risk of unilateral or bilateral sh pain, OR = 1.4 (95% CI 1.0–1.9) for males 60 + .	Perhaps ↑ carotid artery intima-media thickness increases odds of shoulder pain in males 60+
Shoulder pain (internal impingement pain)	Tuite (2007) [72]	Labral length, thick-capsule labrum length, posterior recess angle Labral length: cases > controls, $p = 0.001$. Thick-capsule labrum length: cases > controls, $p < 0.001$. Posterior recess angle: cases > controls, $p = 0.002$. MR arthrogram: greater (dichotomized) glenohumeral internal rotation deficit (GIRD): labral length, thick-capsule labrum length, posterior recess angle, NS.	Yes ↑ labral length in cases ↑ thick capsule labral length in cases ↑ posterior recess angle in cases
Neck/shoulder disorders and symptoms			
Neck/shoulder pain	Hallman (2011) [80]	Muscle blood flow (MBF) During HGT: MBF cases < controls ($p = 0.02$ - ipsi; $p = 0.04$ - contra). After HGT: MBF cases < controls ($p = 0.001$ - ipsi; $p = 0.003$ - contra). During CPT: increase in MBF cases < controls ($p = 0.04$ - ipsi); NS, contra. After CPT: increase in MBF cases < controls ($p < 0.05$ - ipsi); NS, contra.	Yes ↓ MBF in cases during & after HGT in ipsi- and contralateral sides. ↓ increase in MBF during and after CPT in ipsilateral side.
Neck/shoulder pain	Nilsen (2007) [42]	Finger blood flow Finger blood flow: baseline, NS. Response to stressful task: group x time (baseline, 0–10 min, 50–60 min) interaction, $p = 0.02$. Post-hoc comparison: controls vs. cases: $p = 0.35$.	No
Neck/shoulder pain	Shiro (2012) [81]	ΔOHb, ΔHHb, ΔTHb from baseline ΔO2Hb: cases < controls during Relax 3 ($p < 0.01$) & recovery ($p < 0.05$). ΔHHb: NS, cases vs. controls. ΔTHb: cases < controls during Relax 2 & Relax 3 in R trapezius ($p < 0.05$); cases < controls: each Relax & recovery in L trapezius (all $p < 0.05$, except Relax 2 & Relax 3, $p < 0.001$).	Yes ↓ ΔO2Hb in cases during Relax 3 & recovery. ↓ ΔTHb in cases during Relax 2 & Relax 3 in R trapezius; during each Relax & recovery in L trapezius
Neck/shoulder pain	Strøm (2009) [43]	Muscle blood flow At start of work task: cases vs controls, NS difference in blood flow increase in either active or contralateral trapezius. Blood flow during 15 min of recovery in active & contralateral trapezius: cases > controls ($p = 0.05$).	No
Neck/shoulder pain	Takiguchi (2010) [79]	Minimal & maximal standardized uptake values (SUV) of [18F]fluorodeoxyglucose (18F–FDG) Trapezius: mean SUVmax, mean SUVmin: cases < controls, $p < 0.0001$. Presence/absence of neck/shoulder pain and mean SUVmax (R2 = 0.16, $p < 0.0001$), and for SUVmin(R2 = 0.26, $p < 0.0001$), after adjusting for age, gender, smoking status, and diabetes. Gluteus maximus: mean SUVmax, mean SUVmin: NS, cases vs. controls mean. Presence/absence of neck/shoulder pain and mean SUVmax or SUVmin, NS.	Yes
Cervicobrachial pain syndrome	Larsson (1998) [114]	Muscle blood flow Unilateral pain patients: muscle blood flow: painful < asymptomatic side, $p = 0.01$; painful < control, $p = 0.0009$.	Yes ↓ blood flow in painful side in unilateral cases ↓ blood flow in cases

Table 1 Are there quantitative imaging biomarkers associated with the presence of neck and shoulder MSDs? *(Continued)*

Trapezius myalgia	Acero (1999) [74]	Relative blood volume ANOVA - main effect for group, case < control, during 61–120 s of cold pressor stimulation, $p = 0.04$. All other time points group NS.	Yes ↓ relative blood volume in cases during 61–120 s of cold pressor stimulation.
Trapezius myalgia	Andersen (2010) [44]	ΔOHb, ΔHHb, ΔTHb from baseline ANOVA - main effect of time for all 3ΔxHb ($p < 0.0001$), group x time interaction for OHb ($p < 0.05$). Group effect NS for HHb & THb. Group effect *p*-value for OHb not stated. OHb after exercise increase from baseline: cases < controls, $p = 0.05$.	No
Trapezius myalgia	Cagnie (2012) [75]	Oxygen saturation, muscle blood flow Oxygen saturation: MANOVA - main effects of time, muscle part, and interaction muscle part x group ($p = 0.049$). Post hoc cases < controls in L & R middle trapezius at all time points $p = 0.03$, except 40 min for R middle trapezius (NS). Blood flow: MANOVA - main effects of time, muscle part, and no interaction muscle part x group. No group effect.	Yes ↓ oxygen saturation in L & R trapezius at all but 1 time point.
Trapezius myalgia	Flodgren (2010) [76]	Muscle oxygenation Muscle oxygenation percentage decreased during work ($P = 0.02$), and returned to baseline during recovery.	Perhaps No control subjects were included in this study. Authors conclude normal response in these cases when comparing them to a previous similar study with normal subjects (see Flodgren (2005)).
Trapezius myalgia	Peolsson (2008) [45]	Strain rate, strain rate RMS - before provocation, after provocation, difference after - before NS cases vs. controls: strain rate, strain rate RMS - before provocation, after provocation, difference after - before. After factor analysis with strain rate and strain variables (not velocity variables), followed by clustering, distribution of cases and controls differed, $p = 0.05$. Examination of factors indicated that post-provocation – most cases have lower levels of strain rate & strain after pain provocation compared with most controls.	No
Trapezius myalgia	Sjøgaard (2010) [77]	ΔOHb, ΔHHb, ΔTHb from baseline Cases: OHb 35 min after start of peg board task < baseline, $p < 0.05$. Controls: OHb not different from baseline. Other OHb, HHb, and THb similar results for cases and controls.	Yes ↓ OHb (vs. baseline) 35 min after start of peg board task in cases, but no change in controls.

[a]: result significant in 1 of 2 radiologists

patients with unilateral rotator cuff tears with night pain, increased peak systolic velocity and decreased resistance index in the anterior humeral circumflex artery was observed in the symptomatic side in comparison to the asymptomatic side [59].

Initially asymptomatic full-thickness rotator cuff tears were examined in two unique longitudinal cohorts. Increased tear dimension and tear progression rate was found in asymptomatic rotator cuff tears that became symptomatic versus those that remained asymptomatic [33]. In this same cohort, Keener et al. [34] found an increased tear enlargement risk in asymptomatic full-thickness tears and in asymptomatic partial-thickness tears versus those with rotator cuff disease, but no tear. In the other longitudinal study, greater rotator cuff tear size was observed in the anteroposterior plane in tears that became symptomatic at 3-year follow-up, although there was no difference in the tear size at baseline [36]. No such increase was observed in the other planes examined. In a cross-sectional study, there was no difference between symptomatic and asymptomatic rotator cuff tears in subacromial-subdeltoid bursal fluid amount, proportion of full- or partial-thickness tears, or tear size [39].

Concommitant to rotator cuff tears, increased dimensions been observed in particular anatomical structures. Greater rotator cable (a fibrous band spanning the insertions of the supraspinatus and infraspinatus) width and thickness were observed in those with full-thickness rotator cuff tears than in healthy subjects [57]. In full-thickness rotator cuff tears, the biceps long tendon (BLT) showed increased thickness and cross-sectional area, and decreased BLT flattening ratio (width/thickness) in comparison to controls [56]. In the first longitudinal study referred to above, greater rotator cuff tear width at baseline was observed in those with anterior supraspinatus cable disruption vs. those without such disruption [35]. However, no difference in tear width enlargement percentage was observed in a minimum of 2 years later.

Rotator cuff tendinitis (5 studies)

Five studies examined rotator cuff tendinitis [57, 60–63]. Decreased subacromial distance and humerus diameter [60] were observed in cases. Joensen et al. [62] found increased supraspinatus tendon thickness in cases' symptomatic side, while Arend et al. [63] observed a greater maximal supraspinatus tendon thickness in cases. Greater rotator cable width was observed in rotator cuff tendinosis than in healthy subjects [57]. No difference in carotid artery intima-media thickness was seen in rotator cuff tendinitis vs. controls [61].

Adhesive Capsulitis (4 studies)

Four studies examined adhesive capsulitis (frozen shoulder) [64–67]. Increased coracohumeral ligament [64, 66], articular capsule [66], and axillary recess joint capsule thicknesses [65, 67] were observed in cases. Increased axillary recess and rotator interval contrast enhancement, along with axillary recess thickening were observed [65].

Shoulder impingement syndrome (5 studies)

Five studies investigated shoulder impingement syndrome [58, 68–71]. Increased supraspinatus tendon thickness was observed [69]. Decreased acromiohumeral distance (i.e., subacromial distance) was found in one study [68], but not in another [69]. Park et al. [70] found a difference in mean skin temperature between sides (in unilateral shoulder impingement syndrome). Decreased overall supraspinatus blood flow was observed in cases, with less blood flow in specifically in the medial portions of the supraspinatus [58]. Increased subacromial-subdeltoid bursal thickness was observed in one imaging view in cases [71].

Shoulder pain (4 studies)

Four studies examined shoulder pain [40, 41, 61, 72]. As the diagnoses were non-specific, we were unable to place them into one of the other more specific categories. Tuite et al. [72] saw an increased labral length, thick capsule labral length and posterior recess angle in cases. No difference was seen in acromiohumeral distance (AHD) between cases and controls at rest or at 45 degrees abduction [40]. Neither was any difference observed between groups in percent change in trapezius muscle thickness between rest and during muscle contraction with shoulder abduction [41]. Rechardt et al. [61] saw increased carotid artery intima-media thickness in males 60+ with shoulder pain, but not in females or in younger cases.

Trapezius myalgia, cervicobrachial syndrome and other neck/shoulder pain (12 studies)

Seven studies examined trapezius myalgia and cervicobrachial syndrome, in which muscle hemodynamics, muscle oxygenation or muscle velocity biomarkers were assessed in the trapezius [44, 45, 73–77]. Decreased muscle blood flow was observed in cases versus controls and on the painful side in unilateral cases [78]. A decrease was found in muscle relative blood volume during cold pressor stimulation [74], and oxygen saturation was reduced at baseline and in response to typing [75]. In response to an upper extremity physical task, decreased oxygenated hemoglobin (compared to baseline) was observed in the trapezius in cases, but not controls [77]. No difference in change in trapezius blood flow, or in oxygenated or deoxygenated hemoglobin in response to ergometer exercise was found [44]. Lastly, there was no change in trapezius strain rate/strain rate RMS, a muscle velocity measure, between cases and controls in response to a provocative upper extremity exercise [45].

Five studies examined neck/shoulder pain [42, 43, 79–81]. Decreased trapezius blood flow was seen during and after hand grip and cold pressor tests [80]. Decreased trapezius oxygenated hemoglobin and relative blood volume was observed in response to isometric trapezius contractions [81], but no difference in trapezius blood flow was found in response to a computer work task [43]. Nilsen et al. [42] saw no decrease in finger blood flow in response to a stressful task. Minimal and maximal standardized uptake values of [18F]fluorodeoxyglucose (18F–FDG), glucose metabolism indicator evaluated by PET/CT were lower in trapezii of cases versus controls, but no difference was observed in the control gluteus maximus, even after adjusting for age, gender, smoking status and diabetes [79].

In summary, a) neck muscle size appeared to be decreased in neck pain, and b) reduced blood flow, relative blood volume and reduced oxygen saturation was observed in the trapezius at rest and in response to upper extremity tasks with myalgia and neck/shoulder pain.

Are there quantitative imaging biomarkers associated with the severity of neck and shoulder MSDs?

Five of eight studies demonstrated a relationship between MSD severity and quantitative imaging biomarkers

Table 2 Are there quantitative imaging biomarkers associated with the severity of neck and shoulder MSDs?

MSD Classification or diagnosis Author(s)	Biomarker	Severity measure mean & range if available	Symptom duration (mean & SD if available)	Major results (association between biomarker & disease)	Conclusion
Neck disorders and symptoms					
Neck pain Dibai Filho (2012) [37]	Skin temperature	NDI Cases: 8.33 (SD = 2.65) Controls: 2.27 (SD = 1.27)	Unknown	Correlation NDI and skin temperature in right versus left trapezius; thermal asymmetry: NS.	No
Neck pain Elliott (2008) [46]	Fat index indicating fatty infiltration (relative fat)	NDI Cases: 21.9 (SD = 7.5) Controls: 45.5 (SD = 15.9)	Cases: 33.7 (20.6) mo Controls: 20.3 (9.6) mo	Within groups there was no association between NDI and fat levels; total upper fat, $p = 0.15$; total fat, $p = 0.94$. (No description of total vs upper fat in paper)	No
Neck pain Javanshir (2011) [48]	Longus colli muscle CSA, APD, LD, and LD/APD	NDI 33 (SD = 0.5) VAS pain intensity 5.1 (SD = 0.8)	≥ 3 mo[a]	NDI and CSA: rho = −0.45, $p = 0.05$, dominant side; rho = −0.48, $p = 0.03$, non-dominant side. NDI and APD: rho = −0.49, $p = 0.03$, dominant side; rho = −0.45, $p = 0.05$ non-dominant side. NDI and LD or shape ratio, NS. VAS and CSA, APD, LD or shape ratio, NS.	Yes
Shoulder disorders and symptoms					
Rotator cuff tear (partial & full) or rotator cuff disease Keener (2015) [34]	Rotator cuff tear enlargement (see paper for definition), shoulder pain	ASES score - American Shoulder & Elbow Cases: 98.3 (IRQ = 10) Controls: 100(IQR = 0) Surgeons SST score - simple shoulder test (score normalized to 100) Cases: 91.7 (IQR = 33) Controls: 100(IQR = 0) VAS pain intensityCases & controls: 1.0 (IQR = 0)	Unknown	ASES: smaller w. advancing tear type, $p < 0.05$; median decreased by 31.9 points w. new pain, $p < 0.05$. SST: smaller w. advancing tear type, $p < 0.05$; median decreased by 14.8 points w. new pain, $p < 0.05$. VAS: NS. w. advancing tear type; median increased by 3 points w. new pain, $p < 0.05$.	Yes
Shoulder impingement syndrome Park (2007) [70]	Difference in mean skin temperature btwn shoulder sides	VAS pain intensity 6.6 (5.5–9)	22.6 (SD = 40.4) mo	NS differences btwn normal, hypothermic, and hyperthermic cases for VAS (all cases in this analysis, hypothermic defined as abnormally low temperature in involved side vs uninvolved side, hyperthermic defined as opposite of hypothermic).	No

Table 2 Are there quantitative imaging biomarkers associated with the severity of neck and shoulder MSDs? *(Continued)*

Neck/shoulder disorders and symptoms					
Neck/shoulder pain Nilsen (2007) [42]	Finger skin blood flow	VAS pain intensity: maximal pain response, shoulder pain response, neck pain response Maximal pain response: Cases: 25 (SD = 20.0) Controls: 15 (SD = 16.1) Shoulder pain response: Cases: 17 (SD = 16.9) Controls: 10 (SD = 12.6) Neck pain response: Cases: 20 (SD = 20.3) Controls: 9 (SD = 11.1)	> 3 mo [a]	Maximal pain response: correlation w. finger skin blood flow response during first 10 min of the stressful task in cases, (rho = 0.52, p = 0.004), NS in controls (rho = 0.06, p = 0.71.	Yes
Neck/shoulder pain Strøm (2009) [43]	Blood flow	Complaint severity score: neck pain, shoulder pain, musculoskeletal complaint severity index (MCI; mean of 7 pain items). 0 = no complaint; 12 = severe complaint. VAS during experiment: pain intensity and general tension Median (range) cases: neck pain 3 (1–12), shoulder pain 4 (0–12), MCI 2.5 (0.3–4.1) controls: neck pain 0 (0–6), shoulder pain 0 (0–6), MCI 0.5 (0–2.1) These scores are a composite measure of intensity x duration during the 4 weeks preceding the experiment.	3 subjects (2 women) reported having had shoulder and neck pain for less than 12 months, 13 (7 women) for 1–years, three (all men) for 5–10 years, and five (all women) for more than 10 years.	Cases: correlation between pain VAS and blood flow in active trapezius at end of work task (90 min): rho = 0.47, p = 0.03. No correlation at 15 or 45 min into work task, p > 0.05. Controls: no correlation at 15, 45, or 90 min into work task, $p \geq 0.05$. Cases: correlation between pain VAS and blood flow in contralateral trapezius at end of work task (90 min): rho = −0.53, p < 0.01. No correlation at 15 or 45 min into work task, p > 0.05. Controls: similar direction of results, no rho or p-values supplied.	Yes
Neck/shoulder pain Takiguchi (2010) [79]	Minimal & maximal standardized uptake values (SUV) of [18F]fluorodeoxyglucose (18F–FDG)	VAS	> 6 mo, with pain at least 1×/mo[a]	Trapezius: mean SUVs & pain VAS (SUVmax: r = −0.603, p < 0.0001; SUVmin: r = −0.405, p < 0.0001). Gluteus maximus: mean SUVs & pain VAS, NS.	Yes

[a]: inclusion criteria

(Table 2). Four studies investigated a quantitative imaging biomarker in relation to a severity score or disease stage assessment determined during a physical examination. Neck Disability Index (NDI) was negatively correlated with longus colli cross-sectional area (CSA) and anterior-posterior distance in neck pain [48]. No correlation was observed between NDI and trapezius skin temperature [37] or with fat levels in cervical extensor muscles [46]. In rotator cuff tears or rotator cuff disease, American Shoulder and Elbow Score (ASES) was significantly decreased with advancing tear type, and with incident pain in the asymptomatic shoulder [34]. Simple shoulder test score (SST) was similarly reduced.

Six of eight studies solicited pain ratings from participants through a VAS or other means. Three neck/shoulder pain studies investigated pain severity. In Takiguchi et al. [79], minimal and maximal standardized 18F–FDG uptake values, a glucose metabolism measure, were negatively correlated with VAS pain. In one study, maximal pain response was correlated with finger skin blood flow during the first 10 min of a mentally stressful task in cases, but not controls [42]. In another study, in cases (but not controls) pain and blood flow was positively correlated in the active trapezius, and negatively correlated in the contralateral trapezius at the end of a 90 min computer task [43]. No association was observed between pain rating and longus colli CSA, anterior-posterior distance, or other quantitative imaging parameters examined [48]. Neither was VAS pain related to mean skin temperature differences in shoulder impingement syndrome [70].

In summary, very few studies reviewed found associations between quantitative imaging biomarkers and neck and shoulder MSD severity. As might be inferred from results to our first research question, functional impairment in neck pain may be associated with reduced longus colli dimensions. Functional impairment in rotator cuff disease in an asymptomatic shoulder may be correlated with increasing tear type and incident shoulder pain. In neck/shoulder syndromes, increased pain may be associated with reduced glucose metabolism and increased blood flow in the active trapezius in response to a computer task.

Discussion

In this study we have summarized the current state of quantitative medical imaging marker research in neck and shoulder MSDs by conducting a comprehensive systematic review. A critical approach was used to synthesize results for the two research questions: 1) are there quantitative medical imaging markers associated with the presence of neck and shoulder MSDs, and 2) are there quantitative medical imaging markers associated with the severity of neck and shoulder MSDs? Within the studies of sufficient quality, we found associations between quantitative medical imaging biomarkers and neck and shoulder MSDs, and were able to identify several commonalities.

Evidence was found for the following quantitative imaging biomarkers: With respect to referents, decreased neck muscle size was observed in cases with neck pain [47–50, 52]. Reduced trapezius blood flow and relative blood volume [73, 74, 80, 81] and oxygen saturation at rest and in response to upper extremity tasks [75, 77, 81] occurred with trapezius myalgia and neck/shoulder pain. Lastly, reduced blood flow and altered vascular parameters were observed in rotator cuff tears [54, 55, 58, 59].

In contrast to the first research question, associations between biomarkers and the severity of neck and shoulder MSDs were observed in only a few studies. Most notably, minimal and maximal standardized 18F–FDG uptake values, a biomarker of trapezius metabolism in neck/shoulder pain, were inversely correlated with pain, indicating reduced muscle metabolism in this condition. However, this was found in only one study [79]. The small sample size resulting in reduced ranges of severity measures in many studies examining neck and shoulder MSD severity may have hampered the feasibility of detecting statistically significant results for our second research question.

A possible explanation for the decreased size of deep neck muscles in neck pain cases advanced by several articles [47–50] is the development of muscle atrophy due to a long term reduction in muscle activity through either pain or reflex inhibition. This explanation is consistent with a smaller change in multifidus muscle thickness during MVC from rest in those with neck pain in comparison to control subjects [52]. In another study, cases and controls showed different patterns of muscle thickness alterations during MVC when compared with rest [53]. A possible mechanism for activity changes during muscle pain is the redistribution of activity from painful muscles or painful areas to adjacent or synergistic muscles, as described in the pain adaptation model [82]. Subjects with neck pain showed reduction in deep neck muscle activity in the longus colli [49]. This was corroborated by prior studies showing reduced strength and endurance during neck flexion tests in subject with neck pain [83, 84]. However, causal relationships cannot be deduced due to the cross-sectional design of sufficient quality studies.

The pathophysiology associated with reduced blood flow, relative blood volume and oxygen saturation with trapezius myalgia and neck/shoulder pain is not clear. Decreased oxygenation as presented by several studies [75, 77] may be related to a reduction in oxygen delivery to the muscle or to increased muscle oxygen consumption. Previous studies using muscle microdialysis found increased pyruvate and lactate, metabolites related to increased anaerobic energy production, in painful trapezius muscles [77, 85]. Findings of reduced trapezius muscle blood flow in response to physical load [73, 80, 81] or pain induced during an experiment [74, 80] does not oppose the hypothesis of reduced oxygen delivery. Reduced blood flow may be attributed to an imbalance between vasoconstriction and dilatation in muscle arterioles [86]. This imbalance could be due to aberrant activation in the sympathetic nervous system or downregulation of adrenoreceptors in the arteriole epithelium in patients with MSDs [87]. Indeed, in some sufficient quality studies in this review, patients with MSDs show aberrant sympathetic activity compared to asymptomatic controls [75, 77, 80], although adrenoreceptor expression was not investigated. Together, the reduction in blood flow and oxygen saturation may facilitate the production of muscle metabolites like lactate, which are known to influence muscle nociceptor activity.

Limitations of the review

Other techniques besides imaging are available for measuring some of the functional and morphological features or processes addressed in this review. However, these other methods for assessing biomarkers were beyond the scope of the present review. For instance, our inclusion criteria allowed for articles on photoplethysmography to measure blood pressure, but not strain-gauge plethysmography. Although the term "plethysmography" was part of our search string, no papers were found that utilized strain-gauge plethysmography in neck or shoulder MSDs. Studies using plain x-rays to the exclusion of other imaging modalities were excluded. Plain radiographs are best utilized in evaluating osteoarthritis, fractures, dislocations and other bone abnormalities, and are not routinely indicated in soft tissue MSDs [23–26]. However, we may have missed some biomarkers that could be of interest such as calcifications, soft tissue swelling, or acromial abnormalities including variant acromial morphology and acromial spurs.

Methodological limitations in the articles reviewed

Selection bias - response rate

The response rate to participate could be ascertained in only 15 (31%) of the 49 sufficient quality studies. Without response rates, selection bias cannot be adequately assessed. Hence, it is unknown if the cases and controls represent the underlying population, or to what extent they may be comparable. We recommend including response rates for both cases and controls in future quantitative imaging studies.

Confounding

Approximately half of the reviewed sufficient quality studies controlled for potential confounders, either through restriction of study subjects (e.g., by age or gender) or through adjustment in the statistical analysis. With respect to the quantitative imaging parameters reviewed here, muscle oxygenation, including in the trapezius, was found to be greater in males than females in many studies [88–91]. However, gender had no influence on erector spinae oxygenation in a sustained trunk extension test [92]. This latter study also found no difference in relative blood volume with respect to gender. But, literature is sparse in this area. Muscle oxygenation and blood volume responses in limb muscles are significantly influenced by both age [93] and level of exercise training [94], yet no study has looked at the effects on shoulder and neck muscles.

Trapezius muscle size is greater in males than females [91]. In a biopsy study, Lindman et al. [95] found that female trapezius muscle fibers have smaller cross-sectional areas than males, and more type II fibers. Neck muscle size may also differ by gender. Zheng et al. [96] found a greater total neck muscle volume in males versus females. However, the proportion of each muscle volume examined in comparison to total neck muscle volume was similar between genders, except for the sternocleidomastoid, longus capitis, and obliqus capitis inferior. Deep neck posterior muscles and semispinalis capitis cross-sectional areas were larger in males than females, but not after adjusting for body weight [97]. In that study, muscle shape ratio did not differ by gender. Nor were there any differences in muscle dimension by age.

Although several studies suggested that reduced vascularity in the supraspinatus tendon may be associated with rotator cuff tears, two of these studies used much younger controls than cases [55, 58] (see Additional file 7). Due to the design of these studies, it is difficult to determine whether the results were due to age or to pathology. Rudzki et al. [98] found reduced blood flow in the supraspinatus tendon in those over 40 years in their study of asymptomatic rotator cuff tears, which roughly corresponds to the differentiating age between the two groups in the above studies.

The above findings suggest that (minimally) age, gender, exercise frequency, and BMI should be collected from study subjects and controlled for, either during analysis or through selection.

Directions for future research

Despite the similarity of symptoms in neck and neck/shoulder disorders, there is a marked difference in the imaging metrics obtained in studies with these two symptom designations. Muscle dimensions have been researched in neck pain, but not in trapezius myalgia and other neck/

shoulder disorders. Conversely, muscle oxygenation and relative blood volume have been explored in the trapezius, but not in other neck muscles. Future research should examine muscle dimensions in the trapezius, and muscle oxygenation and relative blood volume in other muscles.

The research on muscle dimension, oxygenation and relative blood volume has been conducted in subjects with different MSD labels, i.e., in neck pain, trapezius myalgia and neck/shoulder pain. Here, we used the diagnosis or syndrome name presented in the articles. These diagnoses or syndrome names are based on the painful region. However, the division between neck and shoulder is not clear. For example, when considering functional anatomy, the neck and upper trapezius could be considered as the same region thus rendering definitions of neck and neck/shoulder regions arbitrary. Furthermore, there are suggestions of a possible common pathophysiological mechanism in these syndromes [99].

As mentioned previously, a majority of shoulder studies were conducted in older populations (at least one analysis group with mean age ≥ 50 years), whereas the neck and neck/shoulder studies were conducted in younger populations (mean age < 50 years). This could be due partially to the average age at onset of these disorders. However, given the potential for a possible spectrum effect [100], it would be of interest to study a broader range of ages.

Only 12 of the 49 sufficient quality studies in this review listed the duration of symptoms in patients (range: 9.1–114 months), all of which durations are chronic by definition [36, 38, 40, 41, 46, 47, 64, 66, 68, 70, 73, 76, 80]. One review has determined that blood flow increases to the site of rotator cuff small tears, but that decreased vascularity is observed as tear size increases and the healing response fails [101]. This suggests that varying results in vascularity in the rotator cuff tendons may be influenced by symptom duration. In view of pathophysiological mechanism research, we recommend that quantitative imaging biomarkers be investigated in MSD patients with shorter symptom durations. We further recommend that quantitative imaging biomarker study be report the range of symptoms and their duration.

Although focused on computed tomography imaging methods, animal models would suggest that different quantitative imaging biomarkers and findings are present at different MSD stages [102–105]. In humans, various quantitative imaging biomarkers reflective of underlying musculoskeletal changes are valid at different stages of disease. For instance, the AHD decrease is a late stage phenomenon. It is detectable in large chronic full thickness rotator cuff tears, but not in earlier stages of rotator cuff disease [106]. The question of which imaging modality best captures the particular biomarker under consideration is beyond the scope of this review. Determining the most appropriate imaging modality for a given quantitative imaging biomarker is an essential area for future research.

Heterogeneity – other considerations

Quantitative imaging has the potential to be unbiased and precise, particularly in comparison to ordinal scales such as the Bigliani classification [107] sometimes used in shoulder impingement syndrome. As with all types of biomarkers, optimally, a complete analytical evaluation should be conducted for each quantitative imaging biomarker under consideration. This evaluation should include determination of limit of detection, limit of quantification, reference values in normal subjects, as well as assessing the reliability and validity of any such biomarker [108]. There are unique considerations for quantitative imaging. Sources of variability include the instrument/acquisition system, and the image measurement algorithm, as well as the patient [109]. For instance, patient motion may affect the performance of the imaging acquisition system [110], and image processing software may include a number of steps, each of which requires validation [108]. See Raunig et al. [109] for a thorough review of statistical methods for assessing technical performance in quantitative imaging. These technical considerations must be addressed prior to validating the clinical utility of any suggested quantitative imaging biomarker [108, 109].

Recommendations

Below are our brief recommendations for future quantitative imaging biomarker research:

1. Report the response rate for all analysis groups.
2. Carefully consider and report potential confounders, gather information on these factors from study subjects, and potentially control for them through exclusion or through adjustment in the statistical analysis.
3. Report symptom duration and/or severity in study subjects.
4. Clearly describe MSD case definition criteria, including a description of localization of symptoms.
5. Prioritize quantitative imaging biomarker studies that are longitudinal.

Conclusions

Based on our comprehensive review, there is limited evidence of an association between quantitative medical imaging biomarkers and neck and shoulder MSDs. The most consistent studies suggest that deep neck muscle size holds promise as a biomarker for neck pain, and that trapezius blood flow, relative blood volume, and muscle oxygenation are worthy of consideration as biomarkers for trapezius myalgia and neck/shoulder pain.

Further research is warranted. In the meantime, clinicians may find value in our findings. For instance, radiologists may wish to adjust imaging scan planes to allow better volumetric analysis, and refine protocols to better characterize blood flow. Some quantitative imaging parameters, e.g., muscle size and blood flow, are not routinely included in radiology reports. It may behoov the clinician to do so. Additionally, epidemiologists may wish to include these biomarkers in cross-sectional and prospective studies of neck and shoulder MSDs. Prospective high quality studies are needed as this discipline moves forward. Future testing should be done with regard to MSD symptom duration and severity. Results should be reported with consideration to the effects of potentially confounding factors (minimally including age, gender, and exercise), and response rates of all analysis groups should be described so that potential selection bias may be assessed.

Additional files

Additional file 1: Search terms for musculoskeletal disorders (MSDs) and imaging markers.

Additional file 2: Questions used in the primary screen for exclusion of articles.

Additional file 3: Questions used in the secondary screen for quality assessment.

Additional file 4: PubMed search string.

Additional file 5: Data extraction items.

Additional file 6: Quality scores for each of the reviewed papers in the primary screen, including the papers of sufficient quality (≥70%) and insufficient quality (< 70%) [114–159].

Additional file 7: Overview with descriptive information of included studies, by anatomical region of the disorder.

Abbreviations

18F-FDG: [18F]fluorodeoxyglucose (Glucose analog where one hydoxylgroup has been replaced with a radioacitve fluorine-18 isotope, an indicator of tissue glucose uptake in PET); ADP: Anterior-posterior dimension; AHCA: Anterior humeral circumflex artery; AHD: Acromiohumeral distance; ANOVA: Analysis of Variance; AS: Anterior scalene; ASES: American Shoulder & Elbow Score (A validated instrument to assess shoulder pain and function [111]); Assoc.: Associated; BA: Brachial artery; BLT: Biceps long tendon; BMI: Body mass index (A measure of body fat based on height and weight); C3-C6: Cervical vertebrae; CCFT: Craniocervical flexion test; CHL: Coracohumeral ligament; CI: Confidence interval; CPT: Cold pressor test (A cardiovascular test involving immersion of the dominant hand up to the wrist for 1–3 min in cold water); CSA: Cross - sectional area; HGT: Static hand grip test (A test in which the subject presses a dynamometer with their dominant hand [80]); HR: Hazard ratio; IQR: Interquartile range; Lco: Longus colli muscle; LD: Lateral dimension; LD/ADP: Muscle shape ratio (ratio between lateral and anterior-posterior dimensions); MANOVA: Multivariate analysis of variance; MBF: Muscle blood flow; MCI: Musculoskeletal complaint severity index (Mean value of 7 pain areas [43]); MR: Magnetic resonance; MRI: Magnetic Resonance Imaging; MSTT: Maximal supraspinatus tendon thickness; MVC: Maximum voluntary contraction; NDI: Neck Disability Index (A validated instrument to assess disability due to neck pain [112]); NIRS: Near infrared spectroscopy; NS: Not significant; OHb: Oxygenated hemoglobin; OR: Odds ratio; PET/CT: Positron-emission tomography/computerized tomography; PSV: Peak systolic velocity; RCT: Rotator cuff tear; RI: Resistance index (RI = (PSV (see above) – end diastoic velocity)/PSV); RMS: Root mean square; ROI: Region of interest; SA: Serratus anterior muscle; SCM: Sternocleidomastoid muscle; SD: Standard deviation; SIS: Shoulder impingement syndrome; SST: Simple shoulder test score (An instrument to assess shoulder functional disability [113]); SUV: Standardized uptake values (Measurment for quantification in positron-emission tomography); T6-T10: Thoracic vertebrae; TVI: Tissue velocity imaging; VAS: Visual Analogue Scale; VO2max: Maximal oxygen uptake; ΔHHb: Change in de-oxygenated hemoglobin (Determined through NIRS, from a baseline value); ΔOHb: Change in oxygenated hemoglobin (Determined through NIRS, from a baseline value); ΔTHb: Change in total hemoglobin, interpreted as relative blood volume (Determined through NIRS, from a baseline value)

Acknowledgements
None.

Funding
This study was funded by a grant from the Swedish Research Council for Health, Working Life and Welfare [Forte Dnr. 2009–1761], and by the National Institute of Arthritis and Musculoskeletal and Skin Diseases (NIAMS) of the National Institutes of Health (NIH) under Award Number AR056019 to MFB.

Authors' contributions
JG conceived of the systematic review, led the project, performed primary and secondary scoring, and data extraction, and led the manuscript drafting effort. DH performed primary and secondary scoring, and data extraction, and drafted the initial Methods section and results Tables. FH performed primary and secondary scoring, and drafted sections of the Discussion. AC and MB performed primary and secondary scoring. MFB and SA served as musculoskeletal biomarker and radiology consultants to the project, respectively. JG, DH, FH, AC, MB, SEM, and MFB participated in initial meetings to determine the scope of the review. All authors have read and approved the final manuscript.

Consent for publication
Not applicable.

Competing interests
The author(s) declare that they have no competing interests. No author evaluated their own published article during the review process.

Author details
[1]Centre for Musculoskeletal Research, Department of Occupational and Public Health Sciences, University of Gävle, Gävle, Sweden. [2]Department of Community Medicine and Rehabilitation, Physiotherapy, Umeå University, Umeå, Sweden. [3]Department of Anatomy and Cell Biology, Temple University Medical School, Philadelphia, PA, USA. [4]Department of Radiology, Temple University Medical School, Philadelphia, PA, USA. [5]Gold Standard Research Consulting, 830 Montgomery Ave, Bryn Mawr, PA, USA.

References
1. Hassard J, Teoh K, Cox T, Dewe P, Cosmar M, Grundler R, et al. Calculating the cost of work-related stress and psychosocial risks - a literature review. In: The European Agency for Safety and Health at work. Luxembourg: Publications Office of the European Union; 2014.
2. Huisstede BM, Bierma-Zeinstra SM, Koes BW, Verhaar JA. Incidence and prevalence of upper-extremity musculoskeletal disorders. A systematic appraisal of the literature. BMC Musculoskelet Disord. 2006;7:7. doi:10.1186/1471-2474-7-7.

3. Health and Safety Executive. Cost benefit studies that support tackling musculoskeletal disorders. Research Report 491, 2006. http://www.hse.gov.uk/research/rrpdf/rr491.pdf. Accessed 14 Aug 2017.
4. World Health Organization. Physical Inactivity: A Global Public Health Problem, http://www.who.int/dietphysicalactivity/factsheet_inactivity/en/. 2014. Accessed 8 Oct 2014.
5. Schneider E, Irastorza X. OSH in figures: work-related musculoskeletal disorders in the EU — facts and figures. Luxembourg: Publications Office of the European Union: European Agency for Safety and Health at Work; 2010.
6. Buckle PW, Devereux JJ. The nature of work-related neck and upper limb musculoskeletal disorders. Appl Ergon. 2002;33:207–17.
7. National Academy of Sciences. Panel on musculoskeletal disorders and the workplace commission on behavioral and social sciences and education, National Research Council. Musculoskeletal disorders and the workplace: low back and upper extremities. Washington, D.C.: National Academy Press; 2001.
8. Virta L, Joranger P, Brox JI, Eriksson R. Costs of shoulder pain and resource use in primary health care: a cost-of-illness study in Sweden. BMC Musculoskelet Disord. 2012;13:17. doi:10.1186/1471-2474-13-17.
9. Coyte PC, Asche CV, Croxford R, Chan B. The economic cost of musculoskeletal disorders in Canada. Arthritis Care Res. 1998;11(5):315–25.
10. Bureau of Labor Statistics. The cost of care: new insights into healthcare spending growth. 2017. https://www.bls.gov/opub/btn/volume-6/cost-of-care.htm. Accessed 14 Aug 2017.
11. OSHA. Prevention of work-related musculoskeletal disorders. U.S. Department of Labor, Occupational Safety & Health Administration. 2014. https://www.osha.gov/pls/oshaweb/owadisp.show_document?p_table=UNIFIED_AGENDA&p_id=4481. Accessed 29 July 2014.
12. Viikari-Juntura E. New avenues in research on musculoskeletal disorders. Scand J Work Environ Health. 1999;26(6, special issue):564–8.
13. Punnett L, Gold JE. Work-related upper extremity disorders: epidemiologic findings and unresolved questions. In: Johansson H, Djupsjöbacka M, Windhorst U, Passatore M, Ljubisavljevic M, Blair SJ, editors. Chronic work-related Myalgia: neuromuscular mechanisms behind work-related chronic muscle pain syndromes. Umea: National Institute for Working Life; 2003.
14. Institute of Medicine. Evaluation of biomarkers and surrogate endpoints in chronic disease. Washington, DC: The National Academies Press; 2010.
15. Kessler LG, Barnhart HX, Buckler AJ, Choudhury KR, Kondratovich MV, Toledano A, et al. The emerging science of quantitative imaging biomarkers terminology and definitions for scientific studies and regulatory submissions. Stat Methods Med Res. 2015;24(1):9–26. doi:10.1177/0962280214537333.
16. Mayeux R. Biomarkers: potential uses and limitations. NeuroRx. 2004;1(2):182–8. doi:10.1602/neurorx.1.2.182.
17. Committee on Biological Markers of the National Research Council. Biological markers in environmental health research. Environ Health Perspect. 1987;74:3–9.
18. Mastin JP, Henningsen GM, Fine LJ. Use of biomarkers of occupational musculoskeletal disorders in epidemiology and laboratory animal model development. Scand J Work Environ Health. 1992;18(Suppl 2):85–7.
19. Saxton JM. A review of current literature on physiological tests and soft tissue biomarkers applicable to work-related upper limb disorders. Occup Med (Lond). 2000;50(2):121–30.
20. Gold JE, Hallman DM, Hellstrom F, Bjorklund M, Crenshaw AG, Djupsjobacka M et al. Systematic review of biochemical biomarkers for neck and upper-extremity musculoskeletal disorders. Scand J Work Environ Health. 2015. doi:10.5271/sjweh.3533.
21. Boocock MG, Collier JM, McNair PJ, Simmonds M, Larmer PJ, Armstrong B. A framework for the classification and diagnosis of work-related upper extremity conditions: systematic review. Semin Arthritis Rheum. 2009;38(4):296–311. doi:10.1016/j.semarthrit.2007.10.006.
22. Organization WH. Identification and control of work-related diseases. Geneva: World Health Organization; 1985. Contract No.: 714
23. Seidenberg PH, Howe AH. Musculoskeletal imaging: types and indications. Med Clin North Am. 2014;98(4):895–914, xiv. doi:10.1016/j.mcna.2014.04.003.
24. Aagesen AL, Melek M. Choosing the right diagnostic imaging modality in musculoskeletal diagnosis. Prim Care. 2013;40(4):849–861, viii. doi:10.1016/j.pop.2013.08.005.
25. Bearcroft PW. Imaging modalities in the evaluation of soft tissue complaints. Best Pract Res Clin Rheumatol. 2007;21(2):245–59. doi:10.1016/j.berh.2006.11.003.
26. Bussieres AE, Peterson C, Taylor JA. Diagnostic imaging guideline for musculoskeletal complaints in adults-an evidence-based approach-part 2: upper extremity disorders. J Manip Physiol Ther. 2008;31(1):2–32. doi:10.1016/j.jmpt.2007.11.002.
27. Bruns DE, Huth EJ, Magid E, Young DS. Toward a checklist for reporting of studies of diagnostic accuracy of medical tests. Clin Chem. 2000;46(7):893–5.
28. Altman DG. Statistical reviewing for medical journals. Stat Med. 1998;17(23):2661–74.
29. Downs SH, Black N. The feasibility of creating a checklist for the assessment of the methodological quality both of randomised and non-randomised studies of health care interventions. J Epidemiol Community Health. 1998; 52(6):377–84.
30. Whiting P, Rutjes AW, Reitsma JB, Bossuyt PM, Kleijnen J. The development of QUADAS: a tool for the quality assessment of studies of diagnostic accuracy included in systematic reviews. BMC Med Res Methodol. 2003;3:25. doi:10.1186/1471-2288-3-25.
31. von Elm E, Altman DG, Egger M, Pocock SJ, Gotzsche PC, Vandenbroucke JP, et al. Strengthening the reporting of observational studies in epidemiology (STROBE) statement: guidelines for reporting observational studies. BMJ. 2007;335(7624):806–8. doi:10.1136/bmj.39335.541782.AD.
32. Slavin RE. Best evidence synthesis: an intelligent alternative to meta-analysis. J Clin Epidemiol. 1995;48(1):9–18.
33. Mall NA, Kim HM, Keener JD, Steger-May K, Teefey SA, Middleton WD, et al. Symptomatic progression of asymptomatic rotator cuff tears: a prospective study of clinical and sonographic variables. J Bone Joint Surg Am. 2010; 92(16):2623–33. doi:10.2106/JBJS.I.00506.
34. Keener JD, Galatz LM, Teefey SA, Middleton WD, Steger-May K, Stobbs-Cucchi G, et al. A prospective evaluation of survivorship of asymptomatic degenerative rotator cuff tears. J Bone Joint Surg Am. 2015;97(2):89–98. doi:10.2106/jbjs.n.00099.
35. Keener JD, Hsu JE, Steger-May K, Teefey SA, Chamberlain AM, Yamaguchi K. Patterns of tear progression for asymptomatic degenerative rotator cuff tears. J Shoulder Elb Surg. 2015;24(12):1845–51. doi:10.1016/j.jse.2015.08.038.
36. Moosmayer S, Tariq R, Stiris M, Smith HJ. The natural history of asymptomatic rotator cuff tears: a three-year follow-up of fifty cases. J Bone Joint Surg Am. 2013;95(14):1249–55. doi:10.2106/JBJS.L.00185.
37. Dibai Filho AV, Packer AC, Costa AC, Berni-Schwarzenbeck KC, Rodrigues-Bigaton D. Assessment of the upper trapezius muscle temperature in women with and without neck pain. J Manip Physiol Ther. 2012;35(5):413–7. doi:10.1016/j.jmpt.2012.04.006.
38. Falla D, Jull G, Edwards S, Koh K, Rainoldi A. Neuromuscular efficiency of the sternocleidomastoid and anterior scalene muscles in patients with chronic neck pain. Disabil Rehabil. 2004;26(12):712–7. doi:10.1080/09638280410001704287.
39. Hirano Y, Sashi R, Izumi J, Itoi E, Watarai J. Comparison of the MR findings on indirect MR arthrography in patients with rotator cuff tears with and without symptoms. Radiat Med. 2006;24(1):23–7.
40. Kalra N, Seitz AL, Boardman ND, Michener LA. Effect of posture on acromiohumeral distance with arm elevation in subjects with and without rotator cuff disease using ultrasonography. J Orthop Sports Phys Ther. 2010; 40(10):633–40. doi:10.2519/jospt.2010.3155.
41. O'Sullivan C, McCarthy Persson U, Blake C, Stokes M. Rehabilitative ultrasound measurement of trapezius muscle contractile states in people with mild shoulder pain. Man Ther. 2012;17(2):139–44. doi:10.1016/j.math.2011.11.003.
42. Nilsen KB, Sand T, Westgaard RH, Stovner LJ, White LR, Bang Leistad R, et al. Autonomic activation and pain in response to low-grade mental stress in fibromyalgia and shoulder/neck pain patients. Eur J Pain. 2007;11(7):743–55. doi:10.1016/j.ejpain.2006.11.004.
43. Strøm V, Røe C, Knardahl S. Work-induced pain, trapezius blood flux, and muscle activity in workers with chronic shoulder and neck pain. Pain. 2009; 144(1–2):147–55. doi:10.1016/j.pain.2009.04.002.
44. Andersen LL, Blangsted AK, Nielsen PK, Hansen L, Vedsted P, Sjogaard G, et al. Effect of cycling on oxygenation of relaxed neck/shoulder muscles in women with and without chronic pain. Eur J Appl Physiol. 2010;110(2):389–94. doi:10.1007/s00421-010-1517-4.
45. Peolsson M, Larsson B, Brodin LA, Gerdle B. A pilot study using tissue velocity ultrasound imaging (TVI) to assess muscle activity pattern in patients with chronic trapezius myalgia. BMC Musculoskelet Disord. 2008;9:127. doi:10.1186/1471-2474-9-127.
46. Elliott J, Sterling M, Noteboom JT, Darnell R, Galloway G, Jull G. Fatty infiltrate in the cervical extensor muscles is not a feature of chronic, insidious-onset neck pain. Clin Radiol. 2008;63(6):681–7. doi:10.1016/j.crad.2007.11.011.
47. Fernandez-de-las-Penas C, Albert-Sanchis JC, Buil M, Benitez JC, Alburquerque-Sendin F. Cross-sectional area of cervical multifidus muscle in

females with chronic bilateral neck pain compared to controls. J Orthop Sports Phys Ther. 2008;38(4):175–80. doi:10.2519/jospt.2008.2598.

48. Javanshir K, Rezasoltani A, Mohseni-Bandpei MA, Amiri M, Ortega-Santiago R, Fernandez-de-Las-Penas C. Ultrasound assessment of bilateral longus colli muscles in subjects with chronic bilateral neck pain. Am J Phys Med Rehabil. 2011;90(4):293–301. doi:10.1097/PHM.0b013e31820173e5.
49. Jesus-Moraleida FR, Ferreira PH, Pereira LS, Vasconcelos CM, Ferreira ML. Ultrasonographic analysis of the neck flexor muscles in patients with chronic neck pain and changes after cervical spine mobilization. J Manip Physiol Ther. 2011;34(8):514–24. doi:10.1016/j.jmpt.2011.08.006.
50. Park KN, Kwon OY, Choung SD, Kim SH. Bilateral asymmetry of semispinalis capitis muscle thickness and neck motion during prone neck extension in subjects with unilateral posterior neck pain. J Phys Ther Sci. 2013;25(1):37–40. doi:10.1589/jpts.25.37.
51. Sheard B, Elliott J, Cagnie B, O'Leary S. Evaluating serratus anterior muscle function in neck pain using muscle functional magnetic resonance imaging. J Manip Physiol Ther. 2012;35(8):629–35. doi:10.1016/j.jmpt.2012.09.008.
52. Rahnama L, Rezasoltani A, Zavieh MK, NooriKochi F, Baghban AA. Differences in cervical multifidus muscle thickness during isometric contraction of shoulder muscles: a comparison between patients with chronic neck pain and healthy controls. J Manip Physiol Ther. 2015;38(3): 210–7. doi:10.1016/j.jmpt.2014.11.008.
53. Karimi N, Rezasoltani A, Rahnama L, Noori-Kochi F, Jaberzadeh S. Ultrasonographic analysis of dorsal neck muscles thickness changes induced by isometric contraction of shoulder muscles: a comparison between patients with chronic neck pain and healthy controls. Man Ther. 2016;22: 174–8. doi:10.1016/j.math.2015.12.004.
54. Biberthaler P, Wiedemann E, Nerlich A, Kettler M, Mussack T, Deckelmann S, et al. Microcirculation associated with degenerative rotator cuff lesions. In vivo assessment with orthogonal polarization spectral imaging during arthroscopy of the shoulder. J Bone Joint Surg Am. 2003;85-A(3):475–80.
55. Funakoshi T, Iwasaki N, Kamishima T, Nishida M, Ito Y, Kondo M, et al. In vivo visualization of vascular patterns of rotator cuff tears using contrast-enhanced ultrasound. Am J Sports Med. 2010;38(12):2464–71. doi:10.1177/0363546510375536.
56. Chang KV, Chen WS, Wang TG, Hung CY, Chien KL. Quantitative ultrasound facilitates the exploration of morphological association of the long head biceps tendon with supraspinatus tendon full thickness tear. PLoS One. 2014;9(11):e113803. doi:10.1371/journal.pone.0113803.
57. Choo HJ, Lee SJ, Kim DW, Park YM, Kim JH. Assessment of the rotator cable in various rotator cuff conditions using indirect MR arthrography. Acta Radiol. 2014;55(9):1104–11. doi:10.1177/0284185113512483.
58. Karthikeyan S, Griffin DR, Parsons N, Lawrence TM, Modi CS, Drew SJ, et al. Microvascular blood flow in normal and pathologic rotator cuffs. J Shoulder Elb Surg. 2015;24(12):1954–60. doi:10.1016/j.jse.2015.07.014.
59. Terabayashi N, Watanabe T, Matsumoto K, Takigami I, Ito Y, Fukuta M, et al. Increased blood flow in the anterior humeral circumflex artery correlates with night pain in patients with rotator cuff tear. J Orthop Sci. 2014;19(5): 744–9. doi:10.1007/s00776-014-0604-5.
60. Cay N, Tosun O, Dogan M, Karaoglanoglu M, Bozkurt M. The effect of morphometric relationship between the glenoid fossa and the humeral head on rotator cuff pathology. Acta Orthop Traumatol Turc. 2012;46(5):325–31.
61. Rechardt M, Shiri R, Karppinen J, Jula A, Heliovaara M, Viikari-Juntura E. Lifestyle and metabolic factors in relation to shoulder pain and rotator cuff tendinitis: a population-based study. BMC Musculoskelet Disord. 2010;11: 165. doi:10.1186/1471-2474-11-165.
62. Joensen J, Couppe C, Bjordal JM. Increased palpation tenderness and muscle strength deficit in the prediction of tendon hypertrophy in symptomatic unilateral shoulder tendinopathy: an ultrasonographic study. Physiother. 2009;95(2):83–93. doi:10.1016/j.physio.2008.09.006.
63. Arend CF, Arend AA, da Silva TR. Diagnostic value of tendon thickness and structure in the sonographic diagnosis of supraspinatus tendinopathy: room for a two-step approach. Eur J Radiol. 2014;83(6):975–9. doi:10.1016/j.ejrad.2014.02.021.
64. Li JQ, Tang KL, Wang J, Li QY, Xu HT, Yang HF, et al. MRI findings for frozen shoulder evaluation: is the thickness of the coracohumeral ligament a valuable diagnostic tool? PLoS One. 2011;6(12):e28704. doi:10.1371/journal.pone.0028704.
65. Song KD, Kwon JW, Yoon YC, Choi SH. Indirect MR arthrographic findings of adhesive capsulitis. AJR Am J Roentgenol. 2011;197(6):W1105–9. doi:10.2214/AJR.10.6099.
66. Zhao W, Zheng X, Liu Y, Yang W, Amirbekian V, Diaz LE, et al. An MRI study of symptomatic adhesive capsulitis. PLoS One. 2012;7(10):e47277. doi:10.1371/journal.pone.0047277.
67. Michelin P, Delarue Y, Duparc F, Dacher JN. Thickening of the inferior glenohumeral capsule: an ultrasound sign for shoulder capsular contracture. Eur Radiol. 2013;23(10):2802–6. doi:10.1007/s00330-013-2874-2.
68. Hebert LJ, Moffet H, Dufour M, Moisan C. Acromiohumeral distance in a seated position in persons with impingement syndrome. J Magn Reson Imaging. 2003;18(1):72–9. doi:10.1002/jmri.10327.
69. Leong HT, Tsui S, Ying M, Leung VY, Fu SN. Ultrasound measurements on acromio-humeral distance and supraspinatus tendon thickness: test-retest reliability and correlations with shoulder rotational strengths. J Sci Med Sport. 2012;15(4):284–91. doi:10.1016/j.jsams.2011.11.259.
70. Park JY, Hyun JK, Seo JB. The effectiveness of digital infrared thermographic imaging in patients with shoulder impingement syndrome. J Shoulder Elb Surg. 2007;16(5):548–54. doi:10.1016/j.jse.2006.11.010.
71. Daghir AA, Sookur PA, Shah S, Watson M. Dynamic ultrasound of the subacromial-subdeltoid bursa in patients with shoulder impingement: a comparison with normal volunteers. Skelet Radiol. 2012;41(9):1047–53. doi:10.1007/s00256-011-1295-z.
72. Tuite MJ, Petersen BD, Wise SM, Fine JP, Kaplan LD, Orwin JF. Shoulder MR arthrography of the posterior labrocapsular complex in overhead throwers with pathologic internal impingement and internal rotation deficit. Skelet Radiol. 2007;36(6):495–502. doi:10.1007/s00256-007-0278-6.
73. Larsson R, Cai H, Zhang Q, Oberg PA, Larsson SE. Visualization of chronic neck-shoulder pain: impaired microcirculation in the upper trapezius muscle in chronic cervico-brachial pain. Occup Med (Lond). 1998;48(3):189–94.
74. Acero CO Jr, Kuboki T, Maekawa K, Yamashita A, Clark GT. Haemodynamic responses in chronically painful, human trapezius muscle to cold pressor stimulation. Arch Oral Biol. 1999;44(10):805–12.
75. Cagnie B, Dhooge F, Van Akeleyen J, Cools A, Cambier D, Danneels L. Changes in microcirculation of the trapezius muscle during a prolonged computer task. Eur J Appl Physiol. 2012;112(9):3305–12. doi:10.1007/s00421-012-2322-z.
76. Flodgren GM, Crenshaw AG, Hellstrom F, Fahlstrom M. Combining microdialysis and near-infrared spectroscopy for studying effects of low-load repetitive work on the intramuscular chemistry in trapezius myalgia. J Biomed Biotechnol. 2010;2010:513803. doi:10.1155/2010/513803.
77. Sjogaard G, Rosendal L, Kristiansen J, Blangsted AK, Skotte J, Larsson B, et al. Muscle oxygenation and glycolysis in females with trapezius myalgia during stress and repetitive work using microdialysis and NIRS. Eur J Appl Physiol. 2010;108(4):657–69. doi:10.1007/s00421-009-1268-2.
78. Larsson B, Rosendal L, Kristiansen J, Sjogaard G, Sogaard K, Ghafouri B, et al. Responses of algesic and metabolic substances to 8 h of repetitive manual work in myalgic human trapezius muscle. Pain. 2008;140(3):479–90. doi:10.1016/j.pain.2008.10.001.
79. Takiguchi S, Maekawa K, Ono T, Sasai N, Kaji M, Clark GT, et al. Relationship between a chronically painful trapezius muscle and its metabolic state analyzed with PET/CT. Oral Surg Oral Med Oral Pathol Oral Radiol Endod. 2010;110(1):54–61. doi:10.1016/j.tripleo.2010.02.028.
80. Hallman DM, Lindberg LG, Arnetz BB, Lyskov E. Effects of static contraction and cold stimulation on cardiovascular autonomic indices, trapezius blood flow and muscle activity in chronic neck-shoulder pain. Eur J Appl Physiol. 2011;111(8):1725–35. doi:10.1007/s00421-010-1813-z.
81. Shiro Y, Arai YC, Matsubara T, Isogai S, Ushida T. Effect of muscle load tasks with maximal isometric contractions on oxygenation of the trapezius muscle and sympathetic nervous activity in females with chronic neck and shoulder pain. BMC Musculoskelet Disord. 2012;13:146. doi:10.1186/1471-2474-13-146.
82. Lund JP, Donga R, Widmer CG, Stohler CS. The pain-adaptation model: a discussion of the relationship between chronic musculoskeletal pain and motor activity. Can J Physiol Pharmacol. 1991;69(5):683–94.
83. O'Leary S, Jull G, Kim M, Vicenzino B. Cranio-cervical flexor muscle impairment at maximal, moderate, and low loads is a feature of neck pain. Man Ther. 2007;12(1):34–9. doi:10.1016/j.math.2006.02.010.
84. Ylinen J, Salo P, Nykanen M, Kautiainen H, Hakkinen A. Decreased isometric neck strength in women with chronic neck pain and the repeatability of neck strength measurements. Arch Phys Med Rehabil. 2004;85(8):1303–8. doi:10.1016/j.apmr.2003.09.018.
85. Rosendal L, Larsson B, Kristiansen J, Peolsson M, Sogaard K, Kjaer M, et al. Increase in muscle nociceptive substances and anaerobic metabolism in patients with trapezius myalgia: microdialysis in rest and during exercise. Pain. 2004;112(3):324–34. doi:10.1016/j.pain.2004.09.017.

86. Passatore M, Roatta S. Influence of sympathetic nervous system on sensorimotor function: whiplash associated disorders (WAD) as a model. Eur J Appl Physiol. 2006;98(5):423–49. doi:10.1007/s00421-006-0312-8.
87. Maekawa K, Clark GT, Kuboki T. Intramuscular hypoperfusion, adrenergic receptors, and chronic muscle pain. J Pain. 2002;3(4):251–60.
88. Heiden M, Lyskov E, Djupsjobacka M, Hellstrom F, Crenshaw AG. Effects of time pressure and precision demands during computer mouse work on muscle oxygenation and position sense. Eur J Appl Physiol. 2005;94(1–2):97–106. doi:10.1007/s00421-004-1295-y.
89. Elcadi GH, Forsman M, Crenshaw AG. The relationship between oxygenation and myoelectric activity in the forearm and shoulder muscles of males and females. Eur J Appl Physiol. 2011;111(4):647–58. doi:10.1007/s00421-010-1688-z.
90. Sugisaki M, Misawa A, Ikai A, Young-Sung K, Tanabe H. Sex differences in the hemoglobin oxygenation state of the resting healthy human masseter muscle. J Orofac Pain. 2001;15(4):320–8.
91. Crenshaw AG, Elcadi GH, Hellstrom F, Mathiassen SE. Reliability of near-infrared spectroscopy for measuring forearm and shoulder oxygenation in healthy males and females. Eur J Appl Physiol. 2012;112(7):2703–15. doi:10.1007/s00421-011-2244-1.
92. Maikala RV, Bhambhani YN. Microvascularity of the lumbar erector spinae muscle during sustained prone trunk extension test. Adv Exp Med Biol. 2009;645:67–73. doi:10.1007/978-0-387-85998-9_11.
93. Costes F, Denis C, Roche F, Prieur F, Enjolras F, Barthelemy JC. Age-associated alteration of muscle oxygenation measured by near infrared spectroscopy during exercise. Arch Physiol Biochem. 1999;107(2):159–67. doi:10.1076/apab.107.2.159.4343.
94. Neary JP. Application of near infrared spectroscopy to exercise sports science. Can J Appl Physiol. 2004;29(4):488–503.
95. Lindman R, Eriksson A, Thornell LE. Fiber type composition of the human female trapezius muscle: enzyme-histochemical characteristics. Am J Anat. 1991;190(4):385–92. doi:10.1002/aja.1001900406.
96. Zheng L, Siegmund G, Ozyigit G, Vasavada A. Sex-specific prediction of neck muscle volumes. J Biomech. 2013;46(5):899–904. doi:10.1016/j.jbiomech.2012.12.018.
97. Rankin G, Stokes M, Newham DJ. Size and shape of the posterior neck muscles measured by ultrasound imaging: normal values in males and females of different ages. Man Ther. 2005;10(2):108–15. doi:10.1016/j.math.2004.08.004.
98. Rudzki JR, Adler RS, Warren RF, Kadrmas WR, Verma N, Pearle AD, et al. Contrast-enhanced ultrasound characterization of the vascularity of the rotator cuff tendon: age- and activity-related changes in the intact asymptomatic rotator cuff. J Shoulder Elb Surg. 2008;17(1 Suppl):96S–100S. doi:10.1016/j.jse.2007.07.004.
99. Visser B, van Dieen JH. Pathophysiology of upper extremity muscle disorders. J Electromyogr Kinesiol. 2006;16(1):1–16. doi:10.1016/j.jelekin.2005.06.005.
100. Mulherin SA, Miller WC. Spectrum bias or spectrum effect? Subgroup variation in diagnostic test evaluation. Ann Intern Med. 2002;137(7):598–602.
101. Hegedus EJ, Cook C, Brennan M, Wyland D, Garrison JC, Driesner D. Vascularity and tendon pathology in the rotator cuff: a review of literature and implications for rehabilitation and surgery. Br J Sports Med. 2010;44(12):838–47. doi:10.1136/bjsm.2008.053769.
102. Barbe MF, Gallagher S, Massicotte VS, Tytell M, Popoff SN, Barr-Gillespie AE. The interaction of force and repetition on musculoskeletal and neural tissue responses and sensorimotor behavior in a rat model of work-related musculoskeletal disorders. BMC Musculoskelet Disord. 2013;14:303. doi:10.1186/1471-2474-14-303.
103. Massicotte VS, Frara N, Harris MY, Amin M, Wade CK, Popoff SN, et al. Prolonged performance of a high repetition low force task induces bone adaptation in young adult rats, but loss in mature rats. Exp Gerontol. 2015;72:204–17. doi:10.1016/j.exger.2015.10.014.
104. Barbe MF, Jain NX, Massicotte VS, Popoff SN, Barr-Gillespie AE. Ergonomic task reduction prevents bone osteopenia in a rat model of upper extremity overuse. Ind Health. 2015;53(3):206–21. doi:10.2486/indhealth.2014-0159.
105. Jain NX, Barr-Gillespie AE, Clark BD, Kietrys DM, Wade CK, Litvin J, et al. Bone loss from high repetitive high force loading is prevented by ibuprofen treatment. J Musculoskelet Neuronal Interact. 2014;14(1):78–94.
106. Saupe N, Pfirrmann CW, Schmid MR, Jost B, Werner CM, Zanetti M. Association between rotator cuff abnormalities and reduced acromiohumeral distance. AJR Am J Roentgenol. 2006;187(2):376–82. doi:10.2214/AJR.05.0435.
107. Bigliani LU, Morrison DS, April EW. The morphology of the acromion and its relationship to rotator cuff tears. Orthop Trans. 1986;10:228.
108. Abramson RG, Burton KR, Yu JP, Scalzetti EM, Yankeelov TE, Rosenkrantz AB, et al. Methods and challenges in quantitative imaging biomarker development. Acad Radiol. 2015;22(1):25–32. doi:10.1016/j.acra.2014.09.001.
109. Raunig DL, McShane LM, Pennello G, Gatsonis C, Carson PL, Voyvodic JT, et al. Quantitative imaging biomarkers: a review of statistical methods for technical performance assessment. Stat Methods Med Res. 2015;24(1):27–67. doi:10.1177/0962280214537344.
110. Sullivan DC, Obuchowski NA, Kessler LG, Raunig DL, Gatsonis C, Huang EP, et al. Metrology standards for quantitative imaging biomarkers. Radiol. 2015;142202 doi:10.1148/radiol.2015142202.
111. Richards RR, An KN, Bigliani LU, Friedman RJ, Gartsman GM, Gristina AG, et al. A standardized method for the assessment of shoulder function. J Shoulder Elb Surg. 1994;3(6):347–52. doi:10.1016/S1058-2746(09)80019-0.
112. Vernon H, Mior S. The neck disability index: a study of reliability and validity. J Manip Physiol Ther. 1991;14(7):409–15.
113. Lippitt SB, Harryman DT, Matsen FA. A practical tool for evaluation of function: the simple shoulder test. In: Matsen FA, Fu FH, Hawkins RJ, editors. The shoulder: a balance of mobility and stability. Rosemont: American Academy of Orthopedic Surgery; 1993.
114. Larsson R, Cai H, Zhang Q, Öberg P, Larsson S-E. Visualization of chronic neck-shoulder pain: impaired microcirculation in the upper trapezius muscle in chronic cervico-brachial pain. Occup Med (Lond). 1998;48:189–94.
115. Levy O, Relwani J, Zaman T, Even T, Venkateswaran B, Copeland S. Measurement of blood flow in the rotator cuff using laser Doppler flowmetry. J Bone Joint Surg Br. 2008;90(7):893–8. doi:10.1302/0301-620X.90B7.19918.
116. Cay N, Tosun O, Isik C, Unal O, Kartal MG, Bozkurt M. Is coracoacromial arch angle a predisposing factor for rotator cuff tears? Diagn Interv Radiol. 2014;20(6):498–502. doi:10.5152/dir.2014.14102.
117. De Loose V, Van Den Oord M, Keser I, Burnotte F, Van Tiggelen D, Dumarey A, et al. MRI study of the morphometry of the cervical musculature in F-16 pilots. Aviat Space Environ Med. 2009;80(8):727–31. doi:10.3357/asem.2389.2009.
118. Gokalp G, Algin O, Yildirim N, Yazici Z. Adhesive capsulitis: contrast-enhanced shoulder MRI findings. J Med Imaging Radiat Oncol. 2011;55(2):119–25. doi:10.1111/j.1754-9485.2010.02215.x.
119. Kaymak B, Ozcakar L, Inanici F, Cetin A, Ariyurek M, Tan AA. Forearm bone mineral density measurements in thoracic outlet syndrome. Rheumatol Int. 2008;28(9):891–3. doi:10.1007/s00296-008-0531-x.
120. Kim KC, Rhee KJ, Shin HD. Adhesive capsulitis of the shoulder: dimensions of the rotator interval measured with magnetic resonance arthrography. J Shoulder Elb Surg. 2009;18(3):437–42. doi:10.1016/j.jse.2008.10.018.
121. Lee MH, Ahn JM, Muhle C, Kim SH, Park JS, Kim SH, et al. Adhesive capsulitis of the shoulder: diagnosis using magnetic resonance arthrography, with arthroscopic findings as the standard. J Comput Assist Tomogr. 2003;27(6):901–6.
122. Macarini L, Muscarella S, Lelario M, Stoppino L, Scalzo G, Scelzi A, et al. Rotator cable at MR imaging: considerations on morphological aspects and biomechanical role. Radiol Med. 2011;116(1):102–13. doi:10.1007/s11547-010-0571-7.
123. Manton GL, Schweitzer ME, Weishaupt D, Karasick D. Utility of MR arthrography in the diagnosis of adhesive capsulitis. Skelet Radiol. 2001;30(6):326–30.
124. Moses DA, Chang EY, Schweitzer ME. The scapuloacromial angle: a 3D analysis of acromial slope and its relationship with shoulder impingement. J Magn Reson Imaging. 2006;24(6):1371–7. doi:10.1002/jmri.20763.
125. O'Leary S, Cagnie B, Reeve A, Jull G, Elliott JM. Is there altered activity of the extensor muscles in chronic mechanical neck pain? A functional magnetic resonance imaging study. Arch Phys Med Rehabil. 2011;92(6):929–34. doi:10.1016/j.apmr.2010.12.021.
126. Ahn KS, Kang CH, Oh YW, Jeong WK. Correlation between magnetic resonance imaging and clinical impairment in patients with adhesive capsulitis. Skelet Radiol. 2012;41(10):1301–8. doi:10.1007/s00256-012-1391-8.
127. Ballyns JJ, Turo D, Otto P, Shah JP, Hammond J, Gebreab T, et al. Office-based elastographic technique for quantifying mechanical properties of skeletal muscle. J Ultrasound Med. 2012;31(8):1209–19.
128. Brasseur JL, Lucidarme O, Tardieu M, Tordeur M, Montalvan B, Parier J, et al. Ultrasonographic rotator-cuff changes in veteran tennis players: the effect of hand dominance and comparison with clinical findings. Eur Radiol. 2004;14(5):857–64. doi:10.1007/s00330-003-2116-0.
129. Cholewinski JJ, Kusz DJ, Wojciechowski P, Cielinski LS, Zoladz MP. Ultrasound measurement of rotator cuff thickness and acromio-humeral distance in the diagnosis of subacromial impingement syndrome of the

shoulder. Knee Surg Sports Traumatol Arthrosc : official journal of the ESSKA. 2008;16(4):408–14. doi:10.1007/s00167-007-0443-4.
130. Curry EJ, Matzkin EE, Dong Y, Higgins LD, Katz JN, Jain NB. Structural characteristics are not associated with pain and function in rotator cuff tears: the ROW cohort study. Orthop J Sports Med. 2015;3(5): 2325967115584596. doi:10.1177/2325967115584596.
131. Gokalp G, Yildirim N, Yazici Z, Ercan I. Using chemical-shift MR imaging to quantify fatty degeneration within supraspinatus muscle due to supraspinatus tendon injuries. Skelet Radiol. 2010;39(12):1211–7. doi:10. 1007/s00256-010-0927-z.
132. Jeracitano D, Cooper RG, Lyon LJ, Jayson MI. Abnormal temperature control suggesting sympathetic dysfunction in the shoulder skin of patients with frozen shoulder. Br J Rheumatol. 1992;31(8):539–42.
133. Jung JY, Jee WH, Chun HJ, Kim YS, Chung YG, Kim JM. Adhesive capsulitis of the shoulder: evaluation with MR arthrography. Eur Radiol. 2006;16(4): 791–6. doi:10.1007/s00330-005-0020-5.
134. Lefevre-Colau MM, Drape JL, Fayad F, Rannou F, Diche T, Minvielle F, et al. Magnetic resonance imaging of shoulders with idiopathic adhesive capsulitis: reliability of measures. Eur Radiol. 2005;15(12):2415–22. doi:10. 1007/s00330-005-2830-x.
135. Roidis NT, Motamed S, Vaishnav S, Ebramzadeh E, Karachalios TS, Itamura JM. The influence of the acromioclavicular joint degeneration on supraspinatus outlet impingement and the acromion shape. J Orthop Surg (Hong Kong). 2009;17(3):331–4.
136. Tamai K, Yamato M. Abnormal synovium in the frozen shoulder: a preliminary report with dynamic magnetic resonance imaging. J Shoulder Elb Surg. 1997;6(6):534–43.
137. Toyoda H, Ito Y, Tomo H, Nakao Y, Koike T, Takaoka K. Evaluation of rotator cuff tears with magnetic resonance arthrography. Clin Orthop Relat Res. 2005;439:109–15.
138. Collinger JL, Fullerton B, Impink BG, Koontz AM, Boninger ML. Validation of grayscale-based quantitative ultrasound in manual wheelchair users: relationship to established clinical measures of shoulder pathology. Am J Phys Med Rehabil. 2010;89(5):390–400. doi:10.1097/PHM.0b013e3181d8a238.
139. Dogan M, Cay N, Tosun O, Karaoglanoglu M, Bozkurt M. Glenoid axis is not related with rotator cuff tears–a magnetic resonance imaging comparative study. Int Orthop. 2012;36(3):595–8. doi:10.1007/s00264-011-1356-x.
140. Girometti R, De Candia A, Sbuelz M, Toso F, Zuiani C, Bazzocchi M. Supraspinatus tendon US morphology in basketball players: correlation with main pathologic models of secondary impingement syndrome in young overhead athletes. Preliminary report. Radiol Med. 2006;111(1):42–52.
141. Huang CC, Ko SF, Ko JY, Huang HY, Ng SH, Wan YL, et al. Contracture of the deltoid muscle: sonographic evaluation with MRI correlation. AJR Am J Roentgenol. 2005;185(2):364–70. doi:10.2214/ajr.185.2.01850364.
142. Kaneko K, DeMouy EH, Brunet ME. MR evaluation of rotator cuff impingement: correlation with confirmed full-thickness rotator cuff tears. J Comput Assist Tomogr. 1994;18(2):225–8.
143. Kim HM, Dahiya N, Teefey SA, Middleton WD, Stobbs G, Steger-May K, et al. Location and initiation of degenerative rotator cuff tears: an analysis of three hundred and sixty shoulders. J Bone Joint Surg Am. 2010;92(5):1088–96. doi:10.2106/JBJS.I.00686.
144. Rezasoltani A, Ali-Reza A, Khosro KK, Abbass R. Preliminary study of neck muscle size and strength measurements in females with chronic non-specific neck pain and healthy control subjects. Man Ther. 2010;15(4):400–3. doi:10.1016/j.math.2010.02.010.
145. Rezasoltani A, Ahmadipoor A, Khademi-Kalantari K, Javanshir K. The sign of unilateral neck semispinalis capitis muscle atrophy in patients with chronic non-specific neck pain. J Back Musculoskelet Rehabil. 2012;25(1):67–72. doi:10.3233/bmr-2012-0303.
146. Shinozaki T, Takagishi K, Ichikawa A, Inoue T, Yamaji T, Ishikawa T, et al. Use of 2-[18F]-fluoro-2-deoxy-d-glucose positron emission tomography (FDG PET) imaging for the evaluation of muscle metabolic activity in ruptured rotator cuffs: identification of shoulder muscles by fusion imaging studies involving both FDG PET and magnetic resonance imaging. J Shoulder Elb Surg. 2003;12(6):544–9. doi:10.1016/S1058274603002088.
147. Sundstrom T, Guez M, Hildingsson C, Toolanen G, Nyberg L, Riklund K. Altered cerebral blood flow in chronic neck pain patients but not in whiplash patients: a 99mTc-HMPAO rCBF study. Eur Spine J. 2006;15(8): 1189–95. doi:10.1007/s00586-005-0040-5.
148. MacGillivray JD, Fealy S, Potter HG, O'Brien SJ. Multiplanar analysis of acromion morphology. Am J Sports Med. 1998;26(6):836–40.
149. Tracy MR, Trella TA, Nazarian LN, Tuohy CJ, Williams GR. Sonography of the coracohumeral interval: a potential technique for diagnosing coracoid impingement. J Ultrasound Med. 2010;29(3):337–41.
150. Vecchio PC, Adebajo AO, Chard MD, Thomas PP, Hazleman BL. Thermography of frozen shoulder and rotator cuff tendinitis. Clin Rheumatol. 1992;11(3):382–4.
151. Harrison MF, Neary JP, Albert WJ, Croll JC. Neck pain and muscle function in a population of CH-146 helicopter aircrew. Aviat Space Environ Med. 2011; 82(12):1125–30.
152. Ko JY, Huang CC, Chen WJ, Chen CE, Chen SH, Wang CJ. Pathogenesis of partial tear of the rotator cuff: a clinical and pathologic study. J Shoulder Elb Surg. 2006;15(3):271–8. doi:10.1016/j.jse.2005.10.013.
153. Larsson SE, Bodegard L, Henriksson KG, Oberg PA. Chronic trapezius myalgia. Morphology and blood flow studied in 17 patients. Acta Orthop Scand. 1990;61(5):394–8.
154. McGinley JC, Agrawal S, Biswal S. Rotator cuff tears: association with acromion angulation on MRI. Clin Imaging. 2012;36(6):791–6. doi:10.1016/j. clinimag.2012.04.007.
155. Wallny T, Wagner UA, Prange S, Schmitt O, Reich H. Evaluation of chronic tears of the rotator cuff by ultrasound. A new index. J Bone Joint Surg Br. 1999;81(4):675–8.
156. Leistad RB, Nilsen KB, Stovner LJ, Westgaard RH, Ro M, Sand T. Similarities in stress physiology among patients with chronic pain and headache disorders: evidence for a common pathophysiological mechanism? J Headache Pain. 2008;9(3):165–75. doi:10.1007/s10194-008-0029-7.
157. Di Mario M, Fraracci L. MR study of the intrinsic acromial angle in 74 symptomatic patients. Radiol Med. 2005;110(3):273–9.
158. Mani R, Cooper C, Kidd BL, Cole JD, Cawley MI. Use of laser Doppler flowmetry and transcutaneous oxygen tension electrodes to assess local autonomic dysfunction in patients with frozen shoulder. J R Soc Med. 1989;82(9):536–8.
159. Breidahl WH, Stafford Johnson DB, Newman JS, Adler RS. Power Doppler sonography in tenosynovitis: significance of the peritendinous hypoechoic rim. J Ultrasound Med. 1998;17(2):103–7.

4

Subtalar instability: imaging features of subtalar ligaments on 3D isotropic ankle MRI

Tae Hyung Kim[1], Sung Gyu Moon[1*], Hong-Geun Jung[2] and Na Ra Kim[1]

Abstract

Background: MRI analysis of subtalar ligaments in the tarsal sinus has not been well performed. We retrospectively investigated the appearance of subtalar ligaments using 3D isotropic MRI and compared imaging findings of subtalar ligaments between patients with subtalar instability (STI) and controls.

Methods: Preoperative MRIs of 23 STI patients treated with arthroscopic subtalar reconstruction were compared to MRIs of 23 age- and sex-matched control subjects without STI. Thickness and width of anterior capsular ligament (ACL) and interosseous talocalcaneal ligament (ITCL) as well as thickness of calcaneofibular ligament (CFL) and anterior talofibular ligament (ATFL) were measured. Abnormalities in ACL, ITCL, CFL, ATFL, cervical ligament, and inferior extensor retinaculum were analyzed.

Results: STI patients had significantly smaller ACL thickness and ACL width than controls (ACL thickness: 1.73 mm vs. 2.22 mm, $p = 0.007$; ACL width: 7.21 mm vs. 8.80 mm, $p = 0.004$). ACL thickness of ≤2.1 mm had a sensitivity of 66.7% and a specificity of 66.7% for diagnosis of STI. ACL width of ≤7.9 mm had a sensitivity of 80.0% and a specificity of 76.2% for the diagnosis of STI. However, thickness and width of ITCL, thickness of CFL, or thickness of ATFL was not significantly different between the two groups. Absence or complete tear of ACL was significantly more frequent in STI patients than that in controls (34.8% vs. 8.7%, $p = 0.035$). Complete tear of CFL and ATFL was more common in STI patients than that in controls, although the difference between the two groups was not statistically significant. Abnormalities of ITCL, cervical ligament, or inferior extensor retinaculum were not significantly different between the two groups.

Conclusions: MRI features of thin or narrow ACLs may suggest STI. Absence or complete tear of ACL was significantly more common in STI patients than that in controls.

Keywords: Instability, Subtalar, Ligaments, Ankle, MRI, 3D

Background

Subtalar instability (STI) is a chronic functional talocalcaneal instability characterized by a combination of anterior movement, medialization, and varus tilt of the calcaneus [1, 2]. STI is usually combined with lateral ankle instability (LAI). Incidence of subtalar joint injury has been reported to be as high as 80% in patients with acute lateral ankle sprain. Approximately 10–25% of patients with LAI have STI [3, 4]. Diagnosis of STI is difficult because clinical symptoms of STI are similar to those of LAI. In addition, there is no optimal assessment for STI [1].

Chronic tear and insufficiency of interosseous talocalcaneal ligament (ITCL), cervical ligament (CL), and calcaneofibular ligament (CFL) have been reported as etiologies of STI [5, 6]. However, anatomy and function of subtalar ligaments remain controversial [5]. Some investigators consider ITCL as the most important stabilizer of the subtalar joint. However, inconsistencies occur in morphologies of ITCL. Cadaver studies have shown that there are two distinct ligaments in the tarsal sinus: ITCL and anterior capsular ligament (ACL) [7, 8].

* Correspondence: sgmoon@kuh.ac.kr
[1]Department of Radiology, Konkuk University Medical Center, Konkuk University School of Medicine, 120-1 Neungdong-ro, Gwangjin-gu, Seoul 05030, South Korea
Full list of author information is available at the end of the article

It has been suggested that ITCL and ACL should be considered as two distinct ligaments since they have unique insertion and running patterns.

Despite the association of subtalar ligaments with STI, little attention was paid to the appearance of subtalar ligaments or the ability of MRI to visualize them. MRI analysis of subtalar ligaments in STI patients has not been well performed yet. Therefore, the objective of this study was to retrospectively evaluate the appearance of subtalar ligaments using 3D isotropic MRI and compare imaging findings of subtalar ligaments between STI patients and controls.

Methods

Study population

Our Institutional Review Board approved this retrospective study. The requirement for informed consent was waived due to its retrospective nature. A computerized search of medical and radiological records and clinical chart review identified 47 patients with STI who were surgically treated between January 2013 and August 2015. Twenty-three patients (10 females, 13 males) were selected for final analysis based on the following inclusion criteria: (a) clinical diagnosis of STI, surgical confirmation of the diagnosis, and treatment with subtalar reconstruction; (b) arthroscopic surgery performed less than three months after MRI; (c) MRI performed at our institution according to a standardized protocol; (d) no history of ankle surgery; and (e) aged 17 years or older. A total of 24 patients were excluded, including 15 who underwent preoperative MRI at outside institutions, five who did not undergo surgery within three months after MRI, two patients who had prior history of lateral ankle ligament repair, and two patients who were younger than 17 years.

Mean age of patients included in this study was 31.3 years (range, 17 to 57 years). The mean age of female patients was 32.7 years (range, 17 to 57 years). Mean age of the 13 male patients was 30.2 years (range, 18 to 50 years). Mean height, weight, and BMI of STI patients were 168.6 ± 10.5 cm, 71.1 ± 13.4 kg, and 24.9 ± 3.8 kg/m^2, respectively. Twelve patients were overweight (BMI greater than 25) and two patients were obese (BMI greater than 30). A total of 17 right ankles and 6 left ankles were included. Ten (43.5%) of these 23 ankles also had LAI. All 23 ankles had previous ankle sprain history and preoperative symptomatic recurrent ankle sprain. The mean duration of symptoms was 3.8 years (range, 1 to 11 years). Surgical treatment was performed in patients who did not show symptom improvement despite functional rehabilitation treatment such as peroneal tendon strengthening exercises for ≥3 months.

Preoperative clinical diagnosis of STI was based on the following diagnostic criteria provided by the senior orthopedic surgeon in our hospital [6]: patients who met at least four of the following five features of preoperative diagnostic criteria: 1) recurrent ankle sprain, 2) sinus tarsi pain and tenderness, 3) hindfoot looseness or giving way, 4) hindfoot instability on physical examination, and 5) radiographic STI on ankle and Broden's varus stress radiographic views. Ankle and Broden's varus stress radiographic views were obtained with a Telos SE 2000 stress device (ARD MedizinProdukte GmbH, Marburg, Germany) using 150 Newton of varus stress–force applied at the hindfoot. Positive response on Broden's varus stress view was defined as an ipsilateral subtalar tilt angle of greater than 10 degrees and a subtalar tilt difference of greater than 5 degrees compared to the contralateral ankle [9] (Fig. 1). Preoperative MRI was performed to determine any additional pathologic condition (such as lateral ankle ligament tear and osteochondral lesion of the talus) that could influence surgical procedure.

For surgical confirmation of STI, the ankle was examined using C-arm stress fluoroscopy under general or spinal anesthesia. In all patients, STI was confirmed by marked tilting of the calcaneus against the talus with lateral widening of the talocalcaneal joint and medial displacement of the calcaneus relative to the talus. Subtalar arthroscopic examination was conducted to evaluate the presence of marked subtalar joint laxity, chronic interosseous ligament tear, synovitis, and other features. Chronic interosseous ligament tear was observed in all patients. An intact ligament was diagnosed when the continuity of the ligament was preserved. Ligament dysfunction caused by chronic tear was defined as definite discontinuity of the ligament and adhesion of adjacent tissue. In 10 cases with both STI and LAI, the Broström procedure was performed in addition to the subtalar reconstruction procedure. Eleven (47.8%) patients had ankle synovitis. Thirteen (56.5%) ankles had subtalar synovitis. Debridement and synovectomy were performed for all patients with synovitis. Combined operations were performed for seven ankles. Two ankles had osteochondral lesion of the talus which was treated by arthroscopic debridement and microfracture. Os subfibulare excision was performed for four ankles. Loose-body removal was performed for one ankle. Lateral sliding calcaneal osteotomy was performed for one ankle with cavovarus deformity.

The control group consisted of 23 subjects who underwent ankle MRI based on a standardized protocol in our institution. They did not show any clinical or arthroscopic sign of STI. Matching criteria for control subjects were: age range, 18–55 years; mean age, 31.9 years; age range of women, 18–55 years; mean age of women, 30.0 years; age range of men, 19–52 years; mean age of men, 32.3 years; sex, 10 women and 13 men. Mean

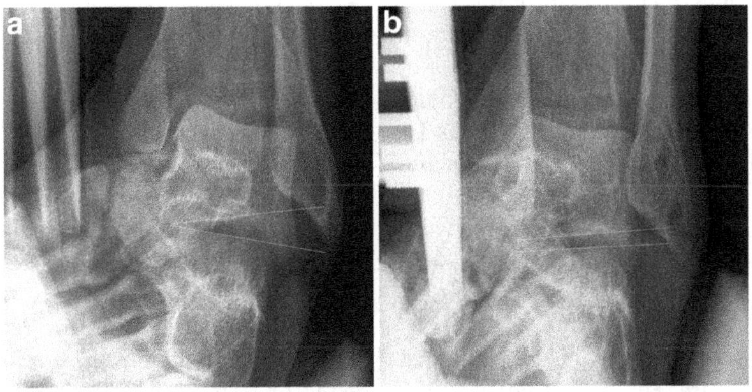

Fig. 1 Subtalar tilt angle on Broden's stress view. Subtalar tilt angle is defined as the angle between lines drawn across the articular surface of the talus and the calcaneus. **a** Preoperative subtalar tilt angle was measured 15 degrees. **b** At 6 months postoperatively, the subtalar tilt angle decreased to 1 degree

height, weight, and BMI of control subjects were 168.5 ± 8.4 cm, 68.0 ± 16.9 kg, and 23.8 ± 4.8 kg/m^2, respectively. Nine subjects were overweight (BMI greater than 25) and three subjects were obese (BMI greater than 30). A total of 13 right ankles and 10 left ankles were included. They were diagnosed as acute ankle sprain ($n = 6$), post-traumatic soft tissue impingement ($n = 4$), osteochondral lesion of the talus (n = 4), inflammatory arthritis (n = 4), achilles tendinopathy ($n = 3$), and peroneus tenosynovitis ($n = 2$). Of these 23 subjects, seven underwent ankle and subtalar arthroscopic examinations. They were confirmed to have no STI. For the control group, the mean follow-up period after ankle MRI was 21 months (range, 6–42 months).

MRI protocol

MR exams were performed using two 3.0-T MRI units with dedicated coils, including a Magnetom Skyra (Siemens Healthcare Diagnostics, Erlangen, Germany) using a sixteen-channel (Siemens Healthcare Diagnostics) ankle coil and a Signa HDxt (GE Healthcare, Milwaukee, WI, USA) with an eight-channel (GE Healthcare) coil. A 3D T2-weighted FSE imaging sequence was used in the sagittal plane without fat suppression. Using Magnetom Skyra, 3D data were acquired with a slice thickness of 0.5 mm using the following imaging parameters: repetition time, 1200 ms; echo time, 155 ms; flip angle, 120°; echo train length, 61; bandwidth, 360 kHz/pixel; field of view, 140 mm; and matrix, 256 × 230. Using Signa HDxt, 3D data acquisition was performed with a slice thickness of 0.4 mm and the following imaging parameters: repetition time, 1250 ms; echo time, 63 ms; flip angle, 90°; echo train length, 34; bandwidth, 195 kHz/pixel; field of view, 140 mm; and matrix, 256 × 224. Subsequently, sagittal images originally acquired from 3D data were reformatted into axial and coronal images with a slice thickness of 0.6 mm without interslice gap. Other 2D imaging sequences including axial and coronal T2-, sagittal T1-, sagittal T2- with fat suppression, and axial, coronal, sagittal T1-weighted images with contrast enhancement were also acquired.

MRI analysis

Quantitative analysis

Schematic illustrations of ligaments in the sinus tarsi are shown in Fig. 2. CL was located in the anterior part of the sinus tarsi, extending from the inferior-lateral aspect of the talar neck to the dorsal surface of the calcaneal neck. ITCL and ACL were located along the posterior wall of the sinus tarsi. On the coronal plane along the posterior wall of the sinus tarsi, ITCL coursed obliquely. However, ACL was vertical like a curtain. This flat thick

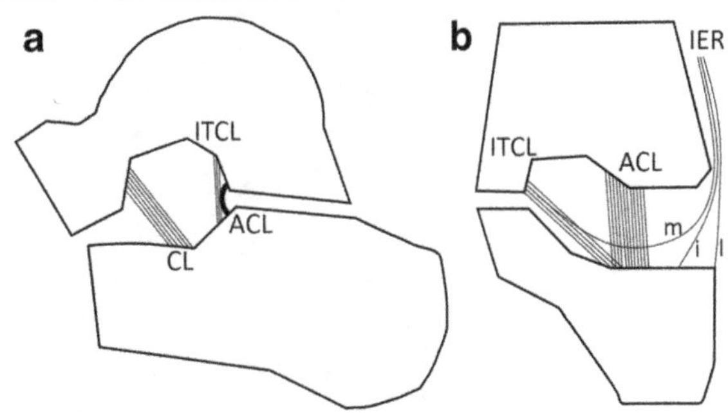

Fig. 2 Schematic illustration of ligaments of the sinus tarsi. **a** On the sagittal plane, cervical ligament is located in the anterior aspect of the tarsal sinus, extending from the undersurface of the talar neck to the back of the calcaneus. Interosseous talocalcaneal ligament and anterior capsular ligament are located along the posterior wall of sinus tarsi. **b** On the coronal plane along the posterior wall of sinus tarsi, interosseous talocalcaneal ligament runs obliquely while anterior capsular ligament is vertical in direction. The inferior extensor retinaculum is more laterally positioned with respect to the anterior capsular ligament and interosseous talocalcaneal ligament. CL, cervical ligament; ITCL, interosseous talocalcaneal ligament; ACL, anterior capsular ligament; IER, inferior extensor retinaculum; m, medial root of IER; i, intermediate root of IER; l, lateral root of IER

ligament was defined as thickened segment of the anterior joint capsule of the posterior talocalcaneal facet. ACL originated at the anterior border of the posterior facet of the talus. It ran vertically across the subtalar joint before attaching to the calcaneus [7]. ITCL was located in the anteromedial side to the ACL. It ran obliquely from the talus in the tarsal canal toward the calcaneus in the tarsal sinus [7]. The space between ITCL and ACL was filled with adipose tissue. Therefore, ACL and ITCL could be clearly distinguished from each other.

Ligament dimensions were measured in the plane that best represented the structure. For ACL, thickness and width were measured on sagittal and axial isotropic 3D T2 weighted images, respectively (Fig. 3). Thickness and width of ITCL were obtained from isotropic 3D T2 weighted images in sagittal and coronal planes, respectively (Fig. 3). Thickness of CFL and ATFL were also measured in axial isotropic 3D T2 weighted image. These measurements were performed at the center of the ligament except for CFL. Thickness of the CFL was measured at the mid-portion between peroneal intersection and calcaneal attachment. Quantitative measurements were obtained thrice by one investigator. Mean values were recorded in millimeters. All measurements were performed using measurement tools included in the PACS computer imaging system.

Qualitative analysis

The following qualitative criteria were evaluated and characterized as present or absent: (a) abnormalities of ACL and ITCL characterized by the absence or complete tear of ligaments, (b) abnormalities of CFL and ATFL characterized by complete tear of ligaments, (c) abnormalities of CL characterized by complete tear, (d) abnormalities of inferior extensor retinaculum characterized by partial or complete absence of three roots of inferior extensor retinaculum. Diagnostic criteria for determining complete tear of the ligament included non-visualization of the ligament, discontinuity, and a wavy or curved contour [10]. MRI was evaluated by two musculoskeletal radiologists (with 17 and 5 years of experience, respectively) who were blinded to the diagnosis. Each reader independently evaluated the status of ligaments and subsequently reviewed them to determine the status in consensus. Additionally, edema or obliteration of tarsal sinus fat, and synovial recess extension into tarsal sinus were evaluated in consensus using 2D imaging sequences with or without contrast enhancement.

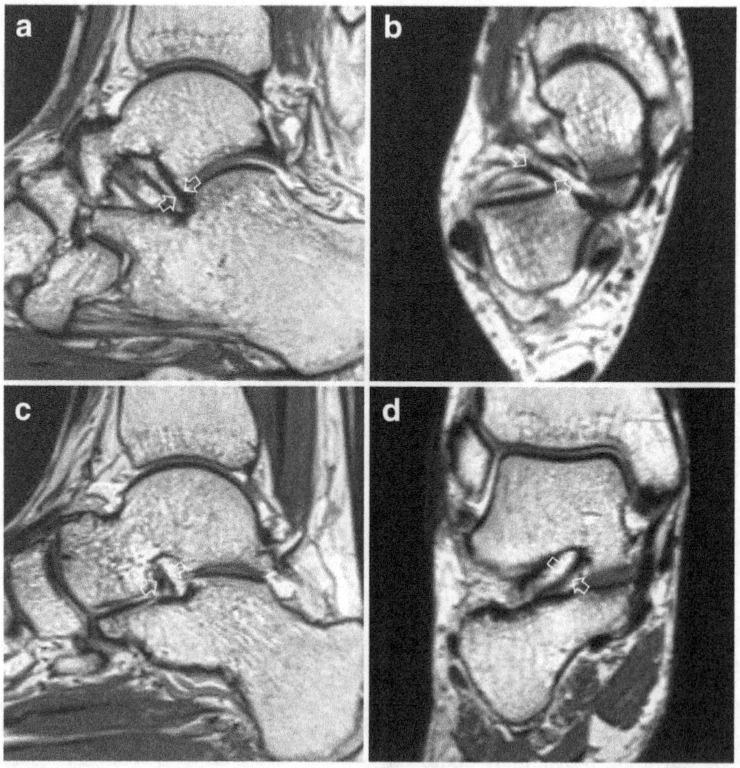

Fig. 3 A 33-year-old woman with ankle sprain. Sagittal (**a**) and axial (**b**) isotropic 3D T2-weighted images demonstrating the thickness and width of anterior capsular ligament (open arrows), respectively. Sagittal (**c**) and coronal (**d**) isotropic 3D T2-weighted images demonstrating the thickness and width of interosseous talocalcaneal ligament (open arrows), respectively

Statistical analysis

Continuous data were analyzed with Mann-Whitney test. Receiver operating characteristic (ROC) analysis was used to determine cutoff values of ACL thickness and width for discrimination between the two groups. Sensitivity and specificity were calculated for quantitative criteria and cutoff values of ACL thickness and width. Fisher's exact test was used to compare qualitative criteria. Interobserver agreement was calculated using kappa statistics based on the following criteria: $\kappa < 0$, no agreement; $0 < \kappa \leq 0.2$, slight agreement; $0.2 < \kappa \leq 0.4$, fair agreement; $0.4 < \kappa \leq 0.6$, moderate agreement; $0.6 < \kappa \leq 0.8$, substantial agreement; $0.8 < \kappa \leq 1$, almost perfect agreement [11]. Statistical analysis was performed using SPSS for Windows version 21.0 (SPSS, Chicago, IL, USA). A p value of less than 0.05 was considered statistically significant.

Results

Mean BMI was 24.9 ± 3.8 kg/m^2 for the STI patient group and 23.8 ± 4.8 kg/m^2 for the control group. There was no significant difference in BMI between STI patient group and the age- and sex-matched control group ($p = 0.223$, Mann-Whitney test).

All patients underwent C-arm stress fluoroscopy under anesthesia. They showed positive STI findings with marked widening of the subtalar joint. Chronic tears in the interosseous ligament were recorded in all cases during subtalar arthroscopy. For 10 cases diagnosed with both LAI and STI, the Broström procedure was also performed in addition to subtalar reconstruction. Semi-tendinous allograft was used to reconstruct anterior and posterior CFL during subtalar reconstruction surgery [6].

Quantitative analysis of MRI findings

The STI patient group had significantly smaller ACL thickness and width than the control group (thickness: 1.73 ± 0.58 mm vs. 2.22 ± 0.49 mm, $p = 0.007$; width: 7.21 ± 1.69 mm vs. 8.80 ± 1.50 mm, $p = 0.004$) (Fig. 4). Thickness of ITCL, width of ITCL, thickness of ATFL, or thickness of CFL was not significantly different between the two groups (Table 1).

Based on ROC analysis of ACL dimensions, a cutoff of 2.1 mm for ACL thickness had a sensitivity of 66.7% and

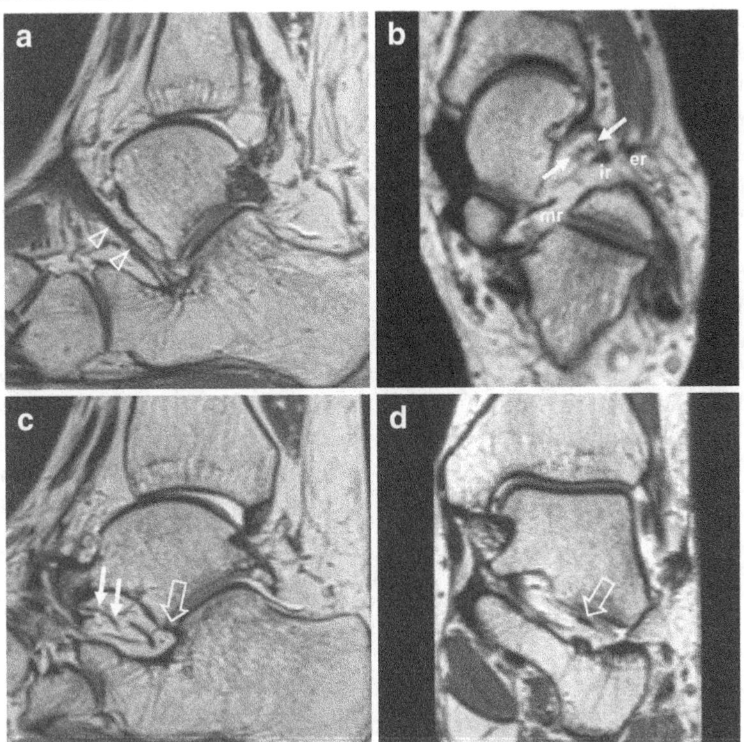

Fig. 4 A 27-year-old woman with subtalar instability. Sagittal (**a**) and axial (**b**) isotropic 3D T2-weighted images demonstrating intact inferior extensor retinaculum (arrowheads). er, ir, and mr indicate external, intermediate, and medial root of inferior extensor retinaculum, respectively. Cervical ligament represents a bundle of fan-shaped striated fibers (solid arrows). Sagittal (**c**) and coronal (**d**) isotropic 3D T2-weighted images demonstrating a thin and narrow anterior capsular ligament (open arrows). Solid arrows indicate cervical ligament with thin sheet-like fan-shaped striped fiber bundles

Table 1 Quantitative analysis of ligaments between subtalar instability patients and controls

Ligaments		Patient (mm)	Control (mm)	*p*-value
ACL	Thickness	1.73 ± 0.58	2.22 ± 0.49	0.007
	Width	7.21 ± 1.69	8.80 ± 1.50	0.004
ITCL	Thickness	2.07 ± 0.96	2.08 ± 0.78	0.860
	Width	2.75 ± 1.07	2.85 ± 1.13	0.991
CFL	Thickness	2.37 ± 1.17	2.34 ± 0.65	0.538
ATFL	Thickness	3.14 ± 1.11	3.63 ± 1.10	0.178

Note. *P* values were determined using Mann-Whitney test. Data are presented as averaged measurement results ± standard deviation
ACL anterior capsular ligament, *ITCL* interosseous talocalcaneal ligament, *CFL* calcaneofibular ligament, *ATFL* anterior talofibular ligament

a specificity of 66.7% (AUC = 0.765; $p = 0.007$) for STI diagnosis while a cutoff of 7.9 mm for ACL width had a sensitivity of 80.0% and a specificity of 76.2% (AUC = 0.778; $p = 0.005$) to distinguish STI patients from controls.

Qualitative analysis of MRI findings

Other ligament abnormalities besides ACL abnormalities were not significantly different between the two groups (Table 2). In the STI patient group, four cases had no ACL while another four had complete tear of ACL (Fig. 5). In the control group, there were two cases without ACL. The absence or complete tear of ACL was significantly more frequent in STI patients compared to that in controls (34.8% vs. 8.7%, $p = 0.035$). Compared to controls, STI patients had more percentages of complete tear of CFL (17.4% vs. 4.3%, $p = 0.173$) and complete tear of ATFL (17.4% vs. 8.7%, $p = 0.333$), although differences between the two groups were not statistically significant. There was no case of absence or complete tear of ITCL in either group. Based on its shape, ITCL was classified into three categories: band type ($n = 38$, 82.6%), fan type ($n = 4$, 8.7%), and split type (n = 4, 8.7%). There was no significant ($p = 0.368$) difference in the type of ITCL shape between STI and control groups. CL was well visualized on coronal and sagittal planes. It was identified 100% in both groups. CL irregularity and thinning were observed in two cases of the STI patient group. The remaining cases in both groups showed fan or band-shape striated fiber bundles. Partial absence of IER was found in two cases of the STI patient group. One of them showed no intermediate or medial root. The other one showed no medial root. However, the lateral root was visualized in all subjects. In all study subjects except two, the medial root was blended with fibers of the ITCL to form a common insertion.

Interobserver agreement between the two readers was considered substantial with kappa values of 0.663 for abnormalities of ACL, 0.726 for ITCL, 0.732 for ATFL, 0.691 for CFL, 0.726 for CL, and 0.646 for IER. Total number of discrepant reads was 18 (six in ACL, three each in ATFL and CFL, and two each in ITCL, CL and IER). All discordantly interpreted cases were re-reviewed to achieve consensus between the two readers. Eleven of them were in favor of reader 1 (four in ACL, one in ITCL, and two each in ATFL, CFL and IER). The rest of them were in favor of reader 2. These two readers were perfectly matched for CL.

Edema of tarsal sinus fat was more frequent in STI patients compared to that in controls (30.4% vs. 21.7%). However, the difference in the percentage of edema of tarsal sinus fat between the two groups was not statistically significant ($p = 0.369$). Synovial recess from the posterior subtalar joint frequently extended into the tarsal sinus, without significant difference between STI patients and controls (47.8% vs. 43.5%, $p = 0.500$). None of all study population demonstrated significant obliteration of tarsal sinus fat.

Discussion

STI tends to be diagnosed late because it is difficult to distinguish it from LAI on physical examination or stress radiography due to complex joint motion and small changes in laxity [12, 13]. Untreated chronic STI can lead to pain, dysfunction, deformity, and potentially degenerative arthritis. Thus, early diagnosis of STI is needed [2]. In addition to bony structures, subtalar

Table 2 Qualitative analysis of ligaments between subtalar instability patients and controls

MRI findings	Patient ($n = 23$)	Control (n = 23)	*p*-value
Absence or complete tear of ACL	8 (34.8%)	2 (8.7%)	0.035
Absence of ITCL	0	0	
Complete tear of CFL	4 (17.4%)	1 (4.3%)	0.173
Complete tear of ATFL	4 (17.4%)	2 (8.7%)	0.333
Irregularity or thinning of CL	2 (8.7%)	0	0.244
Partial absence of IER	2 (8.7%)	0	0.244

Note. *P* values were determined using the Fisher's exact test. Data are presented as number (percent) of patients
ACL anterior capsular ligament, *ITCL* interosseous talocalcaneal ligament, *CFL* calcaneofibular ligament, *ATFL* anterior talofibular ligament, *CL* cervical ligament, *IER* inferior extensor retinaculum

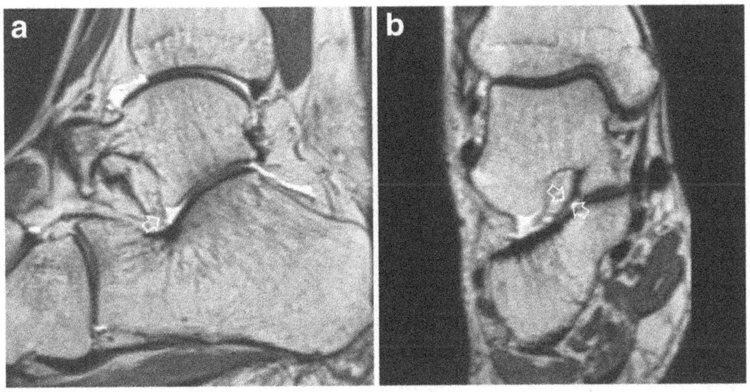

Fig. 5 A 25-year-old women with subtalar instability. **a** Sagittal isotropic 3D T2-weighted image demonstrating the absence of anterior capsular ligament (open arrow). **b** On a coronal image along the posterior wall of sinus tarsi, the interosseous talocalcaneal ligament (open arrow) appears to be intact

ligaments also play an important role in maintaining the stability of the subtalar joint [2, 14].

Subtalar ligaments are known to consist of CL, ITCL, ACL, and three roots of IER. However, controversy remains regarding which ligament is a more important stabilizer [5, 6]. Some reports have indicated that the CFL is the most important primary stabilizer for the subtalar joint while others have indicated that the ITCL or CL is the most important stabilizer [2, 8, 15–17]. Reported description and nomenclature of ligaments have shown many inconsistencies possibly due to subjective differences in the understanding of the anatomy and variation in shapes. Moreover, some of these ligamentous structures might have been confused with each other due to their adjacent positions. The ITCL has been described with different morphologies, including a V shape, an inverted Y shape, a veil extending across the tarsal canal, an oblique band, and a two-layered structure [7, 8, 14, 18]. A consensus on the description of the ITCL is lacking. Nevertheless, ACL and ITCL should be considered as two distinct ligaments based on their unique insertions and running patterns.

A notable subtalar ligament is the ACL. It was initially called an interosseous ligament. Subsequently, it was called an anterior capsular ligament because it was located along the anterior aspect of the posterior talocalcaneal facet [19, 20]. However, this was not mentioned in many later investigations. Recently, Li SY et al. have designated it a posterior capsular ligament because it is found behind the posterior capsule [8]. The ACL has been described as a thick flat ligament connecting the anterior border of the posterior talocalcaneal facet vertically. It is also identified in the same plane as ITCL [7]. Results from cadaver studies have shown the presence of ACL in 78–95% of specimens [7, 8]. To the best of our knowledge, ACL has not been previously described in radiologic literature.

There are relatively few MRI studies involving STI and subtalar ligaments. Previous cadaver studies [7, 8] and MRI studies [21–23] in asymptomatic models have described normal appearances of subtalar ligaments. According to a pediatric study using 3D isotropic proton density MRI [21], ITCL was striated in appearance in all study population with distinct fascicular bundles. CL most often appeared as a striated fiber bundle. It only occasionally demonstrated homogeneous hypo-intensity. The thickness of the CL ranged from 0.6 to 7 mm. Three roots of the IER were distinguishable in all study populations. Root thickness ranged from 0.5 mm to 2 mm. All tarsal sinus ligaments, i.e. CL, ITCL, and IER were well visualized in 3D isotropic proton density MRI. Each ligament had a unique orientation and dimensions with certain variations. Although there were some differences in dimensions, the results of previous studies were mostly consistent with those of our control group.

In the present study, we evaluated imaging features of subtalar ligaments in STI patents using 3D isotropic T2-weighted MRI. In addition, we compared MRI findings of subtalar ligaments between STI patients and controls. Quantitatively, STI patients had significantly smaller ACL in terms of thickness and width. In the control group, ACL width and thickness were 8.80 mm and 2.22 mm, respectively, similar to previous cadaver-study results (width of 10.1 mm and thickness of 2.4 mm) [8]. However, ACL thickness and width were significantly different between STI patient and control groups. Based on ROC analysis of ACL dimensions, a cutoff of 2.1 mm in thickness had a sensitivity of 66.7% and a specificity of 66.7% while a cutoff of 7.9 mm in width showed a sensitivity of 80.0% and a specificity of 76.2% to distinguish between STI and control. Absence or complete tear of the ACL was significantly more common in the STI patient group compared to that in the control group. In the control group, the prevalence of ACL was

91.3%, consistent with previously reported prevalence range of ACL [7].

ITCL thickness or width showed no significant difference between STI and control groups. According to our results, ITCL thickness and width in the control group were 2.08 mm and 2.85 mm, respectively. ITCL thickness of this study was similar to the thickness reported in previous studies. However, ITCL width of this study was much narrower than previously reported. In a cadaver study, ITCL thicknesses has been reported to be 2.3–3.0 mm with width of 8.5–11.0 mm [7]. In addition, medial roots of IER are known to be blended with fibers of ITCL to form a V-shaped large ligamentous lamina in the tarsal sinus [7]. Likewise, we found that the ITCL was mixed with medial roots of the IER in most cases. The reason that the ITCL width was relatively narrower than previously reported might be due to the fact that only main fiber bundles of ITCL that were clearly visualized on 3D isotropic MRI were measured.

Abnormalities of ITCL, CL, and IER characterized by complete or partial tear were not significantly different between the two groups. In most subjects of both groups, the CL was observed in the shape of a fan or band. Only two STI patients showed irregular or thin CL. In the control group, the CL was best visualized in the coronal plane with 100% rate of detection, similar to the detection rate previously reported in normal pediatric population [21]. Three roots of the IER were distinguished in all subjects except two in the present study. The medial root penetrated the tarsal sinus and blended with fibers of the ITCL to form a common insertion. ITCL, CL, and IER were successfully visualized and characterized in three planes at 100% in the control group, supporting the previous report using 3D proton density MRI [21]. Unlike previous reports, our results suggest that ITCL and CL may not be major stabilizers. Instead, ACL might play a more important role in maintaining the stability of the subtalar joint. ACL can be more important in restraining the posterior talocalcaneal joint due to its course. ACL lies closer to the subtalar joint than CL. It travels more laterally than ITCL. Therefore, it can serve as a central core ligament between the front CL and the rear CFL. In contrast, ITCL is located inside the tarsal sinus. It may not play a major role in restraining varus tilt of the talocalcaneal joint.

Quantitatively, the thickness of CFL or ATFL was not significantly different between the two groups. Complete tears of CFL and ATFL were more frequently observed in STI patients than those in controls, although the difference between the two groups was not statistically significant. In our study, 10 cases in the STI patient group were accompanied by LAI. In the control group, 14 cases had history of lateral ankle sprain. Therefore, the inclusion of lateral ankle sprain might have led to the no significant difference in complete tear of CFL or ATFL between the two groups.

Except CL, other subtalar ligaments including ITCL, three roots of IER, and ACL are located in a small space consisting of the tarsal canal and posterior part of the tarsal sinus. This has led to confusion about ligament anatomy. The function of ACL and ITCL in the tarsal sinus remains unclear due to the lack of anatomical studies. Our results indicate that dimensions of ACL are larger than those of ITCL, especially the width. Dimensions may reflect functional requirements. Furthermore, there was a significant difference in ACL dimensions between the two groups. The cutoff of 2.1 mm in thickness and 7.9 mm in width can facilitate the diagnosis of STI. Until recently, ACL has received little attention in the radiologic field. Further research on functional anatomy and imaging is needed.

Edema of tarsal sinus fat was more common in STI patients. However, there was no significant difference between the two groups. Synovial recess from the posterior subtalar joint often extended into the sinus tarsi in both groups. However, none of our study populations demonstrated significant obliteration of tarsal sinus fat. Edema of tarsal sinus fat can be reversible and may be caused by hemorrhage or inflammation with or without tears of the associated ligaments. Edema or obliteration of tarsal sinus fat are known to imply sinus tarsi syndrome, but sinus tarsi syndrome do not mean STI because it can be associated with other ankle diseases as well as STI. Sinus tarsi syndrome usually occurs after inversion injury and is often associated with tear of the lateral collateral ligament [24, 25]. Unlike fat suppression images, 3D isotropic T2-weighted images without fat suppression allowed us to distinguish the ligament boundaries and measure the dimensions because the ligaments had a unique direction and they were more clearly distinguished from the surrounding fat edema. 3D isotropic images provided the additional advantage of anatomical detail by thin section and multiplanar reformation capability, making it easy to track the course and integrity of small structures such as subtalar ligaments.

Our study has several limitations. First, the correlation between clinical and imaging outcomes was not fully evaluated due to the small sample size. In addition, it might be difficult to distinguish between pathologic ligaments and anatomic variations. Anatomic variation is beyond the scope of this study because it needs a large-scale study using normal population. This study focused on STI patients with symptoms rather than asymptomatic ankles, unlike most studies. The aim of this study was to compare STI patients and controls by focusing on subtalar ligaments to find unusual findings that might lead to STI. Second, the patient group consisted of STI patients regardless of LAI combination. More specific results can be obtained by selecting patients with LAI without STI as controls. Further research is needed to address this issue. Third, this study focused on ligamentous structures of the tarsal sinus and lateral ankle. However, other factors such as bony structure might also play a role in maintaining joint stability. Nevertheless, we tried to assess all candidate subtalar ligaments including ACL. Fourth, chronicity of ligament tear that might affect MRI findings was not evaluated in this study. Even though ligaments might appear intact, they could be thinned or thickened by prior partial tears without being detected. This can add bias to the diameters in the current study. Last, due to the retrospective nature of the study, clinical information and radiological evaluation might have introduced a bias.

Conclusions

Thin or narrow ACL MRI findings might suggest STI. Absence or complete tear of ACL was significantly more common in STI patients than that in controls. Since STI is usually combined with LAI, complete tears of CFL and ATFL are common in STI.

Abbreviations

ACL: Anterior capsular ligament; ATFL: Anterior talofibular ligament; CFL: Calcaneofibular ligament; CL: Cervical ligament; ITCL: Interosseous talocalcaneal ligament; LAI: Lateral ankle instability; STI: Subtalar instability

Acknowledgments

Not applicable.

Funding

No funding was obtained for this study.

Authors' contributions

KTH and MSG conceived this study and participated in the study design, data collection, statistical analysis, and manuscript preparation. JHG and KNR participated in data collection and manuscript preparation. All authors read and approved the final manuscript.

Consent for publication

Not applicable.

Competing interests

The authors declare that they have no competing interests.

Author details

[1]Department of Radiology, Konkuk University Medical Center, Konkuk University School of Medicine, 120-1 Neungdong-ro, Gwangjin-gu, Seoul 05030, South Korea. [2]Department of Orthopedic Surgery, Konkuk University Medical Center, Konkuk University School of Medicine, Seoul, South Korea.

References

1. Mittlmeier T, Wichelhaus A. Subtalar joint instability. Eur J Trauma Emerg Surg. 2015;41(6):623–9.
2. Karlsson J, Eriksson BI, Renstrom PA. Subtalar ankle instability. A review. Sports Med. 1997;24(5):337–46.
3. Hertel J. Functional anatomy, Pathomechanics, and pathophysiology of lateral ankle instability. J Athl Train. 2002;37(4):364–75.
4. Meyer JM, Garcia J, Hoffmeyer P, Fritschy D. The subtalar sprain. A roentgenographic study. *Clin Orthop Relat Res*. 1988;226:169–73.
5. Aynardi M, Pedowitz DI, Raikin SM. Subtalar instability. Foot Ankle Clin. 2015;20(2):243–52.
6. Jung HG, Park JT, Shin MH, Lee SH, Eom JS, Lee DO. Outcome of subtalar instability reconstruction using the semitendinosus allograft tendon and biotenodesis screws. Knee Surg Sports Traumatol Arthrosc. 2015;23(8):2376–83.
7. Jotoku T, Kinoshita M, Okuda R, Abe M. Anatomy of ligamentous structures in the tarsal sinus and canal. Foot Ankle Int. 2006;27(7):533–8.
8. Li SY, Hou ZD, Zhang P, Li HL, Ding ZH, Liu YJ. Ligament structures in the tarsal sinus and canal. Foot Ankle Int. 2013;34(12):1729–36.
9. Yamamoto H, Yagishita K, Ogiuchi T, Sakai H, Shinomiya K, Muneta T. Subtalar instability following lateral ligament injuries of the ankle. Injury. 1998;29(4):265–8.
10. Joshy S, Abdulkadir U, Chaganti S, Sullivan B, Hariharan K. Accuracy of MRI scan in the diagnosis of ligamentous and chondral pathology in the ankle. Foot Ankle Surg. 2010;16(2):78–80.
11. Landis JR, Koch GG. The measurement of observer agreement for categorical data. Biometrics. 1977;33(1):159–74.
12. Breitenseher MJ, Trattnig S, Kukla C, Gaebler C, Kaider A, Baldt MM, Haller J, Imhof H. MRI versus lateral stress radiography in acute lateral ankle ligament injuries. J Comput Assist Tomogr. 1997;21(2):280–5.
13. Sijbrandij ES, van Gils AP, van Hellemondt FJ, Louwerens JW, de Lange EE. Assessing the subtalar joint: the Broden view revisited. Foot Ankle Int. 2001;22(4):329–34.
14. Pisani G. Chronic laxity of the subtalar joint. Orthopedics. 1996;19(5):431–7.
15. Martin LP, Wayne JS, Monahan TJ, Adelaar RS. Elongation behavior of calcaneofibular and cervical ligaments during inversion loads applied in an open kinetic chain. Foot Ankle Int. 1998;19(4):232–9.
16. Kjaersgaard-Andersen P, Wethelund JO, Nielsen S. Lateral talocalcaneal instability following section of the calcaneofibular ligament: a kinesiologic study. Foot Ankle. 1987;7(6):355–61.
17. Lee BH, Choi KH, Seo DY, Choi SM, Kim GL. Diagnostic validity of alternative manual stress radiographic technique detecting subtalar instability with concomitant ankle instability. Knee Surg Sports Traumatol Arthrosc. 2016;24(4):1029–39.
18. Frey C, Feder KS, DiGiovanni C. Arthroscopic evaluation of the subtalar joint: does sinus tarsi syndrome exist? Foot Ankle Int. 1999;20(3):185–91.
19. Sarrafian SK. Biomechanics of the subtalar joint complex. Clin Orthop Relat Res. 1993;290:17–26.
20. Cahill DR. The anatomy and function of the contents of the human tarsal sinus and canal. Anat Rec. 1965;153(1):1–17.
21. Thacker P, Mardis N. Ligaments of the tarsal sinus: improved detection, characterisation and significance in the paediatric ankle with 3-D proton density MR imaging. Pediatr Radiol. 2013;43(2):196–201.
22. Beltran J, Munchow AM, Khabiri H, Magee DG, McGhee RB, Grossman SB. Ligaments of the lateral aspect of the ankle and sinus tarsi: an MR imaging study. Radiology. 1990;177(2):455–8.
23. Kier R, Dietz MJ, McCarthy SM, Rudicel SA. MR imaging of the normal ligaments and tendons of the ankle. J Comput Assist Tomogr. 1991;15(3):477–82.
24. Klein MA, Spreitzer AM. MR imaging of the tarsal sinus and canal: normal anatomy, pathologic findings, and features of the sinus tarsi syndrome. Radiology. 1993;186(1):233–40.
25. Rosenberg ZS, Beltran J, Bencardino JT: From the RSNA Refresher Courses. Radiological Society of North America. MR imaging of the ankle and foot. *Radiographics* 2000, 20 Spec No:S153–S179.

5

With axial loading during MRI diurnal T2-value changes in lumbar discs are neglectable

L. Torén[1,4], H. Hebelka[1,4*], I. Kasperska[1], H. Brisby[2,4] and K. Lagerstrand[3,4]

Abstract

Background: Axial loading during MRI (alMRI) combined with T2 mapping recently was shown as a promising method to reveal biomechanical intervertebral disc (IVD) characteristics. This feasibility study aims to investigate whether there is a diurnal variation in the IVD T2-value when using alMRI. This is of importance for the planning of when to perform alMRI investigations and for interpretations of alMRI findings in relation to clinical symptoms.

Methods: Six healthy volunteers (30 lumbar discs), were examined with alMRI at three different sessions during 1 day. To be representative for a low back pain cohort in terms of age and IVD degeneration the included participants had a wide age range (27-63y) and all Pfirrmann grades represented. The T2-values were measured in five IVD regions of interest (ROI). The ROIs were equally large in sagittal plane with ROI1 representing anterior parts of the IVD, ROI5 posterior IVD parts and ROI2–4 the parts in between.

Results: T2-values of the entire IVD varied between 38 and 138 ms at 7 am, 33-143 ms at 11.30 am, and 31-147 ms at 4 pm with large regional IVD variations at all time points. No significant alterations of the T2-values over the day were found, neither for the entire IVD ($p = 0.4$) nor for the various ROIs ($p = 0.2–1.0$). Neither when correlated to Pfirrmann grade, any significant diurnal T2-value changes were found.

Conclusions: With alMRI, only minor diurnal T2-value changes were found in the lumbar discs. Nonsignificant and neglectable diurnal changes are advantageous both for research purposes, as well as in the clinical setting, giving comparable and robust data regardless of at what time-point the alMRI is performed.

Keywords: IVD, Axial loading during MRI (alMRI), T2-value, Diurnal variation, T2 mapping

Background

In spite of extensive research, trying to establish diagnostic methods for detailed assessment of intervertebral disc (IVD) degeneration and spinal pain predictors, current imaging methods are insufficient. Today, the imaging methods used for low back pain (LBP) have low specificity and lack the capacity to identify which anatomical structures are causing the patients pain [1–3]. Furthermore, conventional clinical imaging do not enable objective IVD degeneration classification neither assess detailed information regarding IVD architecture. Chronic LBP, often associated with IVD degeneration [4–6], is a worldwide main health issue causing large suffering on an individual level and high economic cost for the society [7]. Clinical care would therefore benefit from improved imaging diagnostics regarding degenerative disc disease [2].

Combining quantitative magnetic resonance imaging (MRI) of the lumbar back with axial loading during MRI (alMRI), has been shown to be a promising way to improve the imaging diagnostics of degenerative disc disease, and reveal functional IVD characteristics [8]. The alMRI already play an important role in clinical management, such as within spinal stenosis [9–11] where alMRI can reveal occult nerve root compressions not seen with conventional MRI in the supine position [12]. Furthermore, alMRI has been shown to aggravate pain and to instantaneously induce regional IVD changes in LBP

* Correspondence: hanna.hebelka@vgregion.se
[1]Department of Radiology, Sahlgrenska University Hospital, Gothenburg, Sweden
[4]Institute of Clinical Sciences, Sahlgrenska Academy, University of Gothenburg, Gothenburg, Sweden
Full list of author information is available at the end of the article

patients [8, 13], with increased T2-values of the anterior annulus fibrosus (AF) and nucleus pulposus (NP) respectively with decreased T2-values of the posterior AF [8]. Quantitative T2-values are known to correlate to hydration grade with an inverse correlation to degeneration grade of the IVD [8, 14]. Quantitative MRI may, thus, enable early detection of global and regional biochemical changes in the IVD that cannot be seen morphologically with qualitative MRI [15].

The IVDs have been demonstrated to have a dynamic behavior over the day. De Puky et al. showed that on a macroscopic level the diurnal load diminished the height of the IVDs with about 1%, which was then restored during rest [16]. They also found that degenerated IVDs did not alter as much in height as non-degenerated IVDs. Qualitative MRI studies of the IVD have proposed that diurnal load alters the hydration grade of various sub-regions of the IVDs [17]. Quantitative MRI of young volunteers has revealed diurnal changes of T2-values in entire IVDs and in different sub-regions of the IVDs [18–21], indicating a dynamic displacement of water between the sub-regions [18, 19]. To our knowledge, it has not yet been investigated if and how the T2-values vary over the day with alMRI.

Since previous studies indicate that the molecular equilibrium in the IVDs might be different in the compressive state and that the compressive force generated by axial load instantly alters the global biochemical IVD composition [8, 22], one may assume that the diurnal behavior of the alMRI T2-values would be different for the compressive state.

This feasibility study aims to investigate whether there is a diurnal variation in the IVD T2-value when using alMRI.

This is of importance for the planning of when to perform alMRI investigations and for interpretations of alMRI findings in relation to clinical symptoms.

Methods

Participants

In this cross sectional study six healthy volunteers were examined with alMRI, at three time points during 1 day, with 30 lumbar IVDs analyzed. None of the volunteers suffered from any known medical history of back pain or spine related disease. The inclusion of the volunteers aimed to largely reflect a LBP cohort in terms of age and IVD degeneration (four men, mean age: 38y, age range 27-63y and two women, mean age: 37y, age 28–46y), with all Pfirrmann grades represented.

Image acquisition

Each volunteer was investigated at three different sessions during the same day. Every session consisted of one MRI scan with the spine in an unloaded position (referred to as uMRI) instantly followed by one scan with alMRI. The first session was at 07 am, the second at 11.30 am and the last at 04 pm. No restrictions regarding activity were imposed before or between sessions. The alMRI was carried out in supine position with a loading device (DynaWell compression device, Dynawell diagnostics AB, Las Vegas, NV, USA), set at half the body weight of the actual volunteer. During uMRI, the lower leg of the volunteer rested on a foam support of 10 cm height, resulting in slight bending of the hip and knee joints. During alMRI, a cushion of approximately 8 cm height was used between the bed and the lumbar back, creating a lumbar lordosis in order to simulate normal upright position [23].

The MR-images were acquired with a Siemens Magnetom Aera 1,5 T scanner (Erlangen, Germany). The scan protocol consisted of a sagittal turbo spin echo (TSE) T1 weighted (w) sequence, a sagittal TSE T2w sequence and an axial TSE T2w sequence. A sagittal multi echo spin echo (SE) T2-sequence was incorporated at the end of the protocol enabling sagittal T2-maps to be calculated. High quality standardized T2-maps (256×256 matrix, slice thickness 3.5 mm, FOV 220×220 mm^2, NEX: 1) were finally reconstructed.

Image analysis

All image analysis were made by a radiology resident, supervised by an experienced radiologist. Degeneration of the IVDs were graded according to the Pfirrmann classification [24]. To enable further image analysis, multiplanar reconstructions were made from the T1w-sequences. 10 mm thick (in order to enable volumetric IVD analysis) midsagittal slices of sagittal TSE T1w-sequences were fused with sagittal SE T2-mapping sequences using software from syngovia (Siemens, Erlangen Germany).

The entire IVD was delineated in the sagittal plane using the polygonal region of interest (ROI) tool. Craniocaudally, the IVD was delineated by the endplates and anterioposteriorly by the anterior longitudinal ligament and the posterior longitudinal ligament. The entire IVD was further divided into five volumetric sub-regions with equal length in the sagittal plane, referred to as ROI1 to ROI5. Thus, ROI1 corresponded to the anterior parts of the IVD, ROI5 the posterior IVD parts and ROI2–4 the regions in between (Fig. 1).

The mean T2-time and standard deviation of the mean T2-time were assessed for the entire IVDs and for each sub-region, on both alMRI and uMRI. To ensure reliable measurements, blinded inter-rater agreement was performed before initiating the study. This was done on 5 clinical LBP patients, in which both uMRI and alMRI had been performed. 36 IVDs were measured with approximately half evaluated at alMRI. Inter-rater agreement was substantial for ROI1 and almost perfect regarding ROI2–5 (Table 1) [25, 26]. To test the robustness of the scanning, three repeated scans with alMRI and three repeated scans with uMRI were made on one volunteer at the same session.

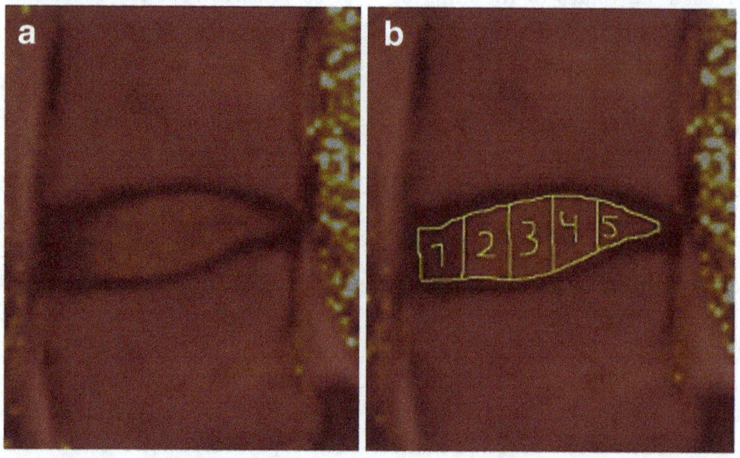

Fig. 1 Typical color setting of the images used for the IVD segmentation (**a**). The images, used for IVD segmentation, were derived by fusing T1-weighted images with T2-map images to enhance the borders of the IVDs. The IVDs were divided in to five subregions (ROI1–5), each with different volume but the same sagittal measure (**b**)

Statistics

If not otherwise stated, all T2-values are expressed as mean. The variation was defined as the standard deviation (SD) of the mean. For comparison between differences in T2-values over day, a parametric paired t test was applied. Non-parametric Spearman rank correlation were used for analyzing T2-values in groups with different Pfirrmann grades. All tests were two-sided, statistical significance was defined as $p < 0.05$. The software used for analyzing data was IBM SPSS Statistics for Windows, Version 22.0 (Armonk, NY: IBM Corp, USA). Reliability of ROI measurements for inter-rater agreement was performed using Intra-class correlation coefficients (ICC), model 2, with 95% confidence intervals (CI). The coefficients were interpreted using Cronbach's alpha. Intra-rater agreement has previously been reported [8].

Results

alMRI T2-values over the day for the entire IVDs and sub-regions

The alMRI T2-value slightly decreased over the day in ROI2 to ROI4, from 102 ms (ROI2), 128 ms (ROI3) and 118 ms (ROI4) in the morning to 94 ms, 121 ms and 111 ms, respectively in the afternoon (Fig. 2/Table 2).

Table 1 ICC measurements for each ROI

ROI ($n = 36$)	ICC	95% CI
1	0.79	0.62–0.89
2	0.95	0.90–0.97
3	0.99	0.97–0.99
4	0.98	0.96–0.99
5	0.86	0.74–0.99

ICC for inter-rater measurements for each ROI with corresponding 95% CI (confidence interval)

Thus, small alterations in absolute numbers of alMRI T2-values over the day were discerned. However, no significant changes were found (Table 2), neither for the entire IVDs nor for the separate sub-regions. For all comparative analyzes, the p-values were larger than 0.2.

uMRI T2-values over the day for the entire IVDs and sub-regions

Neither for the entire IVDs nor for the separate sub-regions were any significant diurnal alterations found with uMRI. P-values larger than 0.2 were found for all comparative analyzes (Fig. 3).

Comparison of T2-values between alMRI and uMRI

When IVDs were compared between alMRI and uMRI, alterations in T2-values were seen for every sub-region both in the morning, at lunchtime and in the afternoon session. For example, mean T2-value for uMRI in ROI1 was 30 ms (SD 11 ms) compared to 35 ms (SD 12 ms) with alMRI, corresponding to an increase of 17%. Likewise, a decrease of 20% in the mean T2-value was seen in ROI5, where the mean T2-value was 59 ms (SD 19 ms) for uMRI and 47 ms (SD 14 ms) for alMRI.

alMRI T2-values over the day in relation to Pfirrmann grading

Among the volunteers investigated IVDs with all Pfirrmann grades were represented (Fig. 4), including one IVD with Pfirrmann grade 5. This IVD, localized at L5-S1, was so severely degenerated that only the most 3 ventral ROIs were enabled to be outlined. Most of the IVDs were Pfirrmann grade 2 (Fig. 4). Large diversity of T2-values were detected between all the investigated IVDs. At the morning session, the alMRI T2-values of the entire IVD varied between 38 and 138 ms, at lunch between 33 and 143 ms, whereas the

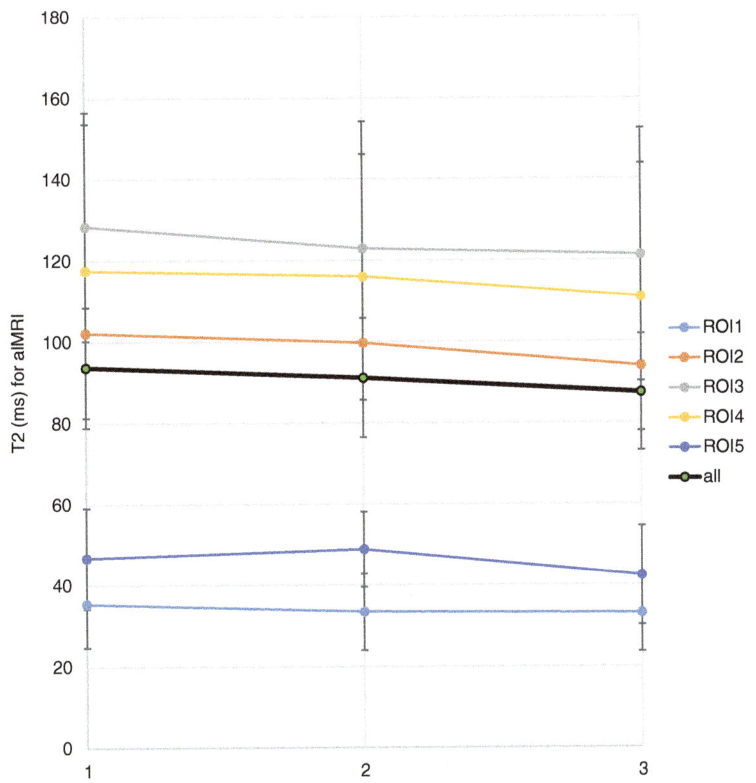

Fig. 2 Mean T2-values for the various subregions of the IVD (ROI1–5) with axial loading during MRI (aIMRI) at the three separate scanning sessions

Table 2 Mean T2-value at all time instances for all sub-regions

	all		ROI1		ROI2		ROI3		ROI4		ROI5	
	mean	SD	mean	SD	mean	SD	mean	SD	mean	SD	mean	SD
uMRI												
7am	92	15	30	8	88	23	124	28	123	35	59	17
11.30am	88	9	28	9	86	25	115	20	116	23	62	18
4pm	85	12	28	7	82	25	111	24	110	21	61	25
aIMRI												
7am	94	15	35	11	102	28	128	28	118	36	47	12
11.30am	91	15	33	9	100	24	123	31	116	30	49	9
4pm	87	14	33	9	94	28	121	31	111	33	42	12
uMRI												
7am vs. 11.30am	$p = 0.8$		$p = 0.4$		$p = 1.0$		$p = 0.7$		$p = 0.6$		$p = 0.8$	
7am vs. 4pm	$p = 0.5$		$p = 0.4$		$p = 0.7$		$p = 0.4$		$p = 0.2$		$p = 0.6$	
11.30am vs. 4pm	$p = 0.5$		$p = 0.8$		$p = 0.8$		$p = 0.6$		$p = 0.4$		$p = 0.6$	
aIMRI												
7am vs. 11.30am	$p = 0.5$		$p = 0.5$		$p = 0.9$		$p = 0.7$		$p = 0.8$		$p = 0.8$	
7am vs. 4pm	$p = 0.4$		$p = 0.9$		$p = 0.6$		$p = 0.5$		$p = 0.6$		$p = 0.2$	
11.30am vs. 4pm	$p = 0.7$		$p = 0.6$		$p = 0.6$		$p = 1$		$p = 0.7$		$p = 0.6$	
uMRI - aIMRI												
7am vs. 11.30am	$p = 0.3$		$p = 0.8$		$p = 0.8$		$p = 0.9$		$p = 0.9$		$p = 0.5$	
7am vs. 4pm	$p = 0.4$		$p = 0.8$		$p = 0.8$		$p = 0.5$		$p = 0.2$		$p = 0.5$	
11.30am vs. 4pm	$p = 0.5$		$p = 0.9$		$p = 0.9$		$p = 0.5$		$p = 0.3$		$p = 1$	

Mean T2-value (ms) at all time instances for all regions of interest (ROI), both with conventional supine MRI (uMRI) and with axial loading during MRI (aIMRI). *P*-value (p) for the T2-value change between all time instances are displayed both with uMRI, aIMRI as well as the change between (uMRI-aIMRI)

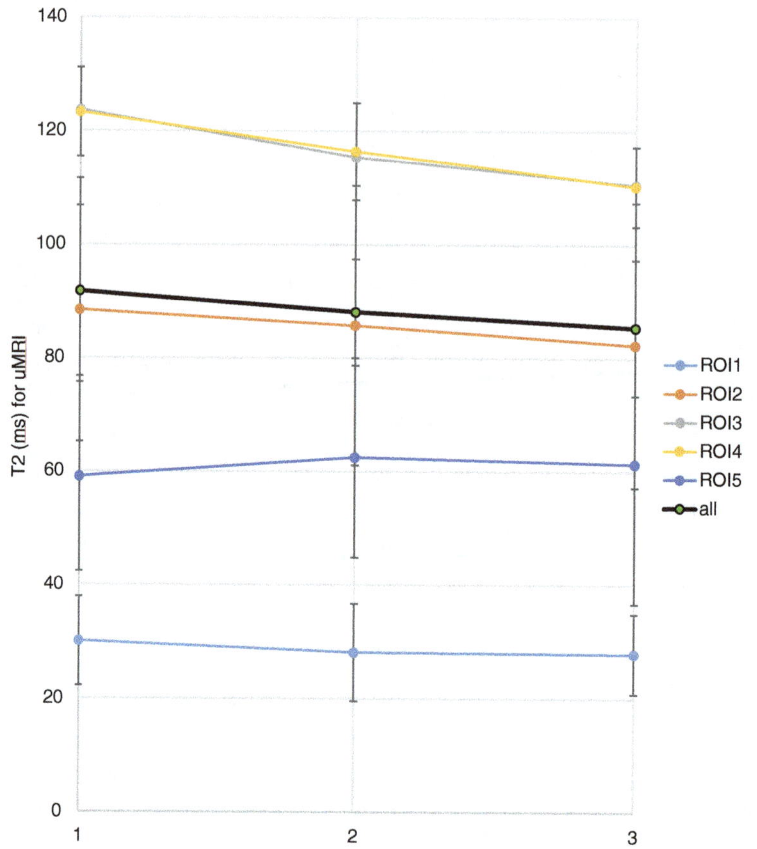

Fig. 3 Mean T2-values for the various subregions of the IVD (ROI1–5) sessions with conventional supine MRI (uMRI) at the three separate scanning sessions

afternoon T2-values varied between 31 to 147 ms. Thus, the difference between the highest and lowest T2-values of the various IVDs were over 300% (Fig. 4). Degenerated IVDs had, in general, lower T2-values. For example, the highest T2-value assessed in an IVD with Pfirrmann grade 5 was 39 ms while the highest value for the entire IVD with Pfirrmann grade 1 was 147 ms. Large regional variations were further seen in non-degenerated IVDs. In a Pfirrmann grade 1 disc for example, the mean alMRI T2-value in the morning was 35 ms in ROI1, 102 ms in ROI2, 128 ms in ROI3, 118 ms in ROI4 and 47 ms in ROI5. In degenerated IVDs, the regional variations were much smaller. In the IVD with Pfirrmann grade 5, the highest T2 value found was 52 ms (ROI3) while the lowest T2 value found was 32 ms (ROI2). When the alMRI T2-values were correlated to Pfirrmann grade, however, no significant changes over the day could be revealed neither on entire IVD level nor within the various sub-regions.

Reliability measurements

Repetitive scans of the same volunteer showed robustness of the scanning with only minor T2-value variations, however, a 10% alteration was seen at one occasion with alMRI at level L5-S1 between scan 1 (36 ms, SD 14 ms) and scan 2 (40 ms, SD 15 ms). Intra-rater measurements are displayed in Table 1.

Discussion

The key findings in this study, investigating the diurnal variations of alMRI T2-values, were the minor changes and lack of significant diurnal alterations in the IVDs, neither for the entire IVD nor in its various sub-regions. It was also found that the diurnal alterations in the examined sub-regions of the IVDs were negligible compared to the large differences in mean T2-values between the sub-regions. These findings are of importance both in the clinical setting and for research purposes since alMRI scans can, based on these findings, be performed at any time of the day.

In several studies, the loading of the spine has been shown to affect quantitative MRI parameters of the IVD [8, 22, 27–29]. For example, Nilsson et al. showed that when the IVDs were compressed the T2-values increased in the ventral parts of the IVDs respectively decreased in its posterior parts [8]. Analogously, Stelzender et al. displayed that when the IVDs were unloaded, the T2-values decreased in the ventral part of the IVD and increased in the posterior part of the IVDs

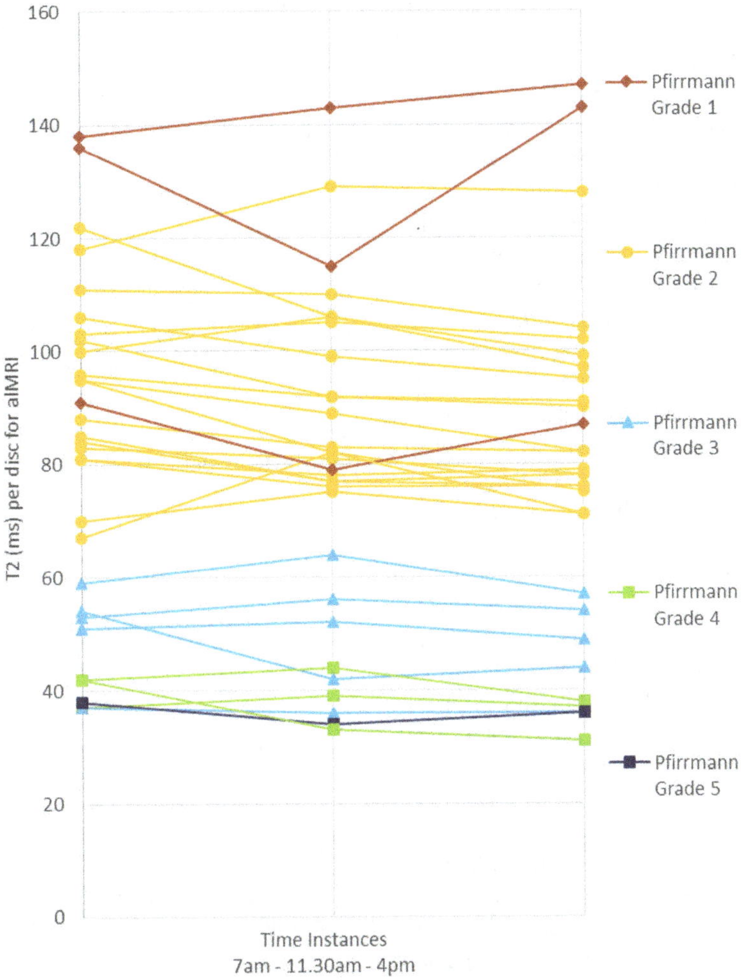

Fig. 4 Mean T2-values for the entire IVDs at the three separate scanning sessions

[30]. Axial loading compresses the IVDs and introduce another microscopic equilibrium within the IVD, i.e. structural alteration between water, collagen and proteoglycans, different from that of the non-compressed state. Furthermore, Mwale et al. displayed that compressive load of the IVD has a greater impact on quantitative MR parameters than matrix degradation (trypsin digestion) while mechanical IVD properties (compressive modulus, hydraulic permeability and swelling pressure), predominantly are affected by matrix degradation [22]. Thus, alMRI combined with quantitative MRI has the potential to reveal functional IVD characteristics and the current study importantly display that there is no need to standardize when to perform such scans.

Contrary to previous studies on young volunteers, in which diminishing T2-values of NP and increasing T2-values of AF have been displayed [18, 19], no significant diurnal alteration of uMRI T2-values were found. These divergent results could partly be caused by small sample size, but are most likely explained by a higher mean age (38 years) and increased degeneration grade in the current cohort, chosen to be representative for LBP patients. For example, Zhu et al. had a mean age of 25 years in their population (20 subjects) with no subject older than 31 years [18] and Ludescher et al. studied no subject older than 29 years (6 subjects) [19]. The lack of significant diurnal T2-value variations with uMRI found in the current study were expected as age and degeneration grade are established as factors diminishing diurnal variations of T2-values with uMRI [21].

In concordance with previous uMRI studies [18, 21], T2-values of entire IVDs were low in degenerated IVDs and displayed less variation between various sub-regions compared to IVDs without degeneration. These findings are anticipated. Macromolecules, as proteoglycans, are key factors for the water holding capacity of the IVDs. In degenerated IVDs, the amount of proteoglycans relative collagen is reduced in general and in the NP in particular. Hence the capacity of holding water is reduced and also, the water is distributed more equally in the degenerated IVDs which is reflected by lower and more uniform T2-values [18, 21, 31].

The current study delineated the entire IVD, also outermost parts near the endplates. In previous studies, various sub-regions have been delineated as preset rectangular or circular areas [18, 21, 31], not following the proper IVD shape. Furthermore 10 mm sagittal slices with mapped T2-values were analyzed compared to 3–5 mm sagittal slices in previous studies [19, 21, 30]. The increased slice thickness, combined with a delineation covering the entire IVD may reduce errors from local irregularities in the IVDs structure. For example, radial or circumferential fissures in the AF may be filled with gelatinous content from the NP pressed out in the periphery when applying axial load on the IVD, influencing the T2-values in an arbitrary way. The predominant theory is that water is pressed out from NP to the AF during diurnal IVD loading [21]. Theoretically, one could argue that a shift of water from the NP to the periphery may not be as obvious when the entire IVD is delineated, as when using smaller regions, since even the craniocaudal parts of the AF are covered. On the other hand, the delineation in the current study is a more fair way to assess the IVDs. Different ways of delineating the IVDs might however aggravate comparisons between various studies.

This study was designed to enable detection of altered alMRI T2-values during the day. To strengthen the study, three scanning sessions were performed over the day, instead of two scanning sessions per day which have previously been used [18, 19]. Another important strength of this study is that the investigated volunteers are representative of a LBP cohort, covering a large age range with a broad spread with respect to IVD degeneration. As such, the study design makes the results applicable in the clinical setting.

Limitations

Only a small number of volunteers were included in the present study. Since there is a lack of similar studies, in which quantitative T2-mapping measurements are performed with alMRI, estimation of the sample size was based on expected changes in regional IVD T2-values over the day for unloaded MRI [19, 25]. With a diurnal effect of 10%, a sample size of 5 individuals and 25 IVDs should be sufficient at 80% power with 95% significance and two sided test. One extra healthy volunteer was included in the study to ensure power. With alMRI, however, the effect size was found to be much smaller and, hence, no statistical significance could be verified. Significant or not, the diurnal changes during alMRI were small and thus likely not clinically relevant. Hence, the alMRI method can be considered as robust over the day. Moreover, the included volunteers were well representative for a LBP cohort, with all degenerations grades represented, and thus these data likely are more clinically relevant compared to results from study cohorts with younger mean age and less degenerated IVDs.

Conclusion

With alMRI, only minor diurnal T2-value changes were found in the lumbar discs. Nonsignificant and neglectable diurnal changes are advantageous both for research purposes, as well as in the clinical setting, giving comparable and robust data regardless of at what time-point the alMRI is performed.

Abbreviations

AF: Annulus fibrosus; alMRI: Axial loading during MRI; CI: Confidence interval; ICC: Intra-class correlation coefficients; IVD: Intervertebral disc; LBP: Low back pain; NP: Nucleus pulposus; ROI: Region of interest; SD: Standard deviation; SE: Spin echo; TSE: Turbo spin echo; uMRI: MRI with the spine in an unloaded position; w: Weighted

Acknowledgements

Not applicable

Funding

The authors acknowledge the financial support from C4I center, Sahlgrenska University Hospital and from Konrad and Helfrid Johanssons fundation. Financial support has been used to cover expenses for examinations and for manuscript writing.

Authors' contributions

KL and HH are responsible for the study design. LT and HH performed the measurement of T2 values. KL performed the statistical analysis. KL, HH, LT, IK and HB analyzed and interpreted the patient data. LT and HH were major contributors in writing the manuscript. IK performed the MRI examinations and was responsible for the administration regarding ethical considerations of the study. All authors read and approved the final manuscript.

Consent for publication

Not applicable

Competing interests

The authors declare that they have no competing interests.

Author details

[1]Department of Radiology, Sahlgrenska University Hospital, Gothenburg, Sweden. [2]Department of Orthopaedics, Sahlgrenska University Hospital, Gothenburg, Sweden. [3]Department of Medical Physics and Techniques, Sahlgrenska University Hospital, Gothenburg, Sweden. [4]Institute of Clinical Sciences, Sahlgrenska Academy, University of Gothenburg, Gothenburg, Sweden.

References

1. Chou R, et al. Imaging strategies for low-back pain: systematic review and meta-analysis. Lancet. 2009;373(9662):463–72.
2. Endean A, Palmer KT, Coggon D. Potential of magnetic resonance imaging findings to refine case definition for mechanical low back pain in epidemiological studies: a systematic review. Spine (Phila Pa 1976). 2011; 36(2):160–9.
3. Manchikanti L, et al. Systematic review of lumbar discography as a diagnostic test for chronic low back pain. Pain Physician. 2009;12(3):541–59.
4. Raj PP. Intervertebral disc: anatomy-physiology-pathophysiology-treatment. Pain Pract. 2008;8(1):18–44.
5. Samartzis D, et al. Novel diagnostic and prognostic methods for disc degeneration and low back pain. Spine J. 2015;15(9):1919–32.
6. Lotz JC, Fields AJ, Liebenberg EC. The role of the vertebral end plate in low back pain. Global Spine J. 2013;3(3):153–64.
7. Dagenais S, Caro J, Haldeman S. A systematic review of low back pain cost of illness studies in the United States and internationally. Spine J. 2008;8(1):8–20.
8 Nilsson M, et al. Axial loading during MRI influences T2-mapping values of lumbar discs: a feasibility study on patients with low back pain. Eur Spine J. 2016;25(9):2856–63.
9 Hiwatashi A, et al. Axial loading during MR imaging can influence treatment decision for symptomatic spinal stenosis. AJNR Am J Neuroradiol. 2004; 25(2):170–4.
10 Kanno H, et al. Changes in lumbar spondylolisthesis on axial-loaded MRI: do they reproduce the positional changes in the degree of olisthesis observed on X-ray images in the standing position? Spine J. 2015;15(6):1255–62.
11 Kim YK, et al. Diagnostic advancement of axial loaded lumbar spine MRI in patients with clinically suspected central spinal canal stenosis. Spine (Phila Pa 1976). 2013;38(21):E1342–7.
12 Saifuddin A, Blease S, MacSweeney E. Axial loaded MRI of the lumbar spine. Clin Radiol. 2003;58(9):661–71.
13 Hebelka H, Brisby H, Hansson T. Comparison between pain at discography and morphological disc changes at axial loaded MRI in patients with low back pain. Eur Spine J. 2014;23(10):2075–82.
14 Watanabe A, et al. Classification of intervertebral disk degeneration with axial T2 mapping. AJR Am J Roentgenol. 2007;189(4):936–42.
15 Perry J, et al. The value of T2 relaxation times to characterize lumbar intervertebral disks: preliminary results. AJNR Am J Neuroradiol. 2006;27(2):337–42.
16 De Puky P. The physiological oscillation of the lenght of the body. Acta Orthop Scand. 1935;1935(6):446–55.
17 Paajanen H, et al. Diurnal fluid changes of lumbar discs measured indirectly by magnetic resonance imaging. J Orthop Res. 1994;12(4):509–14.
18 Zhu T, et al. Segmental quantitative MR imaging analysis of diurnal variation of water content in the lumbar intervertebral discs. Korean J Radiol. 2015; 16(1):139–45.
19 Ludescher B, et al. T2- and diffusion-maps reveal diurnal changes of intervertebral disc composition: an in vivo MRI study at 1.5 Tesla. J Magn Reson Imaging. 2008;28(1):252–7.
20 Roberts N, et al. Quantitative analysis of diurnal variation in volume and water content of lumbar intervertebral discs. Clin Anat. 1998;11(1):1–8.
21 Karakida O, et al. Diurnal T2 value changes in the lumbar intervertebral discs. Clin Radiol. 2003;58(5):389–92.
22 Mwale F, et al. Evaluation of quantitative magnetic resonance imaging, biochemical and mechanical properties of trypsin-treated intervertebral discs under physiological compression loading. J Magn Reson Imaging. 2008;27(3):563–73.
23 Danielson B, Willen J. Axially loaded magnetic resonance image of the lumbar spine in asymptomatic individuals. Spine (Phila Pa 1976). 2001; 26(23):2601–6.
24 Pfirrmann CW, et al. Magnetic resonance classification of lumbar intervertebral disc degeneration. Spine (Phila Pa 1976). 2001;26(17):1873–8.
25 Watson P, Petrie A. Method agreement analysis: a review of correct methodology. Theriogenology. 2010;73(9):1167–79.
26 Landis JR, Koch GG. The measurement of observer agreement for categorical data. Biometrics. 1977;33(1):159–74.
27 Mwale F, Iatridis JC, Antoniou J. Quantitative MRI as a diagnostic tool of intervertebral disc matrix composition and integrity. Eur Spine J. 2008; 17(Suppl 4):432–40.
28 Perie D, et al. Assessment of compressive modulus, hydraulic permeability and matrix content of trypsin-treated nucleus pulposus using quantitative MRI. J Biomech. 2006;39(8):1392–400.
29 Chiu EJ, et al. Magnetic resonance imaging measurement of relaxation and water diffusion in the human lumbar intervertebral disc under compression in vitro. Spine (Phila Pa 1976). 2001;26(19):E437–44.
30 Stelzeneder D, et al. Effect of short-term unloading on T2 relaxation time in the lumbar intervertebral disc–in vivo magnetic resonance imaging study at 3.0 tesla. Spine J. 2012;12(3):257–64.
31 Marinelli NL, Haughton VM, Anderson PA. T2 relaxation times correlated with stage of lumbar intervertebral disk degeneration and patient age. AJNR Am J Neuroradiol. 2010;31(7):1278–82.

6

Utilization of CT scanning associated with complex spine surgery

Vikas V. Patel[1], Gunnar B. J. Andersson[2], Steven R. Garfin[3], Donald L. Resnick[4] and Jon E. Block[5*]

Abstract

Background: Due to the risk associated with exposure to ionizing radiation, there is an urgent need to identify areas of CT scanning overutilization. While increased use of diagnostic spinal imaging has been documented, no previous research has estimated the magnitude of follow-up imaging used to evaluate the postoperative spine.

Methods: This retrospective cohort study quantifies the association between spinal surgery and CT utilization. An insurance database (Humana, Inc.) with ≈ 19 million enrollees was employed, representing 8 consecutive years (2007–2014). Surgical and imaging procedures were captured by anatomic-specific CPT codes. Complex surgeries included all cervical, thoracic and lumbar instrumented spine fusions. Simple surgeries included discectomy and laminectomy. Imaging was restricted to CT and MRI. Postoperative imaging frequency extended to 5-years post-surgery.

Results: There were 140,660 complex spinal procedures and 39,943 discectomies and 49,889 laminectomies. MRI was the predominate preoperative imaging modality for all surgical procedures (median: 80%; range: 73–82%). Postoperatively, CT prevalence following complex procedures increased more than two-fold from 6 months (18%) to 5 years (≥40%), and patients having a postoperative CT averaged two scans. For simple procedures, the prevalence of postoperative CT scanning never exceeded 30%.

Conclusions: CT scanning is used frequently for follow-up imaging evaluation following complex spine surgery. There is emerging evidence of an increased cancer risk due to ionizing radiation exposure with CT. In the setting of complex spine surgery, actions to mitigate this risk should be considered and include reducing nonessential scans, using the lowest possible radiation dose protocols, exerting greater selectivity in monitoring the developing fusion construct, and adopting non-ferromagnetic implant biomaterials that facilitate MRI postoperatively.

Keywords: CT scanning, Spine surgery, Fusion, Instrumentation, Discectomy, Laminectomy, Cancer

Background

The advent and continuous refinement of advanced imaging techniques, specifically computed tomography (CT) and magnetic resonance imaging (MRI), have revolutionized the diagnosis and surgical management of spinal disorders. These imaging techniques provide exquisite detail and characterization of anatomical structures and degenerative changes as well as postoperative evaluation of surgical interventions previously unachievable with standard radiography. Due, in part, to these technical advancements, the rates of advanced spinal imaging have increased markedly over the past several decades [1, 2]. However, it has been estimated that one-third of advanced spinal imaging may be inappropriate or unnecessary, and physician panels convened by the American Board of Internal Medicine Foundation have identified spinal imaging among the top 5 commonly overused procedures [1, 3]. In fact, adults with no back or radicular pain often show spinal abnormalities on advanced imaging and, indeed, the use of these imaging modalities to improve diagnosis has been implicated as a primary factor in the equally dramatic increase in complex spinal surgeries [3–7].

Recognizing the sizable increases in advanced imaging across all areas of medicine [8, 9], the American College of Radiology launched the Image Wisely campaign to curb unnecessary imaging and encourage the use of the

* Correspondence: jb@drjonblock.com
[5]2210 Jackson Street, Ste. 401, San Francisco, CA 94115, USA
Full list of author information is available at the end of the article

minimum amount of radiation needed to perform the indicated test [10]. Unfortunately, the society's appropriateness criteria have had limited impact on reducing the frequency of nonessential imaging due, in part, to the lack of specificity in identifying which imaging studies are appropriate based on the preponderance of clinical data [11].

Reducing the frequency of unnecessary spinal imaging, particularly techniques that expose patients to high levels of ionizing radiation such as CT, hinges on our ability to pinpoint areas of previously unidentified and/or unquantifiable imaging utilization. While much has been published about the rise in preoperative diagnostic spinal imaging, there has been scant mention of the magnitude of spinal imaging that is undertaken postoperatively. The current study was conducted to estimate how often and at what juncture advanced imaging, particularly CT scanning, is utilized to evaluate the postoperative spine.

Methods

The objective of this retrospective cohort study was to examine and quantify the association between spinal surgery and the utilization of advanced imaging, particularly CT and MRI. In addition to determining the prevalence of preoperative diagnostic imaging, we specifically investigated the frequency and timing of postoperative follow-up imaging.

This study utilized an insurance-based administrative database of adjudicated patient claims records (PearlDiver Technologies, West Conshohocken, PA, USA). This electronic database contains procedural volumes and demographics for patients based on specific Current Procedural Terminology (CPT) codes. All data were de-identified and anonymous, and were thus exempt from ethics committee approval [12]. The longitudinal data presented within this report were drawn from actual rates evident within a single managed healthcare system (Humana, Inc., Louisville, KY) representing 8 consecutive years from 2007 through the fourth quarter of 2014. Enrollees within this healthcare system resided mostly in the South (60%) and Midwest (25%) portions of the US. Imaging results are based upon incidence rates for those patients with a full follow-up period available. These files contain patient information identified by CPT coding related to spinal procedures and imaging procedures. All data are Health Insurance Portability and Accountability Act (HIPAA) compliant to protect patient privacy.

Two groups of spine surgery patients were identified by specific CPT codes and segmented based on the complexity of the procedure. "Complex" surgical procedures included cervical fusion, lumbar fusion and other long-segment fusion procedures. The latter group consisted of fusion procedures spanning multiple segments indicated mostly for spinal deformities (e.g., scoliosis, Scheuermann's disease, etc.). All complex procedures involved the concomitant implantation of metallic instrumentation including plates, rods, screws, and interbody devices, often in combination. No distinctions were made regarding surgical approach/technique, i.e., anterior, posterior, interbody, circumferential. "Simple" surgical procedures included discectomy and laminectomy decompression procedures at all levels without instrumentation. Disc arthroplasty procedures were not included as annual procedural counts were less than 200 patients. Specific CPT search codes for each surgical procedure are provided in Additional file 1.

Corresponding imaging events were restricted solely to CT and MRI, and captured using anatomic-specific CPT codes. Advanced imaging CPT search codes are also provided in Additional file 1. To determine preoperative imaging prevalence, an interval of 6 months prior to the index surgical procedure was chosen as this duration corresponds with the period routinely mandated by US federal regulators and medical societies as sufficient to exhaust conservative medical management. Postoperative imaging frequency extended to a period of 5 years after the index surgical procedure.

To adjust for the wide geographic variability in surgical practice patterns [13], estimates of US patient volumes for each surgical or imaging procedure were extrapolated using an algorithm based upon the prevalence of each procedure evident within the Humana patient record set and the Medicare Standard Analytical file for populations under sixty-five and sixty-five plus, respectively. Changes in procedural frequency between 2007 and 2014 were estimated using standard compound annual growth rate (CAGR) computations.

Results

The Humana healthcare database comprised adjudicated claims for 18,620,198 unique patients for the study period of 2007–2014 with an annual median number of enrollees of 6,779,769 (range: 5,412,897–9,434,477). The number of patients (procedures) identified by specific CPT codes for the overall study duration was as follows: cervical fusion, 29,888 (31,121); lumbar fusion, 37,579 (40,199); other long-segment fusion procedures, 63,967 (69,340); discectomy, 38,887 (39,943); and, laminectomy, 49,022 (49,899). Patient demographics are provided in Table 1 for each surgical procedure separately. The largest percentage of surgical interventions occurred in patients > 65 years of age irrespective of operative procedure, with 70% of laminectomy patients included in this age group.

From 2007–2014, the CAGR within the Humana data set for complex surgical procedures was 9.72%, 12.28% and 10.84% for cervical fusion, lumbar fusion and other long-segment fusion procedures, respectively. In comparison, the corresponding CAGR for simple surgical procedures was -1.35% for discectomy and 11.30% for laminectomy.

Table 1 Background Characteristics by Procedure

Variable	Cervical Fusion (N = 31,121)	Lumbar Fusion (N = 40,199)	Other (N = 69,340)	Discectomy (N = 39,943)	Laminectomy (N = 49,889)
Demographics					
Female Sex, n (%)	15,843 (51)	23,524 (59)	38,402 (55)	19,396 (49)	25,101 (50)
Age, n (%), yr					
< 20	0 (0)	125 (0)	595 (1)	109 (0)	181 (0)
20–34	0 (0)	616 (2)	1,166 (2)	2,069 (5)	680 (1)
35–49	5,550 (18)	3,569 (9)	8,671 (13)	7,372 (18)	3,076 (6)
50–64	11,333 (36)	10,996 (27)	21,312 (31)	11,340 (28)	11,145 (22)
65+	13,494 (43)	24,558 (61)	37,094 (53)	19,044 (48)	34,808 (70)

Previous imaging prevalence within 6 months of the index surgical procedure is illustrated in Figure 1. MRI predominated as the primary preoperative advanced diagnostic imaging modality for all surgical procedures (median: 79%; range: 73–82%). Preoperative CT scanning prevalence was notably lower than MRI but, in general, utilization of diagnostic CT was qualitatively higher among patients undergoing complex surgical procedures (median: 30%; range: 28–32%) compared to simple surgical procedures (median: 20%; range: 17–22%).

Postoperative imaging prevalence through 5 years of follow-up for all surgical procedures is illustrated in Figures 2 and 3. For complex surgical procedures, CT scanning prevalence increased more than two-fold from 6 months to 5 years postoperatively, with approximately 30% of patients having at least one follow-up CT scan by 2 years and ≥ 40% of patients having a follow-up CT scan by 5 years (Figure 2). For simple surgical procedures, the prevalence of postoperative CT scanning was lower at all postoperative intervals compared to the prevalence associated with complex procedures (Figure 3). While there was an approximate three-fold increase in CT scanning prevalence over the 5-year follow-up period for simple surgical procedures, the frequency never exceeded 30% at any postoperative interval. For patients having postoperative CT scanning after a complex surgical procedure, the average number of CT imaging events after 5 years of follow-up was 1.97, 2.03 and 2.00 for cervical fusion, lumbar fusion and other long-segment fusion procedures, respectively. The corresponding average number of CT events was 1.68 for both discectomy and laminectomy over the same 5-year follow-up period.

For patients having a postoperative CT scan, Table 2 shows the distribution of CT scan frequency at 6 months postoperatively for each surgical procedure for each study year separately. There is a uniformly steady rise in the number of CT scans over the study observation period (2007 through 2014) with most patients receiving

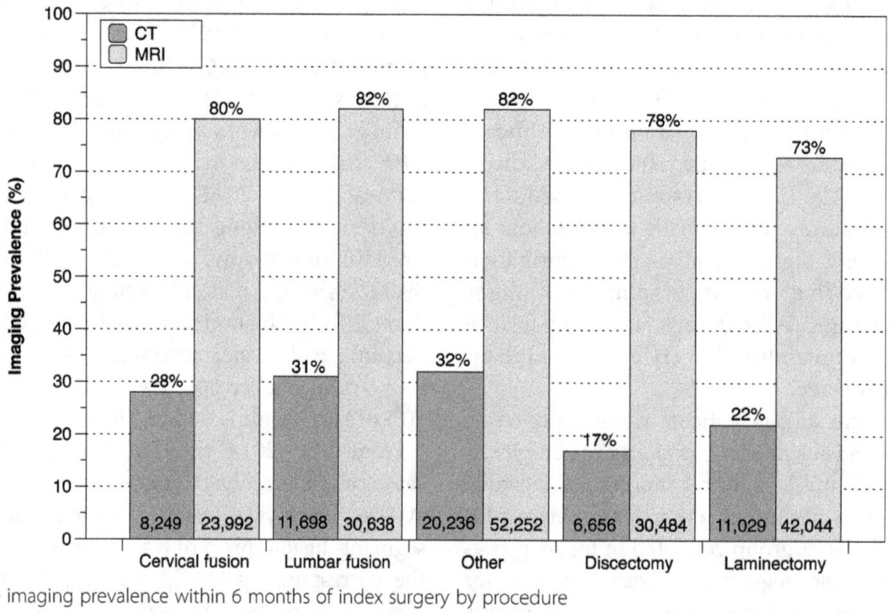

Fig. 1 Preoperative imaging prevalence within 6 months of index surgery by procedure

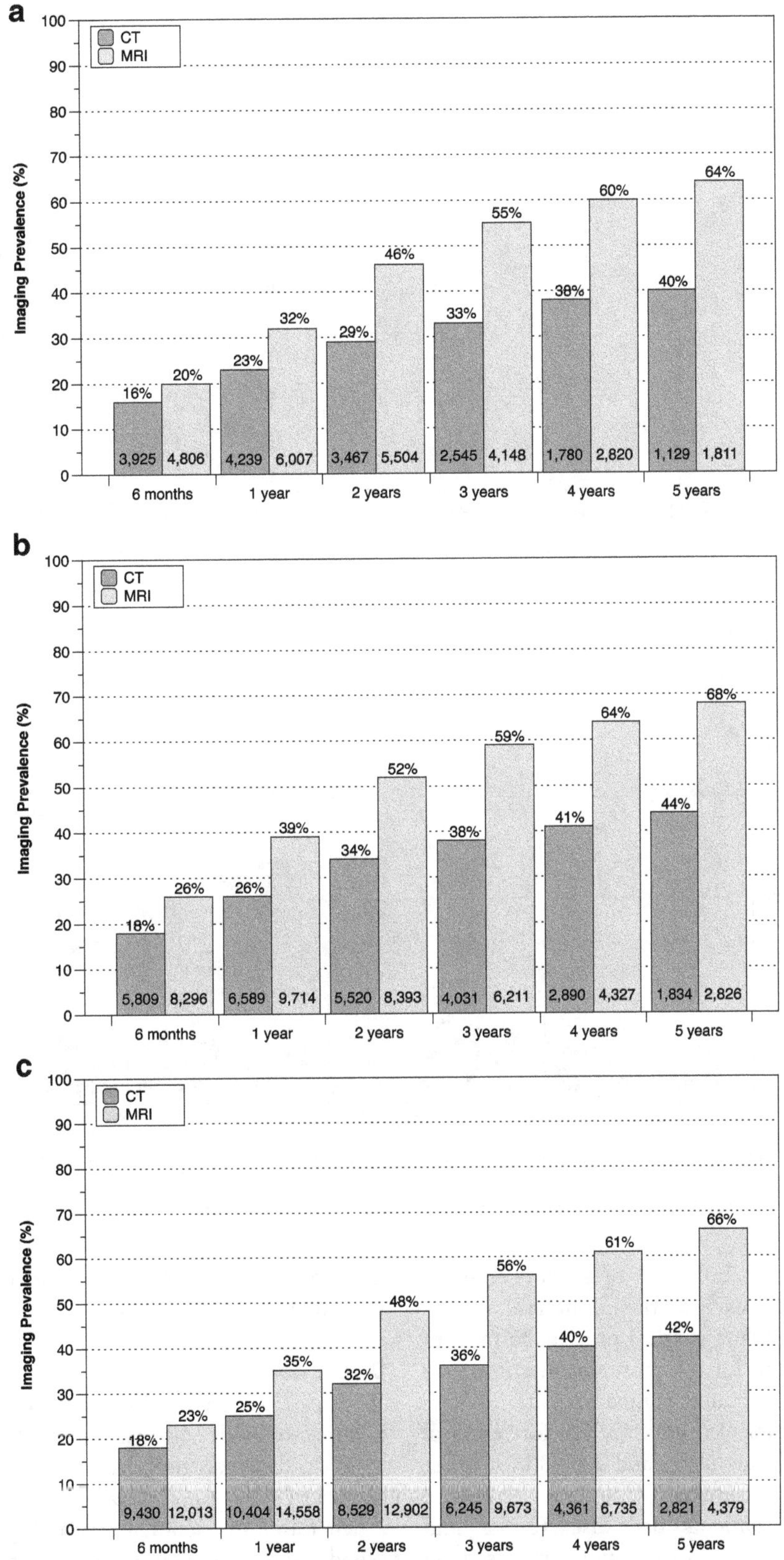

Fig. 2 Postoperative imaging prevalence for complex surgical procedures by follow-up interval for cervical fusion (**a**), lumbar fusion (**b**) and other long-segment fusion procedures (**c**). The corresponding number of imaging events is provided at the bottom of each bar

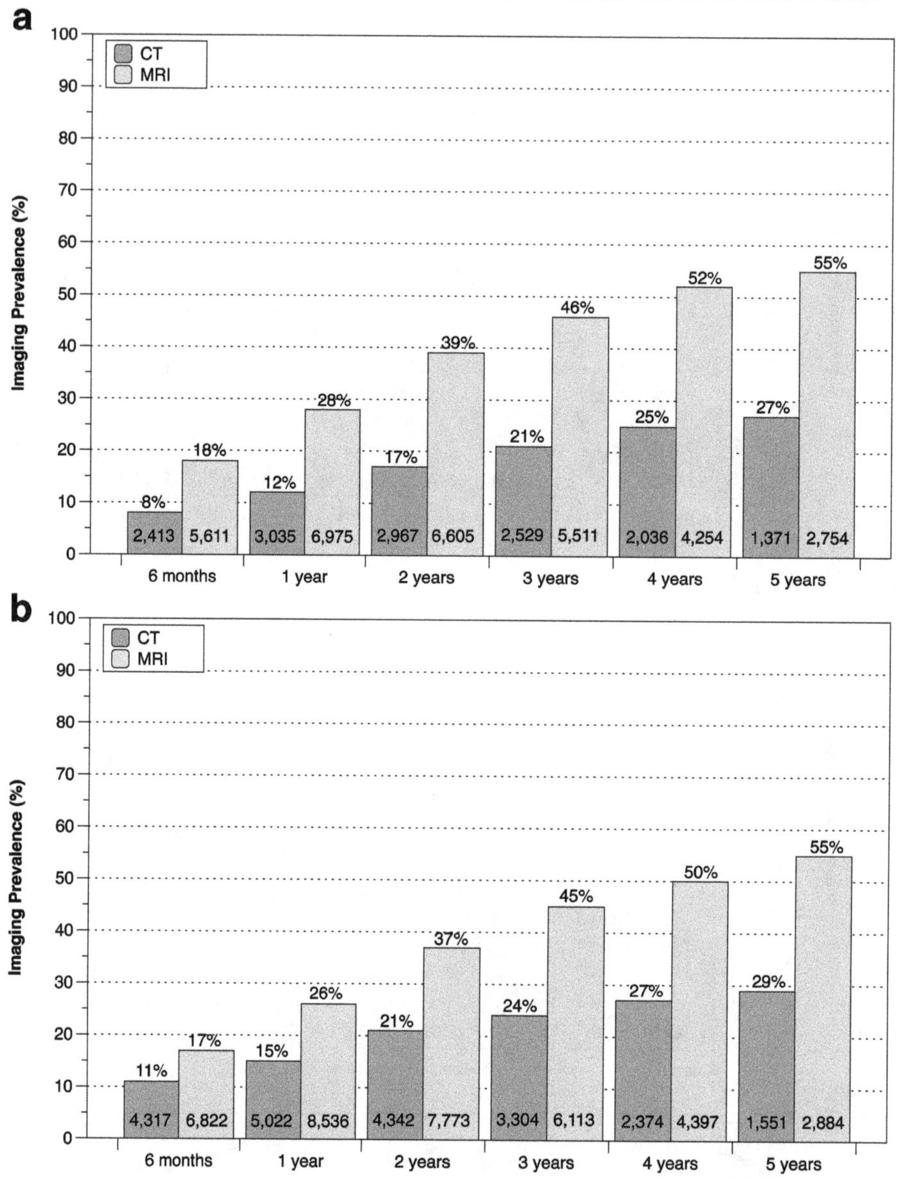

Fig. 3 Postoperative imaging prevalence for simple surgical procedures by follow-up interval for discectomy (**a**) and laminectomy (**b**). The corresponding number of imaging events is provided at the bottom of each bar

one CT scan by 6 months, but > 20% of patients received multiple CT scans at this early follow-up interval.

Extrapolating the Humana surgical prevalence rates to the entire US population for the most recent study year (2014) resulted in an estimated number of patients having complex procedures to be 292,950 for cervical fusion, 298,721 for lumbar fusion and 436,586 for other long-segment fusion procedures. In 2014, an estimated 211,529 and 267,513 patients had discectomies and laminectomies, respectively. Correspondingly, based on the advanced imaging CPT codes used in the current study, the estimated number of all spine-specific preoperative and postoperative CT scans and MRI studies in 2014 in the US for patients undergoing complex spine procedures was 9,180,589 and 8,880,972, respectively.

Discussion

With approximately 80% prevalence, the current study documented that MRI was the predominant imaging modality to diagnose and characterize spinal disorders prior to surgery. Use of preoperative CT scanning occurred with much lower frequency, but was highest among patients scheduled for complex surgical procedures.

While there have been previous reports discussing the unique imaging requirements necessary to evaluate radiographically the postoperative spine [14, 15], this is

Table 2 CT Scan Frequency for each Procedure by Year: All Patients at 6 months Follow-up

Procedure	2007	2008	2009	2010	2011	2012	2013	2014
Cervical Fusion, n (%)	(N = 105)	(N = 135)	(N = 201)	(N = 209)	(N = 249)	(N = 291)	(N = 382)	(N = 339)
No. of Scans 1	81 (77)	107 (79)	142 (71)	156 (75)	174 (70)	214 (74)	297 (78)	274 (81)
2	17 (16)	18 (13)	40 (20)	39 (19)	47 (19)	53 (18)	64 (17)	48 (14)
3	* (*)	* (*)	11 (5)	* (*)	17 (7)	19 (7)	15 (4)	11 (3)
4+	* (*)	* (*)	* (*)	* (*)	11 (4)	* (*)	* (*)	* (*)
Lumbar Fusion, n (%)	(N = 119)	(N = 165)	(N = 220)	(N = 253)	(N = 335)	(N = 413)	(N = 521)	(N = 474)
No. of Scans 1	88 (74)	137 (83)	167 (76)	207 (82)	264 (79)	332 (80)	430 (83)	391 (82)
2	24 (20)	17 (10)	41 (19)	31 (12)	54 (16)	63 (15)	65 (12)	52 (11)
3	* (*)	* (*)	* (*)	* (*)	* (*)	11 (3)	22 (4)	22 (5)
4+	* (*)	* (*)	* (*)	* (*)	* (*)	* (*)	* (*)	* (*)
Other, n (%)	(N = 223)	(N = 305)	(N = 430)	(N = 461)	(N = 563)	(N = 690)	(N = 909)	(N = 798)
No. of Scans 1	169 (76)	246 (81)	317 (74)	358 (78)	420 (75)	528 (77)	722 (79)	646 (81)
2	39 (17)	37 (12)	84 (20)	70 (15)	96 (17)	117 (17)	134 (15)	99 (12)
3	* (*)	15 (5)	14 (3)	20 (4)	24 (4)	31 (4)	41 (5)	37 (5)
4+	* (*)	* (*)	15 (3)	13 (3)	23 (4)	14 (2)	12 (1)	16 (2)
Discectomy, n (%)	(N = 228)	(N = 314)	(N = 313)	(N = 392)	(N = 300)	(N = 264)	(N = 309)	(N = 279)
No. of Scans 1	154 (68)	243 (77)	233 (74)	281 (72)	224 (75)	196 (74)	242 (78)	214 (77)
2	56 (25)	55 (18)	55 (18)	78 (20)	53 (18)	51 (19	42 (14)	48 (17)
3	13 (6)	* (*)	14 (4)	21 (5)	11 (4)	* (*)	15 (5)	* (*)
4+	* (*)	* (*)	11 (4)	12 (3)	12 (4)	* (*)	* (*)	* (*)
Laminectomy, n (%)	(N = 249)	(N = 325)	(N = 419)	(N = 475)	(N = 577)	(N = 695)	(N = 809)	(N = 774)
No. of Scans 1	191 (77)	242 (74)	304 (73)	328 (69)	432 (75)	509 (73)	578 (71)	587 (76)
2	50 (20)	58 (18)	84 (20)	109 (23)	100 (17)	131 (19)	163 (20)	131 (17)
3	* (*)	13 (4)	17 (4)	27 (6)	35 (6)	32 (5)	38 (5)	29 (4)
4+	* (*)	12 (4)	14 (3)	11 (2)	* (*)	23 (3)	30 (4)	27 (3)

*Patient volumes fewer then 11 are denoted with an asterisk (*) to protect patient privacy

the first study to our knowledge to quantify the magnitude and timing of CT scan utilization following simple and complex surgical interventions. The frequency of CT scanning postoperatively was noteworthy with approximately one-quarter of patients undergoing complex spinal procedures having a follow-up CT scan within one year of surgery, with the prevalence exceeding 40% by 5 years postoperatively. Importantly, patients having postoperative CT scans averaged approximately two such imaging events over a 5-year follow-up period, increasing the effects of ionizing radiation exposure. Postoperative CT scan utilization was lower among patients having simple surgical procedures, occurring at about one-half the frequency associated with complex surgical procedures during the initial postoperative year, but still approached almost 30% by 5 years of follow-up.

Why is the prevalence of postoperative CT scanning as high as it is and why is it greater in patients having complex surgical procedures? One reason may be that complex spine surgery invariably involves the implantation of bone graft materials coupled with metallic instrumentation to provide mechanical stability to support fusion as well as surgical insertion of spacers, cages, motion sparing and arthroplasty devices. The dramatically increased utilization of these devices has led to a new field of postoperative imaging assessment to evaluate these implants for breakage, loosening, migration, subsidence, and expulsion as well as to assess the status of the ossifying fusion mass and adjacent level disease [15]. Unfortunately, the presence of metallic instrumentation, often spanning multiple vertebral levels, may necessitate the use of CT scanning to evaluate postoperative neural compression as the image distortion with MRI may be too great [16–19]. This is particularly true for implants composed of stainless steel or cobalt-chrome [20]. Since simple surgical procedures such as discectomy and laminectomy do not involve the concomitant implantation of instrumentation, the CT scanning frequency is correspondingly lower.

With instrumented spinal fusion, CT is often the preferred postoperative evaluation method to elucidate putative sources of residual or worsening symptoms such as screw loosening/breakage and delayed healing/pseudoarthrosis of the developing fusion construct that cannot be visualized adequately with other modalities. However, screw loosening is an infrequent surgical complication and rarely associated with bothersome clinical symptoms [21]. Much of the early-term use of postoperative CT scanning is likely undertaken to confirm healing of the fusion mass. However, pseudoarthrosis is rare and almost all patients inevitably fuse with current interbody techniques, with a solid arthrodesis occurring in greater than 90% of patients [22, 23]. Moreover, fusion status has been shown to be a weak predictor of clinical outcomes with only a modest correlation to back symptoms [24].

Our concern about the marked utilization of postoperative CT scanning is amplified by the growing body of evidence that patients exposed to radiation in the range provided by a single CT scan have an increased cancer risk [25, 26]. Smith-Bindman et al [27] estimated that the lifetime attributable cancer risk from a single CT scan could be as high as 1 in 80 depending on dose and life expectancy. The radiation dose associated with a standard CT study of the spine ranges from 5–8 mSv which equates to approximately 400 to 550 chest X-rays [28].

In the Humana population, the estimated growth rate in complex surgical procedures was approximately 10% per year with almost one million spinal operations being undertaken nationwide when extrapolated to the entire US population. Applying our postoperative imaging prevalence rates to this estimate suggests that about 250,000 patients annually will be subjected to at least a single CT scan within one year of their surgery. Of the 80–100 million CT scans performed in the US annually [29], we estimated that approximately 9 million involve spinal imaging, much of it postoperative follow-up imaging. CT scanning rates overall are also growing at an annual rate of about 10% [29]. This combination of factors should underscore efforts to address this previously unidentified public health concern.

As documented in this study, a healthy percentage of patients having spine surgery are > 65 years of age and, due to their decreased life expectancy, have a lower attributable cancer risk from a single CT scan. However, complex spine surgery for disc degeneration, which affects a far younger cohort typically in their 40s, is growing at a dramatic rate [30]. In this population, the risk of cancer associated with postoperative CT scanning can be very real [31].

Our findings support the adoption of methods to curb nonessential CT scanning after spine surgery and make certain that the lowest possible dose is used to address the clinical question at hand [11, 25, 26]. To accomplish this, we advocate better coordination between surgeons and radiologic staff to ensure that scanning protocols are as parsimonious as possible. We also urge greater selectivity and judiciousness in the use of CT scanning to assess progress of the developing fusion mass or to verify solid fusion in the absence of definitive clinical symptoms. Routine surveillance scanning should be discouraged as a means of assuaging patient anxiety about the success of the procedure and patients should be made aware of the risks and benefits if a CT scan is indicated.

We encourage spine surgeons to choose, when possible, instrumentation and implants that provide excellent visualization on MRI without artifact distortion. This is particularly important in the evaluation of adjacent level disease where MRI is the preferred imaging modality. Devices constructed of titanium offer better MRI visualization and assessment than stainless steel, but characterization of index level changes and pathology can remain blurred using conventional scanner and image acquisition algorithms [32]. Other implant materials, such as polyether ether ketone (PEEK) and bioceramics, have an established history of safe use in other areas of orthopedics and offer excellent MRI visualization [33–35]. Priority should be given to programs investigating the range of MRI compatible biomaterials for more widespread use in the spine to replace ferromagnetic instrumentation and implants.

Due to the retrospective design of our study, we were restricted to computing postoperative imaging event prevalence. Advanced imaging incidence rates could not be computed from this administrative database. However, it is our hope that this foundational work will provide the impetus for future prospective research in different spine surgical indications to estimate postoperative imaging incidence rates.

The findings of this study are also limited by the use of records from a single, geographically-specific healthcare system based on claims identified by anatomic- and imaging-specific CPT codes. It is unclear what impact this has on the generalizability of our findings as use of claims data has been found to underreport imaging utilization [36]. Additionally, since the results of the current study are restricted to CT and MRI prevalence estimates, we could not delineate the reasons why imaging was prescribed. Nonetheless, it remains essential that patient safety be given high priority when selecting the appropriate imaging modality to evaluate the postoperative spine.

Conclusions

We detected a high frequency of CT utilization following complex spine surgery. There is emerging evidence of an increased cancer risk due to ionizing radiation exposure with CT. Thus, in the setting of complex spine surgery, actions to mitigate this risk should be considered and include reducing nonessential scans, using the lowest possible radiation dose protocols, exerting greater selectivity in monitoring the developing fusion construct, and adopting non-ferromagnetic implant biomaterials that facilitate MRI postoperatively.

Abbreviations

CAGR: compound annual growth rate; CPT: current procedural terminology; CT: computed tomography; HIPAA: health insurance portability and accountability act; MRI: magnetic resonance imaging; PEEK: polyether ether ketone; US: United States

Acknowledgements

We thank Scott Ellison at PearlDiver Technologies for conducting the data identification and extraction and are most grateful to Melissa Lui and Jeffrey Polack for helpful suggestions regarding the analysis and manuscript preparation. We appreciate the graphical support of Terry Meredith.

Funding

This study and manuscript development were funded by Simplify Medical (Sunnyvale, CA, USA). No funds were received by VVP, GBJA, SRG, or DLR.

Authors' contributions

JEB conceived the study design and directed the data analysis and interpretation. All authors participated in the development and drafting of the manuscript as well as in critical revision for important intellectual content. All authors read and approved the final manuscript.

Competing interests

JEB is an independent advisor to Simplify Medical (Sunnyvale, CA, USA) and received financial support for the development of this manuscript.

Consent for publication

Not applicable.

Author details

[1]The Spine Center, University of Colorado Hospital, Denver, CO, USA. [2]Midwest Orthopaedics, RUSH University Medical Center, Chicago, IL, USA. [3]Department of Orthopaedic Surgery, University of California, San Diego, CA, USA. [4]Department of Radiology, University of California, San Diego, CA, USA. [5]2210 Jackson Street, Ste. 401, San Francisco, CA 94115, USA.

References

1. Deyo RA, Mirza SK, Turner JA, Martin BI. Overtreating chronic back pain: time to back off? J Am Board Fam Med. 2009;22(1):62–8.
2. Jarvik JG, Hollingworth W, Martin B, Emerson SS, Gray DT, Overman S, Robinson D, Staiger T, Wessbecher F, Sullivan SD, et al. Rapid magnetic resonance imaging vs radiographs for patients with low back pain: a randomized controlled trial. JAMA. 2003;289(21):2810–8.
3. Deyo RA. Real help and red herrings in spinal imaging. N Engl J Med. 2013;368(11):1056–8.
4. Jensen MC, Brant-Zawadzki MN, Obuchowski N, Modic MT, Malkasian D, Ross JS. Magnetic resonance imaging of the lumbar spine in people without back pain. N Engl J Med. 1994;331(2):69–73.
5. Lurie JD, Birkmeyer NJ, Weinstein JN. Rates of advanced spinal imaging and spine surgery. Spine (Phila Pa 1976). 2003;28(6):616–20.
6. Deyo RA, Gray DT, Kreuter W, Mirza S, Martin BI. United States trends in lumbar fusion surgery for degenerative conditions. Spine (Phila Pa 1976). 2005;30(12):1441–5. discussion 1446-1447.
7. Brinjikji W, Luetmer PH, Comstock B, Bresnahan BW, Chen LE, Deyo RA, Halabi S, Turner JA, Avins AL, James K, et al. Systematic literature review of imaging features of spinal degeneration in asymptomatic populations. AJNR Am J Neuroradiol. 2015;36(4):811–6.
8. Drescher FS, Sirovich BE. Use of Computed Tomography in Emergency Departments in the United States: A Decade of Coughs and Colds. JAMA Intern Med. 2016;176(2):273–5.
9. Fazel R, Krumholz HM, Wang Y, Ross JS, Chen J, Ting HH, Shah ND, Nasir K, Einstein AJ, Nallamothu BK. Exposure to low-dose ionizing radiation from medical imaging procedures. N Engl J Med. 2009;361(9):849–57.
10. Brink JA, Amis Jr ES. Image Wisely: a campaign to increase awareness about adult radiation protection. Radiology. 2010;257(3):601–2.
11. Smith-Bindman R, Bindman AB. Imaging More Wisely. JAMA Intern Med. 2016;176(2):168–70.
12. Dokholyan RS, Muhlbaier LH, Falletta JM, Jacobs JP, Shahian D, Haan CK, Peterson ED. Regulatory and ethical considerations for linking clinical and administrative databases. Am Heart J. 2009;157(6):971–82.
13. Weinstein JN, Lurie JD, Olson PR, Bronner KK, Fisher ES. United States' trends and regional variations in lumbar spine surgery: 1992-2003. Spine (Phila Pa 1976). 2006;31(23):2707–14.
14. McLellan AM, Daniel S, Corcuera-Solano I, Joshi V, Tanenbaum LN. Optimized imaging of the postoperative spine. Neuroimaging Clin N Am. 2014;24(2):349–64.
15. Nouh MR. Spinal fusion-hardware construct: Basic concepts and imaging review. World J Radiol. 2012;4(5):193–207.
16. Sekhon LH, Duggal N, Lynch JJ, Haid RW, Heller JG, Riew KD, Seex K, Anderson PA. Magnetic resonance imaging clarity of the Bryan, Prodisc-C, Prestige LP, and PCM cervical arthroplasty devices. Spine (Phila Pa 1976). 2007;32(6):673–80.
17. Sundseth J, Jacobsen EA, Kolstad F, Nygaard OP, Zwart JA, Hol PK. Magnetic resonance imaging evaluation after implantation of a titanium cervical disc prosthesis: a comparison of 1.5 and 3 Tesla magnet strength. Eur Spine J. 2013;22(10):2296–302.
18. Wang JC, Yu WD, Sandhu HS, Tam V, Delamarter RB. A comparison of magnetic resonance and computed tomographic image quality after the implantation of tantalum and titanium spinal instrumentation. Spine (Phila Pa 1976). 1998;23(15):1684–8.
19. Zou YF, Chu B, Wang CB, Hu ZY. Evaluation of MR issues for the latest standard brands of orthopedic metal implants: plates and screws. Eur J Radiol. 2015;84(3):450–7.
20. Fayyazi AH, Taormina J, Svach D, Stein J, Ordway NR. Assessment of Magnetic Resonance Imaging Artifact Following Cervical Total Disc Arthroplasty. Int J Spine Surg. 2015;9:30.
21. Galbusera F, Volkheimer D, Reitmaier S, Berger-Roscher N, Kienle A, Wilke HJ. Pedicle screw loosening: a clinically relevant complication? Eur Spine J. 2015;24(5):1005–16.
22. Kwon BK, Hilibrand AS, Malloy K, Savas PE, Silva MT, Albert TJ, Vaccaro AR. A critical analysis of the literature regarding surgical approach and outcome for adult low-grade isthmic spondylolisthesis. J Spinal Disord Tech. 2005; 18(Suppl):S30–40.
23. Zigler J, Delamarter R, Spivak JM, Linovitz RJ, Danielson 3rd GO, Haider TT, Cammisa F, Zuchermann J, Balderston R, Kitchel S, et al. Results of the prospective, randomized, multicenter Food and Drug Administration investigational device exemption study of the ProDisc-L total disc replacement versus circumferential fusion for the treatment of 1-level degenerative disc disease. Spine (Phila Pa 1976). 2007;32(11):1155–62. discussion 1163.
24. Park Y, Ha JW, Lee YT, Sung NY. The effect of a radiographic solid fusion on clinical outcomes after minimally invasive transforaminal lumbar interbody fusion. Spine J. 2011;11(3):205–12.
25. Smith-Bindman R. Is computed tomography safe? N Engl J Med. 2010;363(1):1–4.
26. Brenner DJ, Hricak H. Radiation exposure from medical imaging: time to regulate? JAMA. 2010;304(2):208–9.
27. Smith-Bindman R, Lipson J, Marcus R, Kim KP, Mahesh M, Gould R, Berrington de Gonzalez A, Miglioretti DL. Radiation dose associated with common computed tomography examinations and the associated lifetime attributable risk of cancer. Arch Intern Med. 2009;169(22):2078–86.
28. Linet MS, Slovis TL, Miller DL, Kleinerman R, Lee C, Rajaraman P, Berrington de Gonzalez A. Cancer risks associated with external radiation from diagnostic imaging procedures. CA Cancer J Clin. 2012;62(2):75–100.
29. Mettler Jr FA, Bhargavan M, Faulkner K, Gilley DB, Gray JE, Ibbott GS, Lipoti JA, Mahesh M, McCrohan JL, Stabin MG, et al. Radiologic and nuclear medicine studies in the United States and worldwide: frequency, radiation dose, and comparison with other radiation sources–1950-2007. Radiology. 2009;253(2):520–31.
30. Yoshihara H, Yoneoka D. National trends in the surgical treatment for lumbar degenerative disc disease: United States, 2000 to 2009. Spine J. 2015;15(2):265–71.

31. Shuryak I, Sachs RK, Brenner DJ. Cancer risks after radiation exposure in middle age. J Natl Cancer Inst. 2010;102(21):1628–36.
32. Ahmad FU, Sidani C, Fourzali R, Wang MY. Postoperative magnetic resonance imaging artifact with cobalt-chromium versus titanium spinal instrumentation: presented at the 2013 Joint Spine Section Meeting, Clinical article. J Neurosurg Spine. 2013;19(5):629–36.
33. Hamadouche M, Sedel L. Ceramics in orthopaedics. J Bone Joint Surg Br. 2000;82(8):1095–9.
34. Kurtz SM, Devine JN. PEEK biomaterials in trauma, orthopedic, and spinal implants. Biomaterials. 2007;28(32):4845–69.
35. Li CS, Vannabouathong C, Sprague S, Bhandari M. The Use of Carbon-Fiber-Reinforced (CFR) PEEK Material in Orthopedic Implants: A Systematic Review. Clin Med Insights Arthritis Musculoskelet Disord. 2015;8:33–45.
36. Dismuke CE. Underreporting of computed tomography and magnetic resonance imaging procedures in inpatient claims data. Med Care. 2005; 43(7):713–7.

7

Change in muscle volume after steroid therapy in patients with myositis assessed using cross-sectional computed tomography

Takashi Nawata[1], Makoto Kubo[1*], Takafumi Nomura[2], Keiji Oishi[1], Kosaku Shiragami[3], Tadayoshi Ikegami[1], Munemasa Okada[2], Shigeki Kobayashi[1] and Masafumi Yano[1]

Abstract

Background: Steroid therapy, a key therapy for inflammatory, allergic, and immunological disorders, is often associated with steroid myopathy as one of the side effects. Steroid therapy is considered the first-line therapy for myositis; however, there have been no reports strictly comparing the muscle mass in patients with myositis before and after steroid therapy. Thus, it is currently unclear whether steroid therapy for such patients affects muscle volume in addition to muscle strength. We aimed to determine the change in muscle mass after steroid therapy via cross-sectional computed tomography (CT) in patients with myositis.

Methods: Data from seven patients with myositis and eight controls, who were all treated with high doses of steroids, were assessed before and after steroid therapy. Clinical factors in patients with myositis included serum muscle enzyme levels and muscular strength. The cross-sectional area of skeletal muscle and the low muscle attenuation rate at the level of the caudal end of the third lumbar vertebra were obtained using CT and measured using an image analysis program for all patients. Data were subjected to statistical analysis using several well-established statistical tests. The Wilcoxon signed-rank test was used for comparing paired data for each patient. The Mann-Whitney U test was used to compare sets of data sampled from two groups. The Spearman's rank correlation coefficient was used for determining the correlations between two variables. Statistical significance was set at $p < 0.05$.

Results: Muscular strength and serum muscle enzyme levels improved following steroid therapy in patients with myositis. In both groups, the cross-sectional areas of skeletal muscles decreased (myositis group: $p = 0.0156$; control group: $p = 0.0391$) and the low muscle attenuation rate tended to increase (myositis group: $p = 0.0781$; control group: $p = 0.0547$). In the myositis group, patients with chronic obstructive pulmonary disease showed a tendency toward muscle volume loss ($p = 0.0571$).

Conclusion: In patients with myositis treated with steroid therapy, muscle mass decreased after steroid therapy suggesting that the improvement in muscle strength was due to factors other than a change in muscle volume. Our study suggests the importance of therapies that not only improve muscle mass but also improve the quality of muscle strength.

Keywords: Computed tomography, Cross section, Steroid, Muscle mass, Myositis

* Correspondence: mkubo@yamaguchi-u.ac.jp
[1]Department of Medicine and Clinical Science, Yamaguchi University Graduate School of Medicine, 1-1-1 Minamikogushi, Ube, Yamaguchi 755-8505, Japan
Full list of author information is available at the end of the article

Background

Steroid therapy is a crucial form of treatment for inflammatory, allergic, and immunological disorders and has been used for > 50 years. Although steroid therapy is useful, there are various side effects, such as an associated increased susceptibility to infection or glucose intolerance [1].

Steroid myopathy is another side effect of steroid therapy, which is induced by the catabolic action of steroids on skeletal muscles [1, 2]. Muscle weakness in steroid myopathy usually begins in the proximal portion of the lower extremities, progresses to the upper proximal extremities, and finally affects the distal extremities [3]. It is known that steroid myopathy occurs in a dose-related manner. It has been reported that muscle strength in patients treated with > 40 mg/day of prednisone was significantly less than that in patients treated with < 40 mg/day [4].

Idiopathic inflammatory myopathies, collectively termed myositis, are autoimmune diseases characterized by skeletal muscle inflammation. Patients with myositis present with muscle weakness and atrophy in the proximal muscles and increases in serum levels of muscular enzymes [5]. Steroid therapy is considered the first-line therapy for myositis. With steroid therapy, patients with myositis show an improvement in muscle strength [6]; however, to our knowledge, there have been no reports strictly comparing the muscle mass of patients with myositis before and after steroid therapy. Therefore, it is unclear whether steroid therapy for patients with myositis improves not only muscle strength but also muscle volume.

Recently, several methods for quantifying muscle mass have been proposed. Bioelectrical impedance analysis and dual X-ray absorptiometry estimate the fat-free mass of the whole body or body segments [7, 8]. Computed tomography (CT) and magnetic resonance imaging (MRI) are also used to measure cross-sectional images that enable the estimation of muscle mass [9, 10]. Yoshizumi et al. reported that the cross-sectional area of skeletal muscle at the caudal end of the third lumbar vertebra, measured using CT, strongly correlated with body surface area [10]. It has been reported that MRI is a useful tool to diagnose muscle disorders. MRI makes it easy to assess not only muscle mass but also muscle quality, especially chemical shift imaging and Dixon based T2W imaging, which are new useful tools to assess fatty infiltration [11]. It has also been proposed that CT allows for the assessment of low attenuation of skeletal muscle (i.e., muscle with increased lipid content) [12]. With regard to the muscle volume of patients with rheumatic diseases, Hosono et al. reported that CT or MRI can estimate the steroid-related skeletal muscle loss in patients with rheumatic diseases more accurately than bioelectrical impedance analysis [13].

In this study, we retrospectively compared the changes in muscle volume before and after steroid therapy in patients with myositis and in steroid-treated patients without myositis by measuring the skeletal muscle area with CT.

Methods

Patients

Seven patients with recent-onset myositis (diagnosed from 2015 to 2017) were included in this study (five patients had dermatomyositis and two had mixed connective tissue disease). All patients fulfilled the diagnostic criteria proposed by Bohan and Peter [14]. The mean age was 55 years (range, 15–95 years) and four patients were female. The myositis group underwent high-dose steroid therapy (maximum dose of corticosteroid was > 0.7 mg/kg/day of prednisolone) (Table 1).

Table 1 Profiles of the patients in the myositis group

Patient	Age (years)	Sex	Diagnosis	Max glucocorticoid (mg/day)[a]	Duration between the start of treatment and second CT (months)[b]	Dose of glucocorticoid at second CT (mg/day)	Cumulative doses of glucocorticoid (g)[c]	MMT (before → after)[d]	Serum level of CK (U/L) (before → after)	Daily intake of protein in hospital (g/day)
1	26	M	DM	mPSL → PSL: 60	3	PSL: 25	PSL: 4.3	3+/3+ → 4+/4	102 → 21	80.0
2	58	F	DM	PSL: 40	2	PSL: 20	PSL: 1.7	4−/4- → 4/4-	500 → 17	54.0
3	74	F	DM	PSL: 45	2.5	PSL: 18	PSL: 2.3	4−/3+ → 4/4	3677 → 55	67.5
4	70	M	DM	mPSL → sPSL: 100	4	PSL: 22.5	PSL: 6.1	3−/3- → 4+/4+	5149 → 22	65.0
5	70	M	DM	PSL: 60	7.5	PSL: 12	PSL: 6.0	4+/4 → 5/5	1119 → 122	75.0
6	15	F	MCTD	PSL: 50	1	PSL: 50	PSL: 1.4	5−/5 → 5/5	876 → 219	70.0
7	69	F	MCTD	PSL: 40	3	PSL: 20	PSL: 2.7	4/4- → 5−/5-	2210 → 69	65.0

M male, *F* female, *DM* dermatomyositis, *MCTD* mixed connective tissue disease, *PSL* prednisolone, *mPSL* methylprednisolone, *sPSL* soluble prednisolone, *MMT* manual muscle test, creatine kinase

[a]Initial mPSL dose was 1 g × 3 d

[b]The first CTs were performed within six weeks before the initial steroid therapy

[c]Steroid taken using steroid pulse was excluded from cumulative doses of glucocorticoid

[d]Muscle strength of the bilateral iliopsoas muscle was evaluated using MMT before and after steroid therapy

Table 2 Profiles of the patients in the control group

Patient	Age (years)	Sex	Diagnosis	Max glucocorticoid (mg/day)[a]	Duration between the start of treatment and second CT (months)[b]	Dose of glucocorticoid at second CT (mg/day)	Cumulative doses of glucocorticoid (g)[c,d]
1	70	M	MCNS	PSL: 40	1.5	PSL: 25	PSL: 1.4
2	66	F	LN	mPSL → PSL: 35	2.5	PSL: 20	PSL: 2.4
3	46	F	LN	mPSL → mPSL: 32	3	mPSL: 12	PSL: 2.2
4	57	F	EPGA	mPSL → PSL: 50	3	PSL: 25	PSL: 3.4
5	80	M	MPA	mPSL → PSL: 30	2.5	PSL: 15	PSL: 1.3
6	86	F	MPA	mPSL → mPSL: 32	1.5	mPSL: 20	PSL: 1.5
7	79	F	MCNS	mPSL: 32	1.5	mPSL: 16 + PSL: 2	PSL: 1.6
8	76	F	HSPN	mPSL: 32	5.0	mPSL: 8	PSL: 2.6

M male, *F* female, *MCNS* minimal change nephrotic syndrome, *LN* lupus nephritis, *EPGA* eosinophilic granulomatosis with polyangiitis, *MPA* microscopic polyangiitis, *HSPN* Henoch-Schönlein purpura nephritis, *PSL* prednisolone, *mPSL* methylprednisolone

[a]Initial mPSL dose was 500 mg × 3 d, except for Patient 3 (1 g × 3 d) and Patients 7 and 8 (reported in table)

[b]The first CTs were performed within 6 weeks before the initial steroid therapy

[c]Steroid taken using steroid pulse was excluded from cumulative doses of glucocorticoid

[d]mPSL 0.8 mg is converted as PSL 1 mg

Eight patients without myositis were also included as a control group. Of these patients, two had lupus nephritis, two had microscopic polyangiitis, two had minimal change nephrotic syndrome, one had eosinophilic granulomatosis with polyangiitis, and one had Henoch-Schönlein purpura nephritis. The mean age of the patients in the control group was 70 years (range, 46–94 years) and six patients were female. The control group also underwent high-dose steroid therapy at the same maximum corticosteroid dose as the myositis group. Patients who experienced disuse syndrome were excluded prior to the inclusion of the final eight patients in the control group (Table 2).

Assessment of muscular strength

The muscular strength of patients with myositis were measured using a manual muscle test (MMT) before and after steroid therapy.

Computed tomography

All patients underwent CT to assess the general involvement before and after steroid therapy, and we retrospectively analyzed the change in muscle mass by comparing the CT findings. The first CT was performed within 6 weeks before the initiation of high-dose steroid therapy. The second CT was performed during the tapering of steroid therapy. CT data, including images of the caudal end of the third lumbar vertebra, were obtained using standard procedures. As indicated by a previous study, we defined values between − 29 and + 150 Hounsfield units (HU) as the skeletal muscle area (Fig. 1). Values between − 29 and + 30 HU were defined as low muscle attenuation [12]. Two radiologists measured the cross-sectional area of the skeletal muscles and the low muscle attenuation rate at the level of caudal end of the third lumbar vertebra. The mean attenuation of the muscles were measured using a semi-automatic image processing program, called "Image J", that was written in Java, which allows the program to be run on Linux, Mac OS X, and Windows (both 32-bit and 64-bit modes) without a license (http://rsb.info.nih.gov/ij/).

Statistical analysis

The inter-reader agreement for measuring the mean attenuation of muscle from the CT image was calculated using Cohen's kappa statistic. The strength of agreement between the two readers was interpreted as poor (< 0.20), fair (0.21–0.40), moderate (0.41–0.60), good (0.61–0.80), or excellent (0.81–0.99) [15]. The Wilcoxon signed-rank test was used to compare paired data for each patient. The Mann-Whitney U test was used to compare two sets of data sampled from the two groups. The Spearman's rank correlation coefficient was used

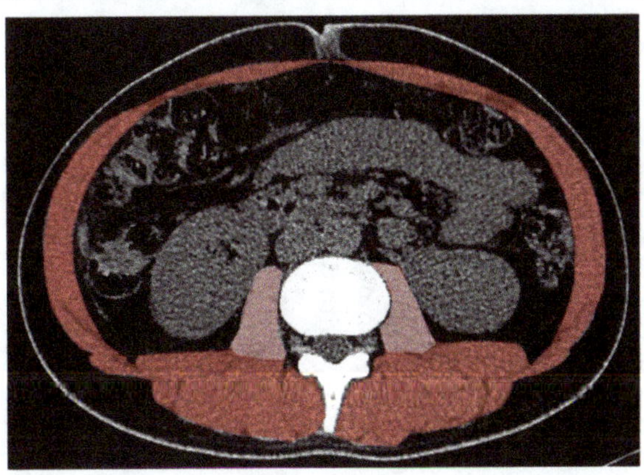

Fig. 1 Measurement of the cross-sectional area of skeletal muscle at the level of the caudal end of the third lumbar vertebra. Muscle volume was measured in the psoas muscle and other muscles

Table 3 Incidence of underlying diseases by group

	Myositis ($n = 7$)	Control ($n = 8$)
COPD	4 (57%)	2 (25%)
ILD	4 (57%)	4 (50%)
CKD	1 (14%)	6 (75%)
Cancer	3 (43%)	0 (0%)

COPD chronic obstructive pulmonary disease, *ILD* interstitial lung disease, *CKD* chronic kidney disease

to assess correlations between two variables. Comparisons were considered statistically significant at $p < 0.05$.

Results

The inter-reader agreement showed excellent correlation between the two readers, ranging from 0.89–0.99, for the mean attenuation of the muscle and the rate of low muscle attenuation.

Seven patients with myositis and eight controls were analyzed in this study. The muscle strength, measured using MMT, improved after steroid therapy in all patients with myositis (Table 1). In addition, the serum level of creatine kinase also improved after steroid therapy in all patients with myositis ([mean ± SD] before: 1948 ± 1855 U/L vs after: 75 ± 74 U/L, $p = 0.0156$, analyzed using the Wilcoxon signed-rank test.) (Table 1). The most frequent underlying diseases in patients with myositis were chronic obstructive pulmonary disease (COPD) and interstitial lung disease followed by cancer (e.g., lung carcinoma, rectal carcinoma, pharyngeal carcinoma). No patients with cancer underwent chemotherapy. All underlying diseases were detected within 2 months of the diagnosis of myositis. Conversely, chronic kidney disease was the most frequent underlying disease in the control group (Table 3).

Muscle mass at the level of the caudal end of the third lumbar vertebra significantly decreased in both groups after steroid therapy ([mean ± SD] myositis group: − 25.6 ± 14.4%, control group: − 12.6 ± 14.6%) (Fig. 2). With regard to the rate of muscle volume change between the groups, although the myositis group showed greater muscle volume loss in comparison to the control group, the difference was not statistically significant (Fig. 3). In the myositis group, patients with COPD also showed a tendency toward muscle volume loss ([mean ± SD] myositis with COPD: − 35.9 ± 9.1%, (myositis without COPD: − 11.9 ± 2.7%). Though the myositis group with cancer showed greater muscle volume loss in comparison to the control group, the difference was not statistically significant ([mean ± SD] myositis with cancer: − 38.1 ± 9.8%, myositis without cancer: − 16.3 ± 9.0%). (Figure 4) in addition, both groups showed a tendency towards an increased low muscle attenuation rate following steroid therapy ([mean ± SD] myositis group: + 7.3 ± 8.5%, control group: + 5.4 ± 6.6%) (Fig. 5). In patients with myositis, correlations between the rate of change of muscle volume and low muscle attenuation and clinical factors (age, serum level of creatine kinase before treatment, cumulative doses of steroid, time between first CT and second CT, time between the start of high-dose steroid and second CT, and daily intake of protein in hospital) analyzed using the Spearman's rank correlation coefficient were not significant.

Discussion

Although all patients with myositis showed improvements in muscle strength and serum muscle enzyme levels after

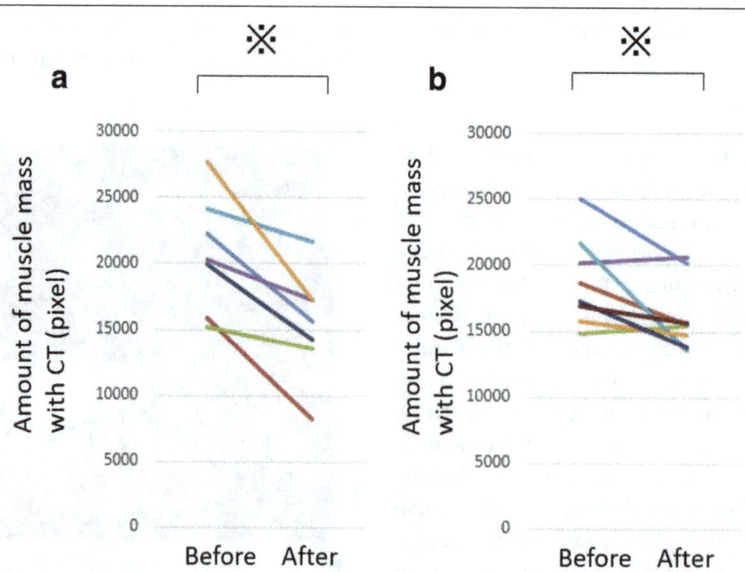

Fig. 2 The muscle mass of both groups significantly decreased after steroid therapy: **a** myositis group: $p = 0.0156$ and **b** control group: $p = 0.0391$. *$p < 0.05$, analyzed using the Wilcoxon signed-rank test. *CT* computed tomography

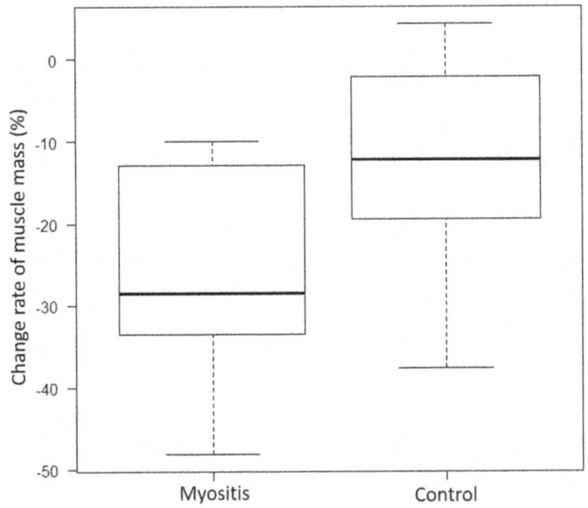

Fig. 3 Though the myositis group showed greater muscle volume loss in comparison to the control group, the difference was not statistically significant ($p = 0.121$); analyzed using the Mann-Whitney U test

steroid therapy, there was a significant loss of muscle volume. The loss of muscle mass is induced by both extrinsic causes and intrinsic causes. Extrinsic causes of focal muscle atrophy often developed after traumatic injury such as Morel-Lavallee syndrome which is a post-traumatic closed degloving injury [16]. Our patients did not have a history of trauma. Therefore, we think that extrinsic causes had little involvement in the change of muscle mass in our patients. With regard to intrinsic causes, previous studies have reported that patients with cancer, COPD, and chronic kidney disease exhibited a loss of muscle volume [17–19]. In the present study, some of the patients had these conditions as underlying diseases. Therefore, the involvement of these underlying diseases may be associated with the observed muscle volume loss in our patients (especially in patients with cancer and COPD in the myositis group). However, the patients with myositis who did not develop these underlying diseases also showed a loss of muscle volume. This suggests that steroid therapy itself decreases muscle volume in patients with myositis. Thus, an improvement in muscle strength in patients with myositis may be attributed to other factors and not to muscle volume change.

Some mechanisms have been proposed to explain the etiology of the loss of muscle volume. One of these mechanisms is an imbalance of protein synthesis and catabolism [20]. Steroid myopathy is induced by the hypercatabolism of skeletal muscle, which might have resulted in the loss of muscle volume in our patients. However, despite the loss of muscle mass, improvement in muscle strength was also observed in patients with myositis who were treated with steroids. As such, we hypothesize that the improvement in muscle strength is influenced by an improvement in mitochondrial function. Currently, a non-immune cell mediated mechanism in myositis has been proposed [21]. It was reported that the endoplasmic reticulum (ER) stress pathways are chronically activated in patients with myositis [21]. Additionally, the biopsy specimens from patients with myositis and mice models of myositis demonstrated an increase in levels of Grp78 (also known as HSPA5), which is an ER stress-related protein [22]. The biopsy specimens from patients with myositis also showed co-localization of MHC class I and the ER marker, calnexin [22]. These results suggest the possibility of the involvement of ER stress in the pathogenesis of myositis. Xiao et al. reported that serum HSPA5 levels significantly decreased after steroid therapy in steroid-responsive patients with myositis. In contrast, serum HSPA5 levels did not change in non-responders [23]. The results of the previous study suggest that steroid therapy reduces ER stress in steroid-responsive patients with myositis. ER stress is known to increase reactive oxygen species, which are closely associated with mitochondrial dysfunction, depressed force generation, and activation of muscle catabolic and autophagy pathways [21]. We speculate that steroid therapy improves muscle strength via the reduction of ER stress and

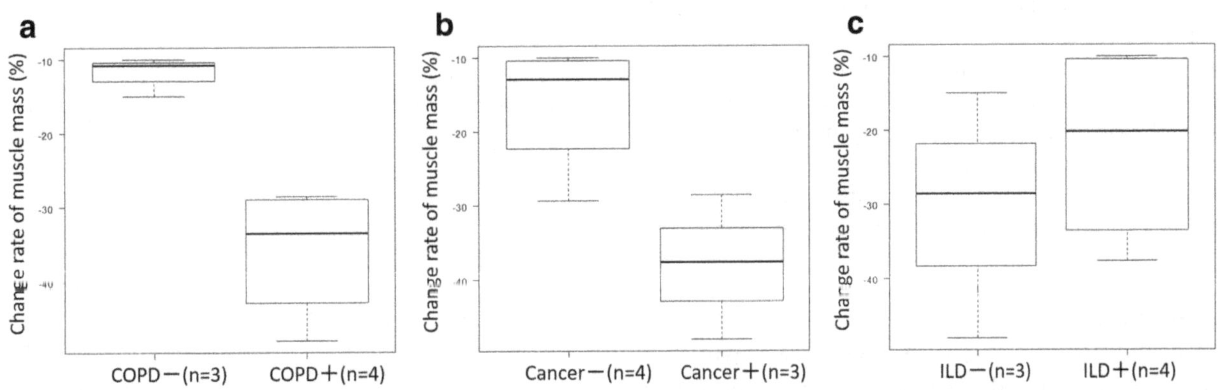

Fig. 4 In the myositis group, patients with chronic obstructive pulmonary disease (COPD) showed a tendency toward muscle volume loss: **a** COPD: $p = 0.0571$; **b** Cancer: $p = 0.114$; **c** interstitial lung disease (ILD): $p = 0.629$, analyzed using the Mann-Whitney U test

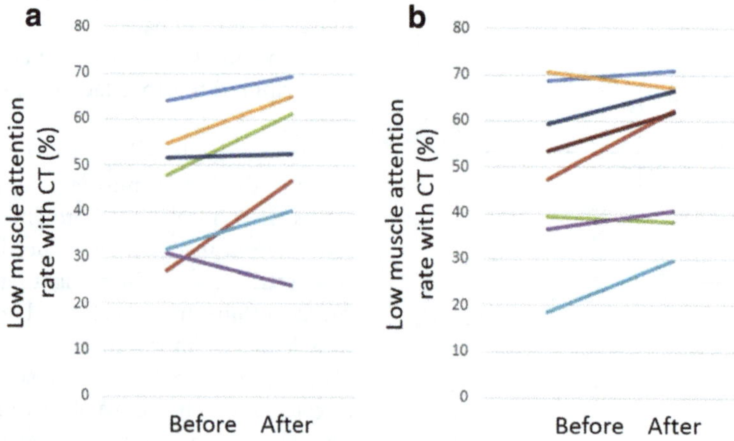

Fig. 5 Both groups showed a tendency toward an increased low muscle attenuation rate after steroid therapy: **a** myositis group: $p = 0.0781$ and **b** control group: $p = 0.0547$, analyzed using the Wilcoxon signed-rank test. *CT* computed tomography

reactive oxygen species followed by an improvement in mitochondrial function. Our study suggests that the improvement in muscle strength after steroid therapy is not influenced by an improvement in muscle volume, but rather by an improvement in other factors, such as amelioration of mitochondrial dysfunction.

Our study has a few limitations. First, this was a retrospective study and the number of patients was small. The non-significant change in the low muscle attenuation rate after steroid therapy and the non-significant change between the rate of change of muscle volume in patients with myositis associated with COPD and cancer may be partly due to the small sample size. Second, the regimens for steroid reduction and the timing of implementation of the second CT were different for each of the patients, which makes it difficult to accurately assess the correlations between muscular changes and clinical factors. Third, though patients who experienced disuse syndrome were excluded from the control group, exact scores from the MMT (muscular strength) of the control group were unknown, which makes it difficult to assess the change of muscle strength in the control group. However, our study suggests the importance of therapies that not only improve muscle mass but also improve the quality of muscle strength for the treatment of myositis. Hence, this study may provide novel insights into therapies for myositis. Nonetheless, further studies are needed to reveal the mechanism and treatment of muscle weakness in patients with myositis.

Conclusions

In patients with myositis treated with steroid therapy, muscle mass decreased after steroid therapy, suggesting that the improvement in muscle strength was due to factors other than changes in muscle volume.

Abbreviations

CKD: Chronic kidney disease; COPD: Chronic obstructive pulmonary disease; CT: Computed tomography; EPGA: Eosinophilic granulomatosis with polyangiitis; ER: Endoplasmic reticulum; HSPN: Henoch-Schönlein purpura nephritis; ILD: Interstitial lung disease; LN: Lupus nephritis; MCSN: Minimal change nephrotic syndrome; MCTD: Mixed connective tissue disease; MMT: Manual muscle test; MPA: Microscopic Polyangiitis; mPSL: Methylprednisolone; MRI: Magnetic resonance imaging; PSL: Prednisolone; ROS: Reactive oxygen species; sPSL: Soluble prednisolone

Acknowledgments

None.

Funding

No funding was obtained for this study.

Authors' contributions

TNawata wrote the manuscript. TNawata, TNomura, KO, TI, MO were involved in study design and analyzing the patients' data. MK, KS, SK, MY contributed to the study design. All authors read and approved the final manuscript.

Consent for publication

Not applicable.

Competing interests

The authors declare that they have no competing interests.

Author details

[1]Department of Medicine and Clinical Science, Yamaguchi University Graduate School of Medicine, 1-1-1 Minamikogushi, Ube, Yamaguchi 755-8505, Japan. [2]Department of Radiology, Yamaguchi University Graduate School of Medicine, 1-1-1 Minamikogushi, Ube 755-8505, Japan. [3]Department of Internal Medicine, Saiseikai Yamaguchi General Hospital, 2-11, Midorimachi, Yamaguchi 753-8517, Japan.

References

1. Schäcke H, Döcke WD, Asadullah K. Mechanisms involved in the side effects of glucocorticoids. Pharmacol Ther. 2002;96:23–43.
2. Schakman O, Gilson H, Thissen JP. Mechanisms of glucocorticoid-induced myopathy. J Endocrinol. 2008;197:1–10.
3. Askari A, Vignos PJ Jr, Moskowitz RW. Steroid myopathy in connective tissue disease. Am J Med. 1976;61:485–92.
4. Bowyer SL, LaMothe MP, Hollister JR. Steroid myopathy: incidence and detection in a population with asthma. J Allergy Clin Immunol. 1985;76:234–42.
5. Lundberg IE, Miller FW, Tjärnlund A, Bottai M. Diagnosis and classification of idiopathic inflammatory myopathies. J Intern Med. 2016;280:39–51.

6. Joffe MM, Love LA, Leff RL, Fraser DD, Targoff IN, Hicks JE, et al. Drug therapy of the idiopathic inflammatory myopathies: predictors of response to prednisone, azathioprine, and methotrexate and a comparison of their efficacy. Am J Med. 1993;94:379–87.
7. Barbosa-Silva MC, Barros AJ. Bioelectrical impedance analysis in clinical practice: a new perspective on its use beyond body composition equations. Curr Opin Clin Nutr Metab Care. 2005;8:311–7.
8. Wang W, Wang Z, Faith MS, Kotler D, Shih R, Heymsfield SB. Regional skeletal muscle measurement: evaluation of new dual-energy X-ray absorptiometry model. J Appl Physiol (1985). 1999;87:1163–71.
9. Cesari M, Fielding RA, Pahor M, Goodpaster B, Hellerstein M, van Kan GA, et al. Biomarkers of sarcopenia in clinical trials-recommendations from the international working group on sarcopenia. J Cachexia Sarcopenia Muscle. 2012;3:181–90.
10. Yoshizumi T, Shirabe K, Nakagawara H, Ikegami T, Harimoto N, Toshima T, et al. Skeletal muscle area correlates with body surface area in healthy adults. Hepatol Res. 2014;44:313–8.
11. Kumar Y, Wadhwa V, Phillips L, Pezeshk P, Chhabra A. MR imaging of skeletal muscle signal alterations: systematic approach to evaluation. Eur J Radiol. 2016;85:922–35.
12. Aubrey J, Esfandiari N, Baracos VE, Buteau FA, Frenette J, Putman CT, et al. Measurement of skeletal muscle radiation attenuation and basis of its biological variation. Acta Physiol (Oxf). 2014;210:489–97.
13. Hosono O, Yoshikawa N, Shimizu N, Kiryu S, Uehara M, Kobayashi H, et al. Quantitative analysis of skeletal muscle mass in patients with rheumatic diseases under glucocorticoid therapy–comparison among bioelectrical impedance analysis, computed tomography, and magnetic resonance imaging. Mod Rheumatol. 2015;25:257–63.
14. Bohan A, Peter JB. Polymyositis and Dermatomyositis (first of two parts). N Engl J Med. 1975;292:344–7.
15. Eliasziw M, Young SL, Woodbury MG, Fryday-Field K. Statistical methodology for the concurrent assessment of interrater and intrarater reliability: using goniometric measurements as an example. Phys Ther. 1994;74:777–88.
16. Diviti S, Gupta N, Hooda K, Sharma K, Lo L. Morel-Lavallee lesions-review of pathophysiology, clinical findings, imaging findings and management. J Clin Diagn Res. 2017;11:TE01–4.
17. Martin L, Birdsell L, Macdonald N, Reiman T, Clandinin MT, McCargar LJ, et al. Cancer cachexia in the age of obesity: skeletal muscle depletion is a powerful prognostic factor, independent of body mass index. J Clin Oncol. 2013;31:1539–47.
18. Bernard S, LeBlanc P, Whittom F, Carrier G, Jobin J, Belleau R, et al. Peripheral muscle weakness in patients with chronic obstructive pulmonary disease. Am J Respir Crit Care Med. 1998;158:629–34.
19. Fahal IH. Uraemic sarcopenia: aetiology and implications. Nephrol Dial Transplant. 2014;29:1655–65.
20. Menconi M, Fareed M, O'Neal P, Poylin V, Wei W, Hasselgren PO. Role of glucocorticoids in the molecular regulation of muscle wasting. Crit Care Med. 2007;35:S602–8.
21. Lightfoot AP, McArdle A, Jackson MJ, Cooper RG. In the idiopathic inflammatory myopathies (IIM), do reactive oxygen species (ROS) contribute to muscle weakness? Ann Rheum Dis. 2015;74:1340–6.
22. Nagaraju K, Casciola-Rosen L, Lundberg I, Rawat R, Cutting S, Thapliyal R, et al. Activation of the endoplasmic reticulum stress response in autoimmune myositis: potential role in muscle fiber damage and dysfunction. Arthritis Rheum. 2005;52:1824–35.
23. Xiao F, Tan JZ, Xu XY, Wang XF. Increased levels of HSPA5 in the serum of patients with inflammatory myopathies–preliminary findings. Clin Rheumatol. 2015;34:715–20.

8

The acutely injured acromioclavicular joint – which imaging modalities should be used for accurate diagnosis?

Jonas Pogorzelski[1], Knut Beitzel[1], Francesco Ranuccio[1], Klaus Wörtler[3], Andreas B. Imhoff[1*], Peter J. Millett[2] and Sepp Braun[1]

Abstract

Background: The management of acute acromioclavicular (AC) joint injuries depends on the degree of injury diagnosed by the Rockwood classification. Inadequate imaging and not selecting the most helpful imaging protocols can often lead to incorrect diagnosis of the injury. A consensus on a diagnostic imaging protocol for acute AC joint injuries does not currently exist. Therefore we conducted a systematic review of the literature considering three diagnostic parameters for patients with acromioclavicular (AC) joint injuries: 1) Assessment of vertical instability; 2) Assessment of horizontal instability; 3) Benefit of weighted panoramic views.

Methods: Internet databases were searched in March 2016 using the terms ("AC joint" OR "acromioclavicular joint") AND (MRI OR MR OR radiograph OR X-ray OR Xray OR ultrasound OR "computer tomography" OR "computed tomography" OR CT). Diagnostic, prospective, retrospective, cohort and cross- sectional studies were included to compare their use of different radiological methods. Case reports, cadaveric studies, and studies concerning chronic AC injuries and clinical outcomes were excluded.

Results: This search returned 1359 citations of which 1151 were excluded based on title, 116 based on abstract and 75 based on manuscript. 17 studies were included for review and were analyzed for their contributions to the three parameters of interest mentioned above. The inter- and intra-observer reliability for diagnosing vertical instabilities of the clavicle using x-ray alone show a high level of reproducibility while for horizontal instabilities the values were much more variable. In general, digitally measured parameters seem to be more precise and reliable between investigators than visual classification alone. Currently, evidence for the value of weighted views and other additional diagnostic imaging to supplement standard x-rays is controversial.

Conclusion: To date there is no consensus on a gold standard for diagnostic measures needed to classify acute AC joint injuries. The inter- and intra-observer reliability for diagnosing vertical instabilities of the clavicle using bilateral projections show a high level of reproducibility while for horizontal instabilities the results are much more inconsistent. There is currently no clear consensus on a protocol for image-based diagnosis and classification of acute AC joint injuries, leading to a lack of confidence in reproducibility and reliability.

Background

Acute injuries of the AC joint are currently treated based on the grade of instability according to Rockwood's classification. This classification was presented by Rockwood [1] in 1998 and is still widely accepted. The higher the Rockwood grade, the higher the severity and extent of injury of surrounding anatomical structures (Table 1).

Successful management of AC joint instability is challenging for many reasons. A variety of non-anatomical and anatomical operative techniques is described, but there is no consensus which should be preferred. Moreover, the distinction between type III and IV injuries is still controversial. A solution to clarify this distinction would streamline treatment choices and may thus lead to more favorable clinical outcomes. As such, it is

* Correspondence: imhoff@tum.de; a.imhoff@lrz.tu-muenchen.de
[1]Department of Orthopaedic Sports Medicine, Hospital Rechts der Isar, University of Munich, Ismaninger Street 22, 81675 Munich, Germany
Full list of author information is available at the end of the article

Table 1 Rockwood classification system for AC joint injuries

Rockwood classification	Type I	Type II	Type III	Type IV	Type V	Type VI
AC ligaments	sprained	disrupted	disrupted	disrupted	disrupted	disrupted
CC ligaments	intact	sprained	disrupted	disrupted	disrupted	disrupted
Deltoid and trapezius muscle	intact	intact	detached from clavicle	detached from clavicle	detached from clavicle	detached from clavicle
Dislocation of the clavicle	none	AC joint widening, CC subluxation	AC joint dislocation, CC interspace 25–100% greater than compared to uninjured side	CC interspace may appear widened, clavicle horizontal unstable with posterior (sub-) luxation	AC joint dislocation, CC interspace more than 100% greater than compared to uninjured side	AC joint dislocation, clavicle displaced inferior to the coracoid

necessary to determine both vertical and horizontal instability with precise and reproducible methods. Radiographs are commonly used as a routine imaging tool in the assessment of shoulder injuries as they are widely available and provide convincing results [2, 3].

However, the literature suggests a broad range of imaging modalities and techniques that can be used to elucidate the extent of the AC joint disruption, including special X-ray images: alternative planes (e.g. bilateral Zanca [4], axillary view, dynamic axillary view), stress imaging, dynamic measures, indices, or additional modalities like ultrasound or MRI. Currently, a standardized protocol to image acute AC joint separations does not exist, rendering proficient and unanimous diagnosis difficult. The purpose of this review was to summarize all relevant available studies dealing with diagnostic imaging of acute AC joint injuries. A focus was set on three questions: 1) Assessment of vertical instability; 2) Assessment of horizontal instability; 3) Importance of weighted panoramic views.

Methods

Inclusion criteria

This systematic review was structured according to the PRISMA Checklist [5]. A literature search was performed focusing on studies reporting diagnostic imaging of acute AC joint injuries (diagnostic imaging within 3 weeks after injury) [6]. We included diagnostic, prospective, retrospective, cohort and cross- sectional studies comparing radiological methods or different applications of the same diagnostic technique. Publications written in English, German and Italian were all included.

Exclusion criteria

We excluded case reports, cadaveric studies and studies on chronic AC injuries and clinical outcomes.

Search strategy

Electronic databases (MEDLINE, COCHRANE Library, and EMBASE) were independently searched by two reviewers (*blinded for review*) on March 15, 2016 using the following search string: ("ac joint" OR "acromioclavicular joint") AND (mri OR mr OR radiograph OR x-ray OR xray OR view OR ultrasound OR "computer tomography" OR "computed tomography" OR ct). In addition, the references of the included fulltext articles and available review articles were searched for additional studies that met the inclusion criteria.

Study selection

In order to include and exclude studies according to the criteria above, two reviewers (*blinded for review*) searched the titles and abstracts of all identified publications and the fulltext of the eligible articles. Divergences were resolved in collaboration with a third reviewer (*blinded for review*).

Data extraction

The data from all included articles were analyzed by two independent reviewers (*blinded for review*). Studies meeting all eligibility criteria were reviewed and the following data were abstracted: study design, level of evidence, type of imaging, number of patients, classification adopted and results. Level of evidence was assigned according to the widely accepted common grading of Evidence Levels for Primary Research. The abstracted data for each study were sorted into one of the following 3 categories: 1) Assessment of vertical instability; 2) Assessment of horizontal instability; 3) Requirement of weighted panoramic views.

Results

Figure 1 demonstrates the results of the literature search. 17 out of 1359 studies were extracted according to the inclusion criteria and are presented in Tables 2, 3 and 4.

All 17 eligible studies were scrutinized three times, each time pertaining to each of the 3 previously asked questions. The results of each question will be discussed separately below.

Assessment of vertical instability

Twelve out of the 17 studies revealed results specifically pertaining to assessment of vertical instability. Of interest in each study were the levels of inter-observer reliability, intra-observer reliability and the preferred diagnostic method. As a general result, the inter- and intra-observer reliability for diagnosing vertical instabilities of the clavicle showed a high level of reproducibility with mostly good to excellent results. In addition, digitally measured results

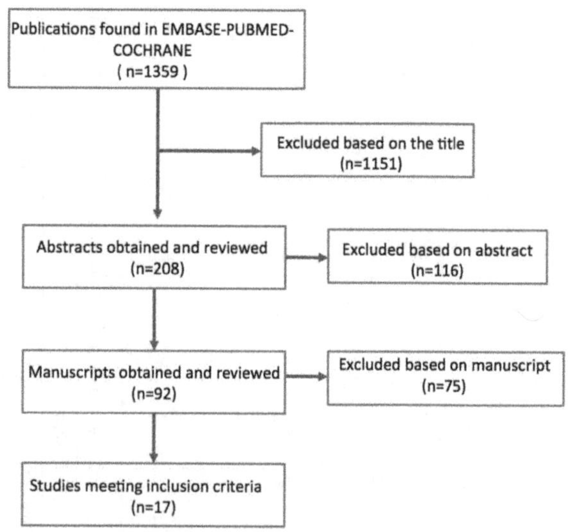

Fig. 1 Flowchart of the study selection process

Table 2 Assessment of vertical instability

Authors	Year of publication	Study design/level of evidence	Number of patients	Classification	Type of imaging	Results (according to classification of Landis/Koch [33])
Kraeutler et al. [34]	2012	Diagnostic study/IV	28	Rockwood	Anteroposterior and axial views: visual classification	Visual (ICC out of 8 investigators): leOR = moderate (0.60) laOR = good (0.69)
Cho et al. [15]	2014	Diagnostic study/I	28	Rockwood	Bilateral plain anteroposterior and axial views: visual classification. Bilateral plain anteroposterior and axial views and 3D–CT: visual classification.	Bilateral plain anteroposterior and axial views: visual (ICC out of 10 investigators): leOR = slight (0.21) laOR = moderate (0.47) Bilateral plain anteroposterior and axial views and 3D–CT: visual (ICC out of 10 investigators): leOR = poor (0.18) laOR = moderate (0.57)
Schneider et al. [7]	2014	Retrospective case series/IV	58	Rockwood	Bilateral panoramic stress and axial views: visual and digitally measured (CCI and HD) classification	Visual (range out of 4 investigators): leOR = good (0.72–0.74) laOR = good to excellent (0.67–0.93) Digitally measured CCI: leOR = excellent (0.85–0.93) laOR = excellent (0.90–0.97)
Gastaud et al. [9]	2015	Diagnostic study/I	15	Rockwood	Bilateral comparative anteroposterior views (Zanca-view [4]), axial views and dynamic axial views (Tauber [8]-protocol): digitally measured (CCI, D/A-ratio, X/Y-ratio, GACA) classification	Digitally measured CCI (range out of 4 investigators): leOR = good to excellent (0.69–0.92) laOR = good (0.60–0.77) Digitally measured D/A-ratio: leOR = good (0.62–0.67) laOR = good to excellent (0.66–0.95)
Schmid and Schmid [23]	1988	Diagnostic study/IV	22	Tossy	Intra-operative findings vs. ultrasound	• Only Tossy III: 100% accordance in classification
Fenkl and Gotzen [21]	1992	Diagnostic study/IV	35	Tossy	Weighted x-ray vs. ultrasound	• 97.2% accordance in classification • 2.8% underestimation of Tossy grade in ultrasound
Matter et al. [16]	1995	Diagnostic study/IV	20	Tossy	Weighted x-ray vs. ultrasound	• Ultrasound: Tossy III: 8.8 ± 2.1 mm AC-distance • Weighted x-ray: Tossy III: 8.4 ± 3.7 mm AC-distance
Kock et al. [35]	1996	Diagnostic study/IV	29	Tossy	Weighted x-ray vs. ultrasound	• Ultrasound: Tossy II: 0.48 ± 0.18 AC-Index Tossy III: 0.20 ± 0.03 AC-Index • Weighted x-ray: Tossy II: 0.50 ± 0.19 AC-Index Tossy III: 0.20 ± 0.03 AC-Index
Iovane et al. [22]	2004	Diagnostic study/IV	18	Rockwood	Weighted x-ray vs. ultrasound	• 100% accordance in classification (only Rockwood I – III)
Schaefer et al. [3]	2006	Diagnostic study/IV	13	Rockwood	Non-weighted x-ray vs. mri	• 84.6% accordance in classification • 15.4% underestimation of Rockwood grade in x-ray

Table 2 Assessment of vertical instability *(Continued)*

Authors	Year of publication	Study design/level of evidence	Number of patients	Classification	Type of imaging	Results (according to classification of Landis/Koch [33])
Takase [18]	2011	Diagnostic study/IV	25	Rockwood	Non-weighted x-ray vs. mri	• 92% accordance in classification • 8% overestimation of Rockwood grade in x-ray
Nemec et al. [19]	2011	Diagnostic study/IV	44	Rockwood	Non-weighted x-ray vs. mri	• 52.2% accordance in classification • 36.4% overestimation of Rockwood grade in x-ray • 11.4% underestimation of Rockwood grade in x-ray

ICC = intraclass correlation coefficient, IeOR = inter-observer reliability, IaOR = intraobserver Reliability, CCI = coracoclavicular index, AC-width index = acromioclavicular-width index [10], D/A-ratio = vertical displacement of the clavicle[9]

Table 3 Assessment of horizontal instability

Authors	Year of publication	Study design/level of evidence	Number of patients	Classification	Type of imaging	Results (according to classification of Landis / Koch [33])
Schneider et al. [7]	2014	Retrospective case series/IV	58	Rockwood	Bilateral panoramic stress and axial views: visual and digitally measured (CCI and HD) classification	Digitally measured HD: IeOR = good to excellent (0.62–0.96) IaOR = good to excellent (0.67–0.98)
Vaisman et al. [10]	2014	Diagnostic study/II	40	Rockwood	Introduction of the AC-width index	Width index of ≥60%: • sensitivity of 95.7% and specificity of 97.5% • positive predictive value of 96.7% and negative predictive value of 95.6% for detecting a Rockwood grade IV injury
Tauber et al. [8]	2010	Diagnostic study/II	25	Rockwood	Introduction of the GACA	Cutoff value of 12.3°: • sensitivity of 93% and specificity of 92% • true-negative in 92% and false-negative in 8% for detecting a Rockwood grade IV injury
Gastaud et al. [9]	2015	Diagnostic study/I	15	Rockwood	Bilateral comparative anteroposterior views (Zanca-view[4]), axial views and dynamic axial views (Tauber[8]-protocol): digitally measured (CCI, D/A-ratio, X/Y-ratio, GACA) classification	Digitally measured X/Y-ratio: IeOR = moderate to good (0.48–0.80) IaOR = moderate to good (0.49–0.72) Digitally measured GACA: IeOR = poor to fair (0.01–0.33) IaOR = poor to fair (0.09–0.38)

AC-width index = acromioclavicular-width index[10], GACA = gleno-acromio-clavicular-angle[8], IeOR = inter-observer reliability, IaOR = intraobserver Reliability, HD = horizontal dislocation

Table 4 Requirement of weighted panoramic views

Authors	Year of publication	Study design/level of evidence	Number of patients	Classification	Kind of imaging? Pro weighted or pro non-weighted?	Justification
Bossart et al. [11]	1988	Diagnostic study/IV	83	Tossy	Weighted vs. non-weighted bilateral comparative x-rays. Pro non-weighted.	„use of weighted radiographs lacks efficacy in unmasking grade III AC sprains on radiograph " [11]
Ibrahim et al. [12]	2015	Retrospective case series/IV	59	Rockwood	Weighted vs. non-weighted bilateral comparative x-rays. Pro weighted.	"value of bilateral weighted views is to 'unmask' a grade V injury" [12]
Izadpanah et al. [13]	2013	Diagnostic study/IV	10	Rockwood	Non-weighted x-ray vs. weighted x-ray and non-weighted mri vs. weighted mri Pro weighted.	"application of stress (...) enables a partial rupture to be dis-tinguished from a complete ligamental rupture" [13]

showed a trend towards superior results compared to those of visually evaluated x-rays. Although radiographs and ultrasound obtained almost identical values and showed comparable measurement accuracy, x-ray remains mandatory to exclude fractures and is examiner-independent. This is why radiographs appear to be superior compared to ultrasound in the diagnosis of the acutely injured AC joint. Further relevant information is presented in Table 2.

Assessment of horizontal instability

Four out of the 17 studies revealed results specifically pertaining to assessment of horizontal instability at the AC joint. Schneider et al. examined the inter- and intra-observer reliability of visual evaluation, which showed mostly good results, and also digitally measured horizontal displacement of the clavicle, which demonstrated superior good to excellent results [7]. Tauber et al. devised the gleno-acromio-clavicular-angle (GACA) to quantify the horizontal clavicular dynamics measured on X-rays [8]. With the help of dynamic views they were able to reveal horizontal instability in six patients, which had previously been classified as "stable" on static axillary views. Gastaud et al. also assessed gleno-acromio-clavicular-angle (GACA) [8] as well as the X/Y-ratio (horizontal displacement of the clavicle), which showed extremely variable inter- and intra-observer reliability from poor to good [9]. Additionally, Vaisman et al. devised the AC-width index (the difference between the AC-width on the injured side and the normal side, subsequently divided by the AC width of the normal side) and suggested an AC-width index value ≥0.6 to be highly predictive of a horizontally unstable AC joint [10]. Further relevant information is given in Table 3.

Requirement of weighted panoramic views

Three out of the 17 studies revealed results discussing the utility of weighted panoramic views. Bossart et al. questioned the routine use of stress views for acutely injured AC joints as they compared weighted and non-weighted views of acutely injured AC joints and could only detect in 3 out of 84 cases (4%) an unmasked Tossy III injury with the help of weighted films [11]. Ibrahim et al. suggested weighted views may be useful because of their ability to uncover Rockwood V injuries [12]. This study reported 10 out of 59 (17%) patient diagnoses increased to Rockwood V injuries when weighted films were used. This was further validated by Izadpanah et al. using MRI with and without stress [13]. In all 10 cases they reported, a precise outline of the CC-ligaments and a differentiation between sprained and torn ligaments could be obtained, suggesting weighted MRI provides a significant diagnostic advantage. Further relevant information is given in Table 4.

Discussion

Our review revealed that only 17 studies, with a low level of evidence varying between level II-IV, met our inclusion criteria. Bilateral panoramic view with digitally measured CC-distance allows for the most accurate diagnosis of vertical instability (type V instability). For the identification of horizontal instability (as seen in type IV instability), data is still insufficient with variable results and multiple diagnostic methods discussed. Due to the heterogeneity of the published literature, no gold standard for the imaging of the AC joint instability can be presented. However, basic principles in the utilized imaging modalities could be identified. In general, radiographs seem to be the preferred diagnostic method due to their wide availability and examiner-independence, which separates it from ultrasound. MRI and CT imaging generally play a subordinate role in the diagnosis of the acutely injured AC joint, mainly due to high costs and poor availability. Moreover, in cases of acute AC joint injuries, the use of MRI and CT might not add additional significant information, as there is normally no need to evaluate bones, nerves or vessels in detail [14].

Assessment of vertical instability

The vertical displacement of the clavicle is found to be reproducible showing strong concordance for intra- and inter-observer reliability. It should be diagnosed as CC-distance rated on bilateral panoramic views. This may be because the coracoid process and the acromion can be easily identified on x-ray and serve as reliable reference points. Since the classification of Rockwood is based on the relative increase of the CC distance compared to the contralateral side, panoramic views allow direct correlation to the uninjured contralateral joint. Results measured digitally seem to be more accurate than those taken visually [7, 9, 15]. One interpretation could be that digitally measuring the extent of the injury is more objective and can be performed with a systematic approach if predetermined diagnostic parameters exist, however visual diagnosis is subjectively based on the experience of the physician.

Several authors have tested alternative imaging modalities such as MRI, ultrasound and computer tomography versus X-ray [3, 13, 15, 16]. The literature suggests that MRI is able to capture superior detail – allowing it to differentiate a sprain from torn ligaments and fascial injury, as well as revealing concomitant intraarticular pathologies of the glenohumeral joint which occur up to 18% of the time [17]. In 2 out of 3 studies, there was a high level of concordance between the results from MRI and X-ray [3, 18]. Only Nemec et al. reported a lack of concordance in Rockwood classification results between MRI and X-ray [19]. However, this may be explained by their patients mainly being graded Rockwood II and III where MRI is most useful because of direct visualization of the AC- and CC-ligaments. Since the patient is examined in the supine position, the weight of the arm does not affect the CC-distance and the scapula will not be able to go into the protracted position, widely encountered in AC-joint instabilities. These factors should also be taken into account, when evaluation MRI in the presentation of an acute AC-joint injury. This mechanical effect is more relevant, if the injury is not acute. In these cases, MRI might demonstrate a ligamentous structure with a structural continuity but without adequate tension of the ligaments.

Ultrasound has been shown to be able to reliably differentiate between sprain and rupture of the AC- and CC-ligaments and is widely available and inexpensive [16, 20, 21]. Therefore it is an interesting addition to the current diagnostic work up which is mainly based on conventional X-ray. Studies evaluating the use of ultrasound for diagnosing AC joint lesions showed results of very good concordance with X-ray and intra-operative findings [20, 22, 23]. The advantage of sonographic evaluation is rather seen in the detection of horizontal instability with the advantage of functional testing to demonstrate the overriding of the lateral clavicle over the acromion. However, ultrasound still provides a rather subjective result and highly depends on the experience of the user. The advantage in conventional X-ray imaging is seen in the possibility to exclude fractures and the direct correlation to Rockwood's criteria.

Using CT, Cho et al. compared intra- and inter-observer reliability, diagnosing acute AC joint injuries with X-ray alone and X-ray augmented with 3D CT [15]. Although the addition of 3D CT improved reliability, it did not reach statistical significance. With the associated radiation exposure and cost, the routine use of 3D CT in clinical practice again may not be justified.

Assessment of horizontal instability

Correct and reliable diagnosis of a horizontal instability is important since the discrimination of a type III injury vs. a type IV injury determines whether the basic treatment recommendation is surgical or non-surgical. It is widely accepted that a horizontally unstable clavicle requires operative management, meaning correct diagnosis of Rockwood IV injuries is imperative [24]. Unfortunately, this diagnosis is often difficult because in most cases, the diagnose of a mainly 3D dynamic pathology has to be made based on a static imaging modality.

Radiographs taken in the axillary projection have been a standard modality to diagnose horizontal instability in the past. The patient is in a supine position (scapula fixed – no effect of bodyweight or scapula position) and the correct projection for good quality requirescompliance of the patient as well an experienced technician. Rahm et al. showed in a cadaver model that using a standard axillary radiograph to diagnose horizontal instability has a very high sensitivity but low specificity, where a variation in axillary views can misguide the examiner to interpret X-Rays to have posterior clavicular translation [25]. Additionally, they found that a small variation in the beam angle has a large effect on measurements taken because of distorted images. Moreover, Barth et al. could show recently that the uninjured AC joint is not perfectly aligned anteriorly and posteriorly in as much as 40% of the cases [26]. This finding might be another explanation for the poor results when interpreting horizontal instability on imaging. As a solution, Vaisman et al. used the AC-width index, a method to detect instability of the clavicle without the need of an axillary view [10]. Even though they presented superior results, there is no further study which could confirm these findings at the present time. Tauber et al. pointed out that a standing or sitting position when taking an axillary view results in dropping the affected shoulder, which subsequently malrotates the scapula, which could potentially conceal the extent of the lesion [8]. They referred to Alexander [27] who described a modification of the axillary view in 1949 with the patient sitting or standing and the shoulders thrusted forward at the time when the x-ray is taken. Thus they recommended removing the vertical forces by taking axillary views in a supine position. They performed a dynamic examination with two lateral views with the arm at 90° of abduction and an additional 60° of flexion or extension to evaluate the horizontal dynamics of the lateral clavicle. The GACA was measured and used to quantify the horizontal instability of the clavicle in terms of angle differences. Although the authors could present very good values for intra- and inter-observer reliability with a sensitivity of 93% and a specificity of 92%, Gastaud et al. could not confirm these results in a study presented in 2015 concluding "that the horizontal displacement was difficult to evaluate on axillary lateral views and that the dynamic instability could not be reproducibly and reliably evaluated" [9]. An explanation may be that lateral axillary views contours overlap, and thus anatomical landmarks could be misinterpreted.

A projection of an axillary X-ray first described by Alexander [27] in 1949 has only been mentioned in the literature, but no study demonstrating its sensitivity or specificity has been published until now [27, 28]. The advantage of this projection is the application of "stress" on the AC joint through the flexion/adduction of the arm. It has been widely suggested by clinicians with increased interest in the last decade, but there is a lack of supporting evidence of their advantage over other views.

Diagnostic value of weighted panoramic views

For decades, surgeons all over the world have debated whether weighted or non-weighted views are more effective in correctly diagnosing AC joint injuries. According to one theory, pain triggered muscle spasm may "mask" the total extent of an injury, making weighted films necessary in order to distract the AC joint [29, 30]. In addition, some authors recommended that the weights should not be held in the hand, but suspended from the wrists to minimize voluntary muscle contraction [31]. Despite no clinical study validating this theory, it remained widely accepted for a long time. The first study challenging the requirement of weighted views was Bossart et al. in 1988 [11]. Using a clinical trial, they showed that in the vast majority of AC joint injuries, weighted films did not change the grade of injury. Due to low diagnostic yield and additional patient discomfort, they recommended weighted views for acute AC joint injuries should be abandoned. This opinion prevailed in the upcoming years, and the use of weighted radiographs became less popular. Yap et al. published a survey showing that a large majority of the specialized American shoulder and elbow community did not use weighted views in daily practice [32]. However, recently, Izadpanah et al. and Ibrahim et al. published studies indicating that stress views provide additional information helping to guide management [12, 13]. Both authors showed a significant increase in the CC distance when weights were applied, sometimes resulting in an upgrading of Rockwood III injuries, potentially changing therapy from conservative to operative treatment. In summary, because so few studies have reported on this topic, it is not possible to confidently advocate whether or not weighted views should be used routinely.

A fundamental problem encountered in most included studies is that the true extent of the injury can only be defined upon assessing the injury intra-operatively. Therefore, when comparing imaging results alone without any intraoperative reference, the assessor can never reliably assess the accuracy of an imaging method. Additionally, by only assessing articles evaluating acute AC joint injuries, following our exclusion criteria, our findings may not be able to be extrapolated to chronic AC joint injuries. Due to this significant lack of evidence, no gold standard for the imaging of AC joint instability can be defined. However, further development of optimal treatment strategies requires a reflected application of a set of all modalities to optimize the information and make the diagnosis as precise as possible. In the authors' current practice, panoramic views in combination with axial and or "Alexander" projections are used. Additional imaging such as MRI or CT is added if further information is required. In addition, current publications try to combine the advantages of clinical examination and imaging through a combined decision-making process. If the patient presents with a high level of pain in the acute phase following trauma, a second evaluation after some days might allow a better diagnose due to less protective muscle activation of the patient [24].

This systematic review has several limitations. First, the partial low level of evidence of the included studies predetermines the level of evidence of our study. Secondly, most of the included studies contain only small patient numbers. Thirdly, some of the publications were based on the Tossy classification, which has largely become obsolete. Despite this, many of these studies provided valuable information justifying their utilization.

Conclusion

A gold standard to investigate and diagnose acute AC joint injuries does not currently exist. The inter- and intra-observer reliability for diagnosing vertical instabilities of the clavicle using bilateral projections show a high level of reproducibility while for horizontal instabilities the results are much more heterogeneous. Currently, the evidence is conflicting over whether weighted views and additional diagnostics can usefully augment results from standard X-ray views. There is currently no consensus on a protocol to view acute AC joint injuries; therefore, classifying these injuries with high levels of confidence, reproducibility and reliability remains difficult. To improve clinical outcomes it may be of high importance to precisely diagnose AC injuries, which asks for an easily feasible, reproducible and safe diagnostic measure.

Abbreviations

AC: Acromioclavicular; CC: Coracoclavicular; CCI: Coracoclavicular index; CT: Computed tomography; D/A-ratio: Vertical displacement of the clavicle; GACA: Gleno-acromio-clavicular angle; MRI: Magnetic resonance imaging

Acknowledgements

Not applicable.

Funding

This work was supported by the German Research Foundation (DFG) and the Technical University of Munich within the funding programme Open Access Publishing.

Authors' contributions

JP participated in the design of the study, performed the literature search and drafted the manuscript. KB checked on all papers of the included literature and drafted the manuscript. FR performed the literature search and helped drafting the manuscript. KW was the supervising radiologist, drafted the manuscript and checked on all images. ABI coordinated the study and helped to draft the manuscript. PJM participated in the design of the study and checked on the manuscript. SB participated in the design of the study, drafted the manuscript and was the supervisor for all surgical belongings. All authors read and approved the final manuscript.

Consent for publication

All authors gave their consent for publishing the above reported paper with his name on it.

Competing interests
Sepp Braun,MD, Knut Beitzel,MD are consultants for Arthrex®.
Peter J. Millett,MD,MSc is a consultant for Arthrex®, Medbridge and Springer Publishing. He also has stock options for GameReady and VuMedi.
Prof. Andreas B. Imhoff,MD is a consultant for Arthrex® and Arthrosurface®.
Prof. Klaus Wörtler,MD, Francesco Ranuccio, MD, and Jonas Pogorzelski,MD declare no conflict of interest.

Author details
[1]Department of Orthopaedic Sports Medicine, Hospital Rechts der Isar, University of Munich, Ismaninger Street 22, 81675 Munich, Germany. [2]Orthopaedic Surgery, The Steadman Clinic, Vail, CO, USA. [3]Department of Radiology, Hospital Rechts der Isar, University of Munich, Munich, Germany.

References

1. Rockwood CJ WG, Young D. Disorders of the acromioclavicular joint. *Rockwood CJ, Matsen FA III, eds. The Shoulder. 2nd ed. Philadelphia: WB Saunders.* 1998:483–553.
2. Alyas F, Curtis M, Speed C, Saifuddin A, Connell D. MR imaging appearances of acromioclavicular joint dislocation. Radiographics 2008;28:463–479; quiz 619.
3. Schaefer FK, Schaefer PJ, Brossmann J, Hilgert RE, Heller M, Jahnke T. Experimental and clinical evaluation of acromioclavicular joint structures with new scan orientations in MRI. Eur Radiol. 2006;16:1488–93.
4. Zanca P. Shoulder pain: involvement of the acromioclavicular joint. (analysis of 1,000 cases). Am J Roentgenol Radium Therapy, Nucl Med. 1971;112:493–506.
5. Moher D, Liberati A, Tetzlaff J, Altman DG, Group P. Preferred reporting items for systematic reviews and meta-analyses: the PRISMA statement. BMJ. 2009;339:b2535.
6. Flint JH, Wade AM, Giuliani J, Rue JP. Defining the terms acute and chronic in orthopaedic sports injuries: a systematic review. Am J Sports Med. 2014;42:235–41.
7. Schneider MM, Balke M, Koenen P, et al. Inter- and intraobserver reliability of the Rockwood classification in acute acromioclavicular joint dislocations. Knee Surg Sports Traumatol Arthrosc. 2014;24(7):2192–6.
8. Tauber M, Koller H, Hitzl W, Resch H. Dynamic radiologic evaluation of horizontal instability in acute acromioclavicular joint dislocations. Am J Sports Med. 2010;38:1188–95.
9. Gastaud O, Raynier JL, Duparc F, et al. Reliability of radiographic measurements for acromioclavicular joint separations. Orthop Traumatol Surg Res. 2015;101:S291–5.
10. Vaisman A, Villalon Montenegro IE, Tuca De Diego MJ, Valderrama Ronco JA. Novel radiographic index for the diagnosis of posterior acromioclavicular joint dislocations. Am J Sports Med. 2014;42:112–6.
11. Bossart PJ, Joyce SM, Manaster BJ, Packer SM. Lack of efficacy of 'weighted' radiographs in diagnosing acute acromioclavicular separation. Ann Emerg Med. 1988;17:20–4.
12. Ibrahim EF, Forrest NP, Forester A. Bilateral weighted radiographs are required for accurate classification of acromioclavicular separation: an observational study of 59 cases. Injury. 2015;46:1900–5.
13. Izadpanah K, Winterer J, Vicari M, et al. A stress MRI of the shoulder for evaluation of ligamentous stabilizers in acute and chronic acromioclavicular joint instabilities. J Magn Reson Imaging. 2013;37:1486–92.
14. Kumar Y, Hayashi D. Role of magnetic resonance imaging in acute spinal trauma: a pictorial review. BMC Musculoskelet Disord. 2016;17:310.
15. Cho CH, Hwang I, Seo JS, et al. Reliability of the classification and treatment of dislocations of the acromioclavicular joint. J Shoulder Elb Surg. 2014;23:665–70.
16. Matter HP, Gruber G, Harland U. Possibilities of ultrasound diagnosis in Tossy type III acromioclavicular joint injuries in comparison with loaded roentgen images. Sportverletz Sportschaden. 1995;9:14–20.
17. Tischer T, Salzmann GM, El-Azab H, Vogt S, Imhoff AB. Incidence of associated injuries with acute acromioclavicular joint dislocations types III through V. Am J Sports Med. 2009;37:136–9.
18. Takase KMRI. Evaluation of coracoclavicular ligament injury in acromioclavicular joint separation. Eur J Orthop Surg Traumatol. 2011;21:563–8.
19. Nemec U, Oberleitner G, Nemec SF, et al. MRI versus radiography of acromioclavicular joint dislocation. AJR Am J Roentgenol. 2011;197:968–73.
20. Fenkl R, Gotzen L. Sonographic diagnosis of the injured acromioclavicular joint. A standardized examination procedure. Unfallchirurg. 1992;95:393–400.
21. Kock HJ, Jurgens C, Hanke J, Schmit-Neuerburg KP. Standardized ultrasound examination for classification of instability of the acromioclavicular joint. Unfallchirurgie. 1994;20:66–71.
22. Iovane A, Midiri M, Galia M, et al. Acute traumatic acromioclavicular joint lesions: role of ultrasound versus conventional radiography. Radiol Med. 2004;107:367–75.
23. Schmid A, Schmid F. Use of arthrosonography in the diagnosis of Tossy injuries of the shoulder joint. Aktuelle Traumatol. 1988;18:134–8.
24. Beitzel K, Cote MP, Apostolakos J, et al. Current concepts in the treatment of acromioclavicular joint dislocations. Arthroscopy. 2013;29:387–97.
25. Rahm S, Wieser K, Spross C, Vich M, Gerber C, Meyer DC. Standard axillary radiographs of the shoulder may mimic posterior subluxation of the lateral end of the clavicle. J Orthop Trauma. 2013;27:622–6.
26. Barth J, Boutsiadis A, Narbona P, et al. The anterior borders of the clavicle and the acromion are not always aligned in the intact acromioclavicular joint: a cadaveric study. J Shoulder Elb Surg. 2017;26:1121–7.
27. Alexander OM. Dislocation of the acromioclavicular joint. *Radiography.* 1949;15:260, illust.
28. Waldrop JI, Norwood LA, Alvarez RG. Lateral roentgenographic projections of the acromioclavicular joint. Am J Sports Med. 1981;9:337–41.
29. Allman FL Jr. Fractures and ligamentous injuries of the clavicle and its articulation. J Bone Joint Surg Am. 1967;49:774–84.
30. Post M. Current concepts in the diagnosis and management of acromioclavicular dislocations. Clin Orthop Relat Res. 1985;200:234–47.
31. Harrison RB, Riddervold HO, Willett ED, Stamp WG. Acromio-clavicular separation masked by muscle spasm. Va Med. 1980;107:377–9.
32. Yap JJ, Curl LA, Kvitne RS, McFarland EG. The value of weighted views of the acromioclavicular joint. Results of a survey. Am J Sports Med. 1999;27:806–9.
33. Landis JR, Koch GG. The measurement of observer agreement for categorical data. Biometrics. 1977;33:159–74.
34. Kraeutler MJ, Williams GR Jr, Cohen SB, et al. Inter- and intraobserver reliability of the radiographic diagnosis and treatment of acromioclavicular joint separations. Orthopedics. 2012;35:e1483–7.
35. Kock HJ, Jurgens C, Hirche H, Hanke J, Schmit-Neuerburg KP. Standardized ultrasound examination for evaluation of instability of the acromioclavicular joint. Arch Orthop Trauma Surg. 1996;115:136–40.

9

Methodological considerations in region of interest definitions for paraspinal muscles in axial MRIs of the lumbar spine

David B. Berry[1], Jennifer Padwal[2], Seth Johnson[3], Callan L. Parra[3], Samuel R. Ward[1,3,4] and Bahar Shahidi[3,4*]

Abstract

Background: Magnetic Resonance Imaging (MRI) is commonly used to assess the health of the lumbar spine and supporting structures. Studies have suggested that fatty infiltration of the posterior lumbar muscles is important in predicting responses to treatment for low back pain. However, methodological differences exist in defining the region of interest (ROI) of a muscle, which limits the ability to compare data between studies. The purpose of this study was to determine reliability and systematic differences within and between two commonly utilized methodologies for ROI definitions of lumbar paraspinal muscle.

Methods: T2-weighted MRIs of the mid-L4 vertebrae from 37 patients with low back pain who were scheduled for lumbar spine surgery were included from a hospital database. Fatty infiltration for these patients ranged from low to high, based on Kjaer criteria. Two methods were used to define ROI: 1) segmentation of the multifidus and erector spinae based on fascial planes including epimuscular fat, and 2) segmentation of the multifidus and erector spinae based on visible muscle boundaries, which did not include epimuscular fat. Total cross sectional area (tCSA), fat signal fraction (FSF), muscle cross sectional area, and fat cross sectional area were measured. Degree of agreement between raters for each parameter was assessed using intra-class correlation coefficients (ICC) and area fraction of overlapping voxels.

Results: Excellent inter-rater agreement (ICC > 0.75) was observed for all measures for both methods. There was no significant difference between area fraction overlap of ROIs between methods. Method 1 demonstrated a greater tCSA for both the erector spinae (14–15%, $p < 0.001$) and multifidus (4%, $p < 0.016$) but a greater FSF only for the erector spinae (11–13%, $p < 0.001$).

Conclusion: The two methods of defining lumbar spine muscle ROIs demonstrated excellent inter-rater reliability, although significant differences exist as method 1 showed larger CSA and FSF values compared to method 2. The results of this study confirm the validity of using either method to measure lumbar paraspinal musculature, and that method should be selected based on the primary outcome variables of interest.

Keywords: Fatty infiltration, MRI, Lumbar spine, Low back pain, Multifidus, Erector spinae

* Correspondence: bshahidi@ucsd.edu
[3]Department of Orthopaedic Surgery, University of California San Diego, 9500 Gilman Drive (MS 0863), La Jolla, CA 92093, USA
[4]Department of Radiology, University of California San Diego, 9500 Gilman Drive (MS 0863), La Jolla, CA 92093, USA
Full list of author information is available at the end of the article

Background

Low back pain (LBP) is a highly prevalent condition, affecting 65–85% of the general population at some point throughout their lifetime [1]. Magnetic resonance imaging (MRI) is a diagnostic tool that is frequently utilized for evaluation of underlying anatomical pathology, as well as to obtain quantitative measures of spinal kinematics, muscle quality, and size, or injuries such as disc herniation, stenosis, or nerve root compression. Recent studies have highlighted the importance of muscle quality (ie. fatty infiltration) and size (cross sectional area or volume) of the lumbar paraspinal musculature in predicting LBP related disability [2, 3], prognosis for recurrence [4–7], and response to exercise [4]. However, these data are confounded by methodological variation across studies, and as such, the interpretation of results are difficult.

One important source of variation in MRI-based measures of muscle size and quality is differences between region of interest (ROI) definitions of muscle compartments. Specifically, there is debate about whether or not to include the epimuscular fat "tent" between muscle and the fascial plane in a ROI [8]. Although several studies demonstrate that intra-class correlation coefficient (ICC) values between and within raters is high for a single method [9, 10], reliability and systematic differences across methods have not been established. There is also potential for different methods to result in systematic error in the extremes of the spectrum of muscle quality (i.e. when there are large amounts of fatty infiltrate) due to the differences in methods for determining fascial boundaries between muscles. For example, some ROI definitions may provide high ICC values in cases with low levels of muscle fatty infiltration, but when the muscle has large amounts of fatty infiltrate, the fascial boundaries may become less obvious and potential for error could increase (Fig. 1).

One important consideration related to these methodological differences is that the basis for these ROI definitions could affect interpretation of the underlying physiological processes thought to be occurring with LBP pathologies. Recent studies have supported the idea that pathological changes in muscle are more related to muscle quality, or fatty infiltration, as compared to just muscle size or cross sectional area (CSA) [11, 12]. The underlying biological process related to muscle atrophy is thought to be a result of disuse or decreased metabolic demand [13], which leads to decreases in the size of the muscle compartment. However, fatty infiltration is associated with an accumulation of fat, both within the muscle compartment (intrafascicular fatty infiltration), and outside the epimyseal border (epimuscular fatty infiltration) [14]. These fatty infiltration measures typically quantify fat signal fraction within a defined ROI, and may be largely influenced by the definition of this ROI. Therefore, understanding the magnitude of differences between commonly utilized methods will allow not only for more accurate comparisons of data across studies, but also will allow a more informed interpretation of the underlying physiological changes as a result of pathology. Therefore, the purpose of this study is to determine reliability and systematic differences within and between two commonly utilized methodologies for ROI definitions of the paraspinal muscles in the lumbar spine.

Methods

Study participants

MRIs from 37 patients were selected from a larger cohort of 236 patients, who were identified based on current procedural terminology (CPT) codes for lumbar spine surgical procedures between 2005 and 2015 at UC San Diego hospitals. Inclusion criterion for this cohort have been previously described [15]. The patients selected in this study were patients with LBP chosen to represent the full range

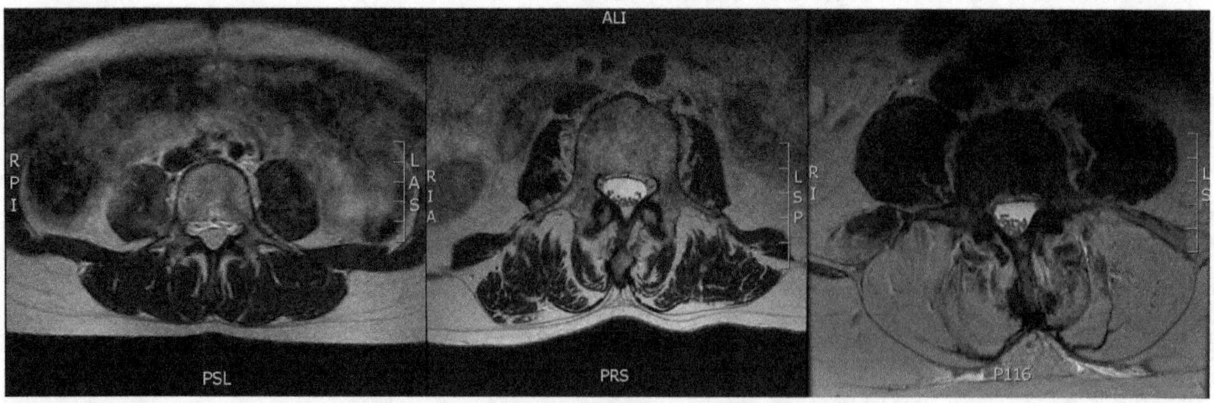

Fig. 1 T2 weighted axial MR images of the lumbar spine. Images represent Kjaer grade [16] 0 (left), 1 (center), and 2 (right) muscles of the lumbar spine. All images are from patients undergoing surgery for low back pain related pathology

of muscle fatty infiltrations observed in patients with Kjaer grades 0–2 [16]. All images analyzed in this study were obtained from T2-weighted MRIs at the mid L4 vertebrae to standardize lumbar spine level across patients [17].

Region of interest definition

Regions of interest (ROIs) for both the multifidus and erector spinae muscles were segmented bilaterally using OsiriX software [18]. Two methods of identifying the posterior boundary of the regions of interest were used:

1. Method 1 – Muscle ROI definitions were based on fascial plane separation using the facet joint as a landmark between the multifidus and erector spinae, and the lumbosacral fascia posteriorly. When a large fat-filled "tent" was observed between the longissimus and illiocostalis, this region was *included* in the ROI because it uses the posterior fascial plane as a border (Fig. 2). Additionally, fat tents lateral to the illiocostalis and under the lumbosacral fascial plane were *included* in the region of interest. This technique has previously been defined in Shahidi et al. [15].
2. Method 2 – Segmentation was based on the fascial plane separation using the facet joint as a landmark between the multifidus and erector spinae, and the epimyseal border posteriorly. When a large fat-filled tent was observed between the longissimus and illiocostalis, this region was *excluded* from the ROI (Fig. 2). Additionally, fatty regions lateral to the illiocostalis and under the fascial plane were *excluded* in the region of interest. This technique has previously been defined in detail in Crawford et al. [8].

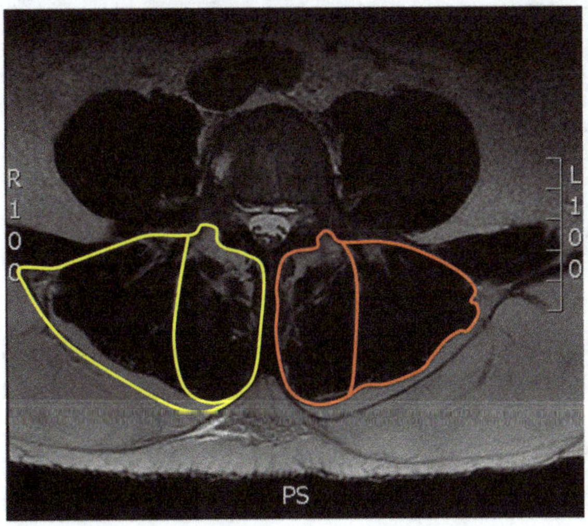

Fig. 2 Sample region of interest definitions of the erector spinae and multifidus muscles using Method 1 (yellow) and Method 2 (red)

Three raters with varying levels of experience with lumbar spine muscle ROI measurements (J.P., S.J., B.S.) underwent standardized training based on the strict criteria noted above for both methods. ROI measurements for each method were randomized for each rater and each rater was blinded to prior ROI definitions.

ROIs were then imported into a custom written Matlab software (Mathworks, Natick, MA) to measure total cross sectional area (tCSA), fat signal fraction (FSF), muscle cross sectional area (mCSA), and fat cross sectional area (fCSA). Pixels were identified as either fat or muscle by fitting a two-term Gaussian model to the histogram of pixel intensities from segmented regions of interest, and finding the intersection of the Gaussian distributions. Pixel values above the intersection were classified as fat, and pixels below were classified as muscle. This thresholding method has been previously described in detail [15]. Total cross sectional area was defined as the total area of the ROI for each muscle. tCSA (Eq. 1), FSF (Eq. 2), mCSA (Eq. 3) and fCSA (Eq. 4) were defined as:

$$tCSA = \sum pixels_{fat} + \sum pixels_{muscle} \tag{1}$$

$$FSF = \frac{npixels_{fat}}{npixels_{fat} + npixels_{muscle}} \tag{2}$$

$$mCSA = tCSA\text{–}tCSA * FSF \tag{3}$$

$$fCSA = tCSA * FSF \tag{4}$$

Statistical analysis

The level of agreement between raters for tCSA, FSF, mCSA, and fCSA was assessed using ICC's for each muscle and method. ICC estimates and their 95% confidence intervals were based on a mean rating (k = 3), absolute agreement, 2-way mixed effects model. Interpretations of ICC results were based on the guidelines proposed by Cicchetti 1994 [19]: less than 0.40 = poor agreement, 0.40–0.59 = fair agreement, 0.60–0.74 = good agreement, > 0.75 = excellent agreement. In order to assess the how similar the masks drawn by each rater were to each other, area fraction overlap was calculated (Eq. 5), defined as the number of voxels overlapping across all 3 rater masks, divided by the cumulative masked area (Figs. 3 and 4).

$$Area\ fraction\ overlap = \frac{\sum common\ voxels}{total\ area\ of\ voxels\ across\ raters} \tag{5}$$

A paired samples t-test was performed to identify any differences between the overlapping area fractions in the masks (tCSA, FSF, mCSA, and fCSA) of the two methods for each muscle on each side. The relationship

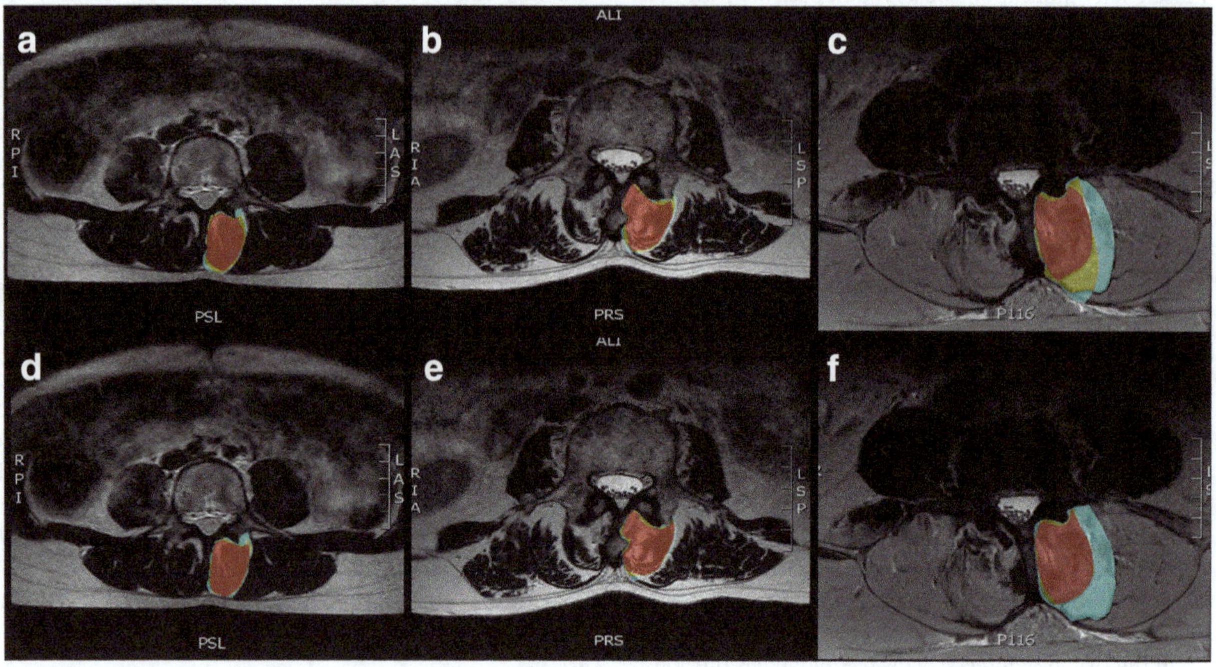

Fig. 3 Examples of overlapping regions of interest defined by all 3 raters (red), 2 raters (yellow), or 1 rater (blue) for the multifidus muscle using region of interest definitions from method 1 (**a-c**) and method 2 (**d-f**) for muscles with Kjaer grade 0 (**a**, **d**), 1 (**b**, **e**), and 2 (**c**, **f**)

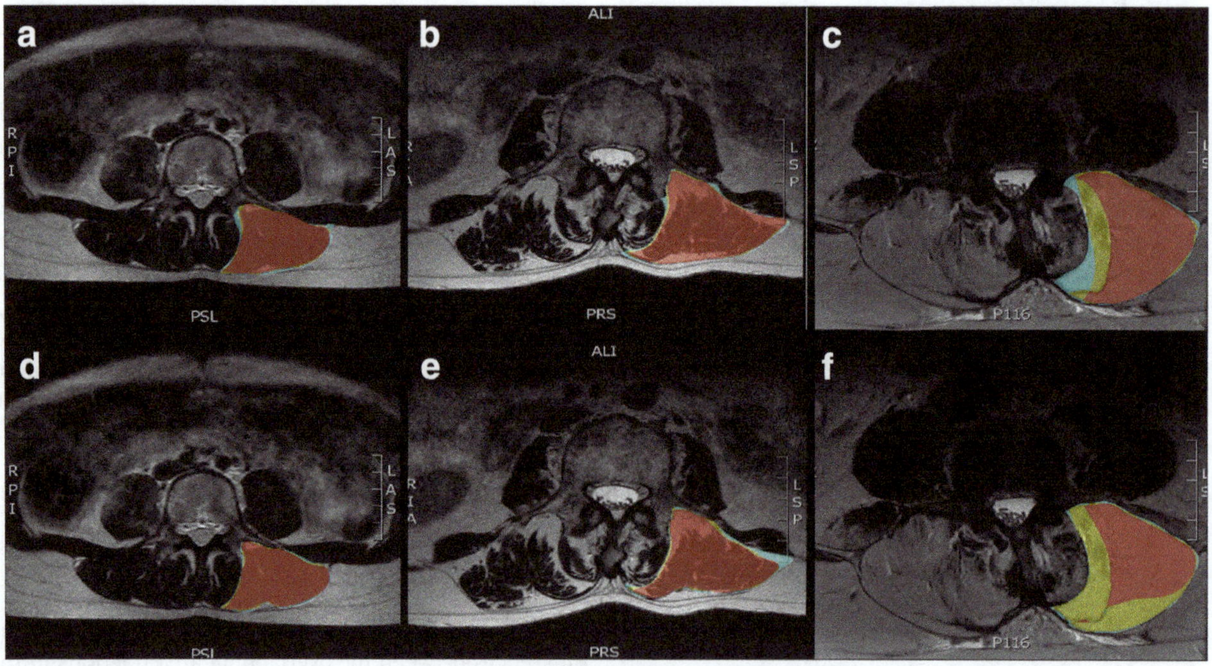

Fig. 4 Examples of overlapping regions of interest defined by all 3 raters (red), 2 raters (yellow), or 1 rater (blue) for the erector spinae muscles using region of interest definitions from method 1 (**a-c**) and method 2 (**d-f**) for muscles with Kjaer grade 0 (**a**, **d**), 1 (**b**, **e**), and 2 (**c**, **f**)

between inter-rater coefficients of variation (CV) and absolute tCSA, FSF, mCSA, or fCSA was assessed by linear regression for each muscle and method. All statistics were performed using SPSS Statistics (Version 21, IBM, Armonk, NY). All data are reported as mean ± standard deviation.

Results

Excellent inter-rater agreement (ICC > 0.75) was observed for all measures for both methods (Table 1). Comparisons between the three raters consistently demonstrated high ICC, with the lowest ICC found for left multifidus tCSA (ICC 0.879; 95% CI 0.761–0.938) and the highest ICC found for right erector spinae FSF (ICC 0.997; 95% CI 0.994–0.998). The ICC's for method 1 ranged from 0.879 (0.761–0.938) to 0.997 (0.994–0.998) for the left multifidus tCSA and right erector spinae FSF, respectively. The ICC's for method 2 ranged from 0.928 (0.861–0.963) to 0.995 (0.960–0.997) for the right multifidus tCSA and left erector spinae mCSA, respectively.

The area fraction overlap included in all three ROIs ranged from 0.72–0.85 for method 1 and 0.73–0.83 for method 2. There were no significant differences in the area fraction overlap between methods ($p = 0.071–0.543$). However, a trend was identified for the right erector

Table 1 ICC results

Measure	Method	Side	Muscle	ICC	95% confidence interval	
					Lower bound	Upper bound
tCSA	1	Left	Multifidus	0.879	0.761	0.938
			Erector Sp.	0.973	0.951	0.986
		Right	Multifidus	0.886	0.771	0.942
			Erector Sp.	0.971	0.948	0.984
	2	Left	Multifidus	0.946	0.897	0.972
			Erector Sp.	0.979	0.951	0.99
		Right	Multifidus	0.928	0.861	0.963
			Erector Sp.	0.968	0.931	0.984
FSF	1	Left	Multifidus	0.987	0.978	0.993
			Erector Sp.	0.996	0.994	0.998
		Right	Multifidus	0.982	0.969	0.99
			Erector Sp.	0.997	0.994	0.998
	2	Left	Multifidus	0.994	0.99	0.997
			Erector Sp.	0.992	0.976	0.997
		Right	Multifidus	0.980	0.965	0.989
			Erector Sp.	0.991	0.978	0.996
mCSA	1	Left	Multifidus	0.939	0.883	0.968
			Erector Sp.	0.981	0.966	0.99
		Right	Multifidus	0.935	0.882	0.965
			Erector Sp.	0.982	0.969	0.99
	2	Left	Multifidus	0.981	0.961	0.99
			Erector Sp.	0.995	0.990	0.997
		Right	Multifidus	0.972	0.948	0.985
			Erector Sp.	0.994	0.989	0.997
fCSA	1	Left	Multifidus	0.954	0.905	0.977
			Erector Sp.	0.992	0.985	0.995
		Right	Multifidus	0.962	0.905	0.982
			Erector Sp.	0.987	0.975	0.993
	2	Left	Multifidus	0.969	0.945	0.984
			Erector Sp.	0.981	0.944	0.992
		Right	Multifidus	0.953	0.913	0.975
			Erector Sp.	0.963	0.915	0.983

Erector Sp. Erector Spinae

spinae group, with method 2 having less overlap than method 1 (– 0.05; $p = 0.071$).

There were systematic differences in tCSA, FSF, mCSA, and fCSA between method 1 and method 2 (Table 2). As expected, tCSA was 14–15% larger in the erector spinae ($p < 0.001$) and 4% larger in the multifidus ($p < 0.016$) in method 1 than method 2 because of the inclusion of the lumbosacral fascial border in the ROI definition (Table 2). The inclusion of the posterior fat tent in method 1 also resulted in a 11–13% increase in the overall fat signal fraction for the erector spinae (p < 0.001). Additionally, method 1 measures of erector spinae mCSA and fCSA increased by 5 and 30% respectively ($p < 0.011$). Of note is that while a 6–8% increase in mCSA was measured in the multifidus with method 1 ($p < 0.037$), no increase in fCSA was found ($p > 0.603$).

Overall CV between raters was similar using method 1 (0.08 ± 0.10, range: 0.001–0.77) and method 2 (0.08 ± 0.08, range: 0.001–0.62) for all measures for all muscles. Between-rater error decreased with increased fCSA ($p = 0.0102$, $R^2 = 0.17$) and FSF ($p = 0.0002$, $R^2 = 0.33$) for in the left multifidus and increased FSF ($p = 0.0032$, $R^2 = 0.22$) in the left erector spinae for method 2 (Fig. 5). Additionally, between-rater error was found to decrease with increased FSF ($p = 0.0114$, $R^2 = 0.17$) for method 1 only in the right erector spinae muscle, with no other significant relationships between error and outcomes.

Discussion

This study determined that the reliability for two commonly utilized ROI methods for measuring paraspinal muscle in the lumbar region is high, however there are systematic differences in cross sectional area and fat fraction between the two methods. Method 1, not surprisingly, demonstrates larger CSA and FSF values as compared to method 2. This discrepancy is due to the inclusion of the fatty region between the lumbosacral fascia and the epimysium of the multifidus and erector spinae muscles in method 1, which is excluded in method 2. For both methods, muscle and side specific errors in FSF and fCSA between raters were found to decrease as level of fatty infiltrate increased. This may be due to inherent FSF asymmetry that exists in most patients, which is likely reflected in the anatomical structure and myofascial borders of the muscles of the patients included in this study. Finally, no discrepancy in whole ROI definition (tCSA) was observed between sides using either method.

Muscle volume is a primary input variable for measuring physiological cross sectional area of muscle [20], which is correlated to muscle force generating capacity [20–22]. Muscle CSA is often measured as it is related to muscle volume, and it is relatively easy to measure a single slice across a muscle as compared to the entire volume. As the area fraction of functional contractile tissue decreases, it follows that whole muscle force generating capacity declines, which may result in decreased overall functional capacity. As the erector spinae and multifidus muscles undergo atrophy, the CSA of individual muscle fibers and fascicles decreases, and fat accumulates between the perimysial layers (fascicle atrophy) and epimysium and lumbosacral fascia as a result. In pathological muscle, this atrophy is often accompanied by intrafascicular fatty infiltration, which involves interdigitation of adipocytes throughout the muscle within the perimysial and epimyseal borders [14, 16].

As such, determination of the appropriate method for defining ROI's in lumbar paraspinal musculature should be dependent on the desired feature of muscle anatomy and physiology to be measured. Prior literature supporting the exclusion of the fatty region in-between the lumbosacral fascia and the epimysium uses the rationale that calculations of muscle area and fatty infiltration

Table 2 Average tCSA, FSF, mCSA, and fCSA measured using both methods

Side	Muscle	tCSA (mm^2)			FSF		
		Method 1	Method 2	*p*-value	Method 1	Method 2	*p*-value
Left	Erector Sp.	18.54 ± 4.97	16.17 ± 4.06	< 0.001	0.42 ± 0.14	0.38 ± 0.14	< 0.001
	Multifidus	9.08 ± 2.59	8.73 ± 2.44	0.016	0.47 ± 0.18	0.48 ± 0.18	0.216
Right	Erector Sp.	17.88 ± 5.31	15.71 ± 4.23	< 0.001	0.43 ± 0.16	0.38 ± 0.16	< 0.001
	Multifidus	9.14 ± 2.77	8.77 ± 2.48	0.003	0.46 ± 0.18	0.48 ± 0.17	0.209
Side	Muscle	mCSA (mm^2)			fCSA (mm^2)		
		Method 1	Method 2	*p*-value	Method 1	Method 2	*p*-value
Left	Erector Sp.	10.63 ± 3.80	10.09 ± 3.65	0.001	7.92 ± 4.08	6.08 ± 2.98	< 0.001
	Multifidus	4.90 ± 2.29	4.62 ± 2.18	0.037	4.18 ± 1.87	4.11 ± 1.71	0.603
Right	Erector Sp.	10.25 ± 4.24	9.85 ± 4.07	0.011	7.62 ± 3.54	5.86 ± 2.88	< 0.001
	Multifidus	4.91 ± 2.32	4.55 ± 2.03	0.011	4.23 ± 2.15	4.22 ± 1.99	0.907

Erector Sp. Erector Spinae

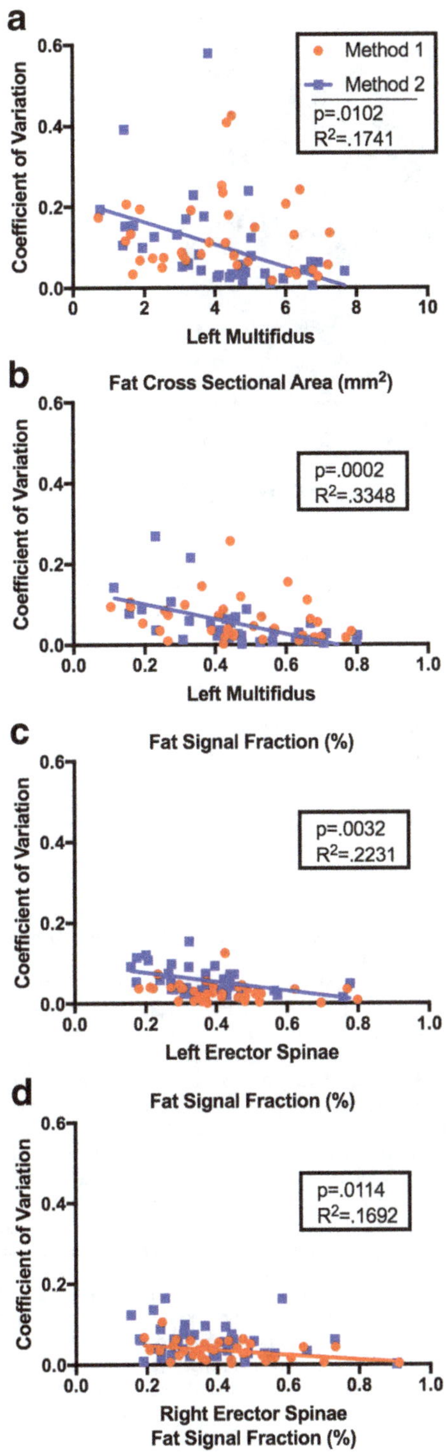

Fig. 5 Between-rater error (Coefficient of Variation) decreased with increased left multifidus fCSA (**a**), left multifidus FSF (**b**), and left erector spinae FSF (**c**), for method 2 (blue). Between rater error decreased with increased right erector spinae FSF (**d**) for method 1 (red)

should only include the region of tissue within the epimysial border [8]. This definition is likely to provide different information about atrophy versus intrafascicular fatty infiltration. For example, in the normal healthy lumbar spine, the paraspinal epimyseal borders approximate the lumbosacral fascia, and some of the fibers of the multifidus even originate in the lumbosacral fascia [23–25]. As the apparent area between the lumbosacral facial plane and epimyseal border is infiltrated by fat (increased epimuscular fatty infiltration), muscle tCSA would decrease, without a concurrent increase in FSF when measured by method 2 (Fig. 6). Therefore, this method can provide an accurate measurement of intramuscular fatty infiltration in the absence of epimuscular fatty changes. This may be helpful in determining muscle quality within the epimyseal borders, and still yields an accurate measure of mCSA.

In contrast, the inclusion of the epimuscular fat compartment in method 1 would reflect an overall increase in fatty infiltration (both intra- and epi-muscular), which may be a more accurate representation of atrophy for a given individual, based on the observations that in normal healthy muscle (in the absence of atrophy), the epimyseal border and the lumbosacral fascia should approximate each other. However, it would not necessarily provide information distinguishing intramuscular and epimuscular fat. It is unknown currently whether there are biological and functional differences between epimuscular and intramuscular fatty infiltration processes, however, literature suggests that muscle quality, not size, is a more relevant predictor of muscle pathology in individuals with LBP [5, 12, 15]. Importantly, weight does not seem to have an influence on fat fraction when including the epimuscular fat, further suggesting that this is a feature that is independently related to muscle health [15]. Future research is needed to determine whether there are distinct biological processes that differentiate the functional consequences of epimuscular versus intramuscular fatty infiltration.

Conclusions

In this study, excellent agreement was found between two common methods used to define the regions of interest of the multifidus and erector spinae muscle from axial MRIs. Inclusion of the fat in-between the epimyseal border and the fascial plane results in larger values for tCSA, FSF, fCSA and mCSA when compared to excluding the area of fat, with no differences in variance. The decision to include or exclude the fat area from a region of interest measurement of the lumbar muscles should be made based on the primary outcome a researcher is interested in measuring. Inclusion of the fat area results in a more gross measure of fatty

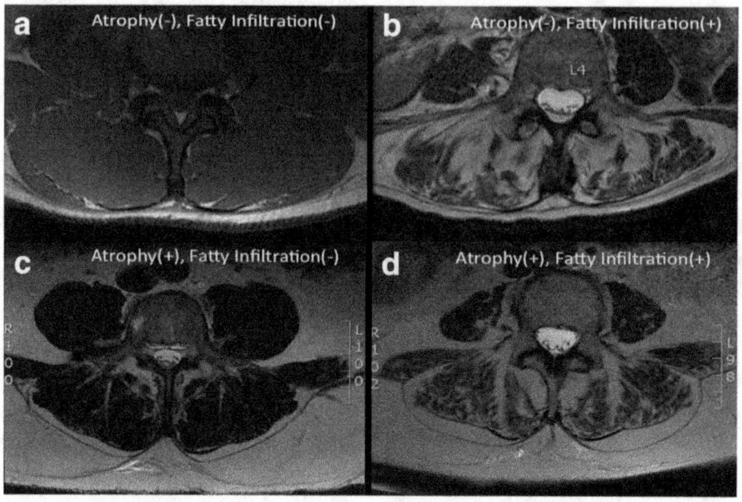

Fig. 6 Example MRI axial cross-sections illustrating differences in presentation of muscle quality and size across patients. Panel **a** illustrates a healthy patient with no atrophy or fatty infiltration, demonstrating approximation of the epimyseum and border of the lumbosacral fascia. Panel **b** demonstrates an individual with no epimuscular fatty infiltration, but significant fatty deposition within the muscle compartment. Panel **c** represents a patient with very little muscle fatty infiltration within the epimyseal border, and epimuscular fat accumulation between the lumbosacral fascia and the paraspinal muscle compartments. Panel **d** demonstrates an individual with both intramuscular and epimuscular fatty infiltration

accumulation as a result of atrophy, whereas exclusion of the fatty area may be a more specific measure of muscle tissue quality and possibly degenerative changes within the epimyseal border. Future research is needed to explore the biological mechanisms and functional implications of epimuscular and intramuscular fatty infiltration.

Abbreviations

CPT: Current procedural terminology; CV: Coefficient of variation; fCSA: Fat cross-sectional area; FSF: Fat signal fraction; ICC: Intra-class correlation coefficients; LBP: Low back pain; mCSA: Muscle cross-sectional area; MRI: Magnetic resonance imaging; ROI: Region of interest; tCSA: Total cross-sectional area

Funding

S.R.W. is supported by grants from the National Institute of Health (R01AR070830, R01HD073180, R01HD088437) and Department of Defense (PR120576). B.S. is supported by grants from the National Institute of Health (R01HD088437, R03HD094598, and TL1TR001443). These funding bodies provided funding for data acquisition and collection only, with no contribution to analysis, study design, interpretation, or manuscript preparation.

Authors' contributions

DB designed the experiment, analyzed the MRI data, and was a major contributor in writing the manuscript. JP was a major contributor in writing the manuscript and analyzed the MRI data. SJ analyzed the MRI data. CP analyzed the MRI data and contributed to writing the manuscript. SRW designed the experiment and revised the manuscript. BS designed the experiment, analyzed the MRI data, and was a major contributor in writing the manuscript. All authors read and approved the final manuscript.

Competing interests

The authors declare that they have no competing interests.

Author details

[1]Department of Bioengineering, University of California San Diego, La Jolla, CA, USA. [2]Department of Medicine, University of California San Diego, La Jolla, CA, USA. [3]Department of Orthopaedic Surgery, University of California San Diego, 9500 Gilman Drive (MS 0863), La Jolla, CA 92093, USA. [4]Department of Radiology, University of California San Diego, 9500 Gilman Drive (MS 0863), La Jolla, CA 92093, USA.

References

1. Andersson GB. Epidemiological features of chronic low-back pain. Lancet. 1999;354(9178):581–5.
2. Hicks GE, Simonsick EM, Harris TB, Newman AB, Weiner DK, Nevitt MA, Tylavsky FA. Trunk muscle composition as a predictor of reduced functional capacity in the health, aging and body composition study: the moderating role of back pain. J Gerontol A Biol Sci Med Sci. 2005;60(11):1420–4.
3. Alaranta H, Tallroth K, Soukka A, Heliövaara M. Fat content of lumbar extensor muscles and low back disability: a radiographic and clinical comparison. J Spinal Disord. 1993;6(2):137–40.
4. Hides JA, Jull GA, Richardson CA. Long-term effects of specific stabilizing exercises for first-episode low back pain. Spine. 2001;26(11):E243–8.
5. D'hooge R, Cagnie B, Crombez G, Vanderstraeten G, Dolphens M, Danneels L. Increased intramuscular fatty infiltration without differences in lumbar muscle cross-sectional area during remission of unilateral recurrent low back pain. Man Ther. 2012;17(6):584–8.
6. Lee HI, Song J, Lee HS, Kang JY, Kim M, Ryu JS. Association between cross-sectional areas of lumbar muscles on magnetic resonance imaging and chronicity of low back pain. Ann Rehabil Med. 2011;35(6):852–9.
7. Barker KL, Shamley DR, Jackson D. Changes in the cross-sectional area of multifidus and psoas in patients with unilateral back pain: the relationship to pain and disability. Spine (Phila Pa 1976). 2004;29(22):E515–9.
8. Crawford RJ, Cornwall J, Abbott R, Elliott JM. Manually defining regions of interest when quantifying paravertebral muscles fatty infiltration from axial magnetic resonance imaging: a proposed method for the lumbar spine with anatomical cross-reference. BMC Musculoskelet Disord. 2017;18(1):25.
9. Ranson CA, Burnett AF, Kerslake R, Batt ME, O'Sullivan PB. An investigation into the use of MR imaging to determine the functional cross sectional area of lumbar paraspinal muscles. Eur Spine J. 2006;15(6):764–73.
10. Fortin M, Battié MC. Quantitative paraspinal muscle measurements: inter-software reliability and agreement using OsiriX and ImageJ. Phys Ther. 2012; 92(6):853–64.

11. Shahidi B, Johnson CL, Curran-Everett D, Maluf KS. Reliability and group differences in quantitative cervicothoracic measures among individuals with and without chronic neck pain. BMC Musculoskelet Disord. 2012;13:215.
12. Teichtahl AJ, Urquhart DM, Wang Y, Wluka AE, Wijethilake P, O'Sullivan R, Cicuttini FM. Fat infiltration of paraspinal muscles is associated with low back pain, disability and structural abnormalities in community-based adults. Spine J. 2015;15(7):1593–601.
13. Bonaldo P, Sandri M. Cellular and molecular mechanisms of muscle atrophy. Dis Model Mech. 2013;6(1):25–39.
14. Gibbons MC, Singh A, Anakwenze O, Cheng T, Pomerantz M, Schenk S, Engler AJ, Ward SR. Histological evidence of muscle degeneration in advanced human rotator cuff disease. J Bone Joint Surg Am. 2017;99(3):190–9.
15. Shahidi B, Parra CL, Berry DB, Hubbard JC, Gombatto S, Zlomislic V, Allen RT, Hughes-Austin J, Garfin S, Ward SR. Contribution of lumbar spine pathology and age to Paraspinal muscle size and fatty infiltration. Spine (Phila Pa 1976). 2016;42(8):616–23.
16. Kjaer P, Bendix T, Sorensen JS, Korsholm L, Leboeuf-Yde C. Are MRI-defined fat infiltrations in the multifidus muscles associated with low back pain? BMC Med. 2007;5:2.
17. Shahidi B, Hubbard JC, Gibbons MC, Ruoss S, Zlomislic V, Allen RT, Garfin SR, Ward SR. Lumbar multifidus muscle degenerates in individuals with chronic degenerative lumbar spine pathology. J Orthop Res. 2017;35(12):2700–6.
18. Rosset A, Spadola L, Ratib O. OsiriX: an open-source software for navigating in multidimensional DICOM images. J Digit Imaging. 2004;17(3):205–16.
19. Cicchetti DV. Multiple comparison methods: establishing guidelines for their valid application in neuropsychological research. J Clin Exp Neuropsychol. 1994;16(1):155–61.
20. Powell PL, Roy RR, Kanim P, Bello MA, Edgerton VR. Predictability of skeletal muscle tension from architectural determinations in guinea pig hindlimbs. J Appl Physiol Respir Environ Exerc Physiol. 1984;57(6):1715–21.
21. Fortin M, Macedo LG. Multifidus and paraspinal muscle group cross-sectional areas of patients with low back pain and control patients: a systematic review with a focus on blinding. Phys Ther. 2013;93(7):873–88.
22. Demoulin C, Crielaard JM, Vanderthommen M. Spinal muscle evaluation in healthy individuals and low-back-pain patients: a literature review. Joint Bone Spine. 2007;74(1):9–13.
23. Hides JA, Stanton WR, McMahon S, Sims K, Richardson CA. Effect of stabilization training on multifidus muscle cross-sectional area among young elite cricketers with low back pain. J Orthop Sports Phys Ther. 2008; 38(3):101–8.
24. Wallwork TL, Stanton WR, Freke M, Hides JA. The effect of chronic low back pain on size and contraction of the lumbar multifidus muscle. Man Ther. 2009;14(5):496–500.
25. Willard FH, Vleeming A, Schuenke MD, Danneels L, Schleip R. The thoracolumbar fascia: anatomy, function and clinical considerations. J Anat. 2012;221(6):507–36.

10

Measurements of the trapezius and erector spinae muscles using virtual touch imaging quantification ultrasound-Elastography

Anne Heizelmann[1], Sümeyra Tasdemir[1], Julian Schmidberger[1], Tilmann Gräter[2], Wolfgang Kratzer[1*] and Beate Grüner[3]

Abstract

Background: This study uses virtual touch imaging quantification (VTIQ) technology for the first time to conduct measurements of the trapezius and erector spinae muscles in a large study population. The significance of various influencing factors, such as age and sex, are also examined.

Method: The study population comprised 278 subjects. The Siemens Acuson S3000 and VTIQ technology were used for measurements of the trapezius and erector spinae muscles (Siemens Healthcare, Erlangen, Germany).

Results: The following mean values ± standard deviation were calculated: left trapezius: males 2.89 ± 0.38 m/s, females 2.71 ± 0.37 m/s; right trapezius: males 2.84 ± 0.41 m/s, females 2.70 ± 0.38 m/s; left erector spinae: males 2.97 ± 0.50 m/s, females 2.81 ± 0.57 m/s; right erector spinae: males 3.00 ± 0.52 m/s, females 2.77 ± 0.59 m/s. A significant difference between male and female subjects was demonstrated both for the shear wave velocities of the trapezius and erector spinae as well as for the thickness of the trapezius muscle ($p < 0.05$). There was also a significant difference in muscle elasticity between subjects over 60 years of age and those under 60 ($p < 0.05$). Furthermore, the results indicate that regular physical activity has an effect on muscle elasticity.

Conclusions: Our results demonstrate significantly different results between male and female subjects and between under- and over-sixty-year-old subjects. This means that sex-related and age-adapted considerations are obviously needed for further studies.

Keywords: Virtual touch imaging quantification, Muscles, Ultrasound Elastography, Trapezius, Erector spinae

Background

Tissue elasticity can be affected by pathological processes such as inflammation or tumours and is of diagnostic significance for many diseases [1]. The elasticity of muscle tissue is also subject to change due to various diseases, resulting for example in fatty depositions or fibrosis [2]. An increase in collagen fibres is also found, for example, in cases of sarcopoenia [3–6]. Several studies have shown that the elasticity of muscle tissue is affected both in congenital and acquired muscle diseases [6–10].

The possibility of measuring and quantifying these changes in the elasticity of muscle tissue can provide further information about the pathogenesis and pathophysiology of muscular disorders and can be used in a clinical setting for establishing a diagnosis, following up on the disease course and monitoring therapy [6, 11, 12].

Ultrasound elastography was developed in 1991 by Ophir et al. and represents a method for determining and measuring changes in tissue elasticity more exactly [13]. Virtual touch imaging quantification technology is a form of shear wave elastography and was used in this

* Correspondence: wolfgang.kratzer@uniklinik-ulm.de
[1]Department of Internal Medicine I, Ulm University Hospital, Albert-Einstein-Allee, 23 89081 Ulm, Germany
Full list of author information is available at the end of the article

study to measure shear wave propagation velocity in tissue. Tissue elasticity can be determined based on the fact that shear wave velocity increases with progressive stiffness of the tissue [6, 11, 14].

We examined the trapezius and erector spinae muscles in this study because muscle pain and stiffness commonly present in the back and neck regions [12]. Myofascial trigger points are often found in the trapezius, but the present state of research in this field has not entirely understood their pathophysiology and pathogenesis. Further research is also made difficult by the lack of objective examination methods, as currently there is no other recognised diagnostic criterion apart from simple palpation [7, 11, 12, 15, 16]. Shear wave elastography represents a further possible examination method in addition to B-mode ultrasound imaging, in which trigger points are displayed by their reduced echogenicity. Shear wave elastography is able to measure objectively the mechanical properties of trigger points, which appear harder in comparison with non-affected muscle [7, 8, 12, 16]. The role of the muscles of the back (such as, for example, the erector spinae) and of the fasciae in the development of pain in the region of the lower back is the subject of an increasing number of research projects [17], since low back pain is very common with a lifetime prevalence of 75–84% [18]. Possible examination methods for assessing lumbar muscles include, for example, magnetic resonance imaging and computed tomography [19]. Thus, a number of studies were able to show that increased fat content in the erector spinae or multifidus is associated with pain in the lower part of the back [20–23]. At present, there are no studies available which have examined the erector spinae muscle of patients with low back pain using shear wave elastography, and the question arises as to whether pathological alterations in the erector spinae of patients with low back pain can also be detected by shear wave elastography.

The aim of this study was to conduct measurements of the trapezius and erector spinae muscles using virtual touch imaging quantification technology in a large study population to obtain reference ranges which can be used as a basis for further studies. Furthermore, these values were to be assessed for the effect of any influencing factors such as sex, age, BMI, physical activity and right- or left-handedness.

Methods

Study design

The study was conducted between March 2013 and August 2013 in the Ultrasound Department of Ulm University Hospital. Exclusion criteria included previous surgery, fractures and injuries of the spinal region or shoulder joint area, intervertebral disc prolapse within the last ten years, use of anabolic agents, pregnancy, diabetes mellitus, osteoporosis, rheumatic disorders, inadequate depiction of the trapezius and erector spinae muscles on B-mode ultrasound imaging, and poor quality of the elasticity measurements. The entire study population comprised 324 subjects, 46 of which were excluded because of the mentioned exclusion criteria. The final study population therefore comprised 278 subjects between the ages of 18 and 73 years (110 males and 168 females). The average BMI of the subjects was 22.94 ± 2.81 and the average age was 35.51 ± 14.93 years.

Ultrasound device and measuring method

The Siemens Acuson S3000 (Siemens Healthcare, Erlangen, Germany) and virtual touch imaging quantification (VTIQ) technology were used for this study, allowing a quantitative and qualitative assessment of tissue elasticity in one single measurement.

Study design

The subjects were given a subject information sheet, an informed consent form and a questionnaire which asked them to give relevant information about themselves, such as age, sex, BMI, previous illnesses, operations, injuries, right- or left-handedness, and the extent of physical activity. In addition they were also asked about frequent backache and headache. Examination of the back muscles was conducted with the subjects positioned prone with their arms at the side of their body. The examination couch had a recess at the top end so that the subjects did not need to turn their head to one side and could lie in a relaxed manner. The subjects had to lie resting for three minutes on the examination couch before the measurements were started to allow the muscles to be as relaxed as possible at the time of measuring. Ten different examiners familiar with the use of B-mode ultrasound imaging examined the subjects.

Erector spinae muscle

To examine the erector spinae muscle, the transducer was placed transversely immediately adjacent to the spine, on the right and left side, at the level of the iliac crest, without applying pressure to the skin. The measurements were made successively, each along the lateral tract of the erector spinae muscle. Firstly, a B-mode image was obtained, after which the ROI box for the subsequent elasticity measurement was placed approx. 5 mm below the superficial lamina of the thoracolumbalis fascia. Next, the VTIQ measurements were carried out: a colour-coded elastogram (blue = soft tissue; red = hard tissue) was created and eight ROIs were placed within the previously defined box for the quantitative measurement of the propagation velocities of the shear waves. The ROI box was divided into four quadrants, with two ROIs placed in each quadrant (Fig. 1).

Trapezius muscle

To examine the trapezius muscle, the transducer was placed transversely from a dorsal approach on the right and left side at the level of the vertebra prominens and the mid-clavicular line. The thickness of the right and left trapezius was measured on the B-mode image and the transducer was aligned longitudinally to the muscle fibres within the transverse part of the trapezius muscle. The ROI box was adjusted on the right and left, depending on the thickness of the trapezius, and positioned. Subsequently, the VTIQ measurements were performed, for which purpose eight ROIs were positioned, each on the right and left side, with again two ROIs per box quadrant.

Statistical evaluation

The statistical analysis system (SAS) Version 9.2 of the North American SAS Institutes, Cary, North Carolina, was used for calculating absolute and relative frequencies and for calculating t-tests (normally distributed) and Wilcoxon two-sample tests (not normally distributed). The Shapiro-Wilk test was used to test the data for normal distribution. A significance level of alpha = 0.05 was chosen. The graphs were created using the table calculation program Microsoft Excel 2013 by Microsoft Corporation, Redmond, USA, based on the statistics obtained from the SAS.

Results

Mean values and 95% confidence intervals

The mean values ± standard deviation and 95% confidence interval were calculated for the shear wave velocities of the trapezius and erector spinae muscles and for the thickness of the trapezius. Calculating the 95% confidence interval provides a reference range for the present study (Table 1).

Sex

There was a significant difference between male ($n = 110$) and female subjects ($n = 168$). Male subjects had significantly higher values for shear wave velocity for the trapezius and erector spinae muscles as well as for the thickness of the trapezius muscle ($p < 0.0001$) (Fig. 2).

Age

The study population was divided into one group with subjects ≤60 years of age ($n = 254$) and a second group with subjects >60 years ($n = 24$ (17 ♂, 7♀)). There was a significant difference between these two groups regarding shear wave velocities of the right and left erector spinae muscles and of the right trapezius; the shear wave velocities were higher in the over-sixty-year-olds (Table 2).

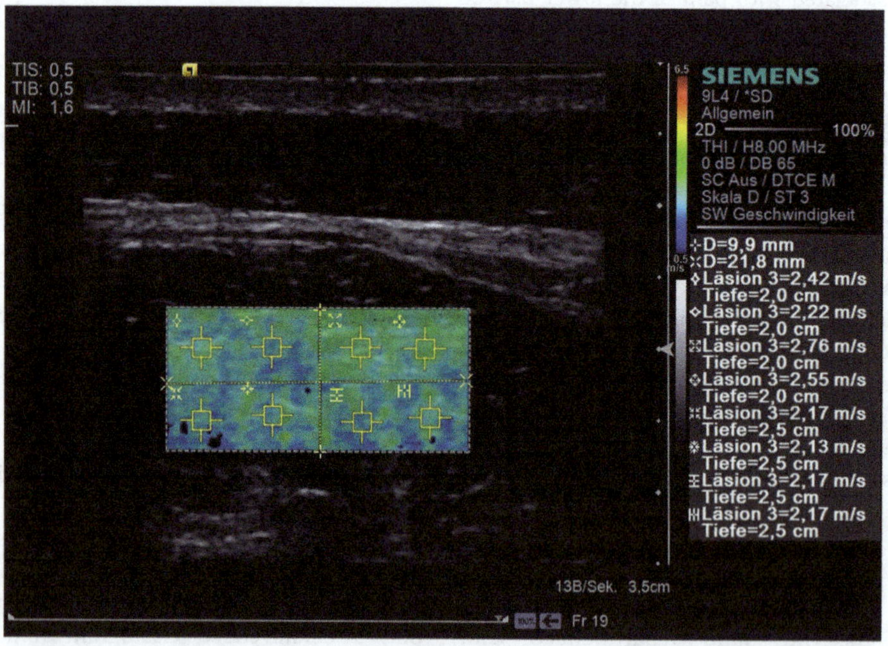

Fig. 1 Examination of the erector spinae muscle. Qualitative and quantitative measurements of the shear wave velocities using virtual touch tissue imaging quantification (Acuson S3000, Siemens) of the erector spinae muscle (shear wave speeds ranging from 0.5 m/s – 6.5 m/s: *blue* = low shear wave velocities, *green* = moderate shear wave velocities, *red* = high shear wave velocities) (Ulm University Hospital, 2013)

Table 1 Mean values ± standard deviation and 95% confidence intervals

		Total (n = 278)	Males (n = 110)	Females (n = 168)
Left trapezius [m/s]	Mean ± SD	2.78 ± 0.38	2.89 ± 0.38	2.71 ± 0.37
	95% confidence interval	[2.73–2.83]	[2.81–2.96]	[2.65–2.77]
Right trapezius [m/s]	Mean ± SD	2.75 ± 0.37	2.84 ± 0.41	2.70 ± 0.38
	95% confidence interval	[2.71–2.80]	[2.76–2.92]	[2.64–2.76]
Left erector spinae [m/s]	Mean ± SD	2.87 ± 0.55	2.97 ± 0.50	2.81 ± 0.57
	95% confidence interval	[2.80–2.93]	[2.87–3.06]	[2.72–2.89]
Right erector spinae [m/s]	Mean ± SD	2.86 ± 0.57	3.00 ± 0.52	2.77 ± 0.59
	95% confidence interval	[2.80–2.93]	[2.90–3.10]	[2.68–2.86]
Thickness left trapezius [mm]	Mean ± SD	11.94 ± 3.05	13.47 ± 3.07	10.93 ± 2.59
	95% confidence interval	[11.58–12.30]	[12.89–14.05]	[10.54–11.32]
Thickness right trapezius [mm]	Mean ± SD	11.95 ± 2.88	13.21 ± 3.03	11.13 ± 2.44
	95% confidence interval	[11.61–12.29]	[12.64–13.79]	[10.75–11.50]

Physical activity of the participants

A subgroup was formed comprising subjects aged 18–30 years (n = 155). Physical activity, specified in hours per week, correlated with the shear wave velocities of the erector spinae muscle (left: p = 0.0021, right: p = 0.0187). No significant correlation was evident in the trapezius muscle (left: p = 0.2024, right: p = 0.3902). Physical activity of the subjects was subdivided into ≤6 h per week (n = 131) and >6 h (n = 24). A significant difference in the thickness of the trapezius was demonstrated on comparing the two groups: (left: p = 0.0249, right: p = 0.0230) and in the shear wave velocities of the erector spinae muscle (left: p = 0.0280 and right: p = 0.0055) (Fig. 3). No significant difference was evident in the trapezius muscle (left: p = 0.6497, right: p = 0.3272).

Correlation between the thickness of the trapezius and muscle elasticity

The thickness of the trapezius muscle correlated with the of the erector spinae. A slight correlation was found in the trapezius muscle only between the thickness of the right trapezius and the shear wave speeds of the right trapezius (Table 3). Calculation of the correlation between shear wave velocities and BMI did not produce any unequivocal results. A significantly negative correlation was evident between the shear wave velocities of the erector spinae and BMI (p < 0.05). There were no

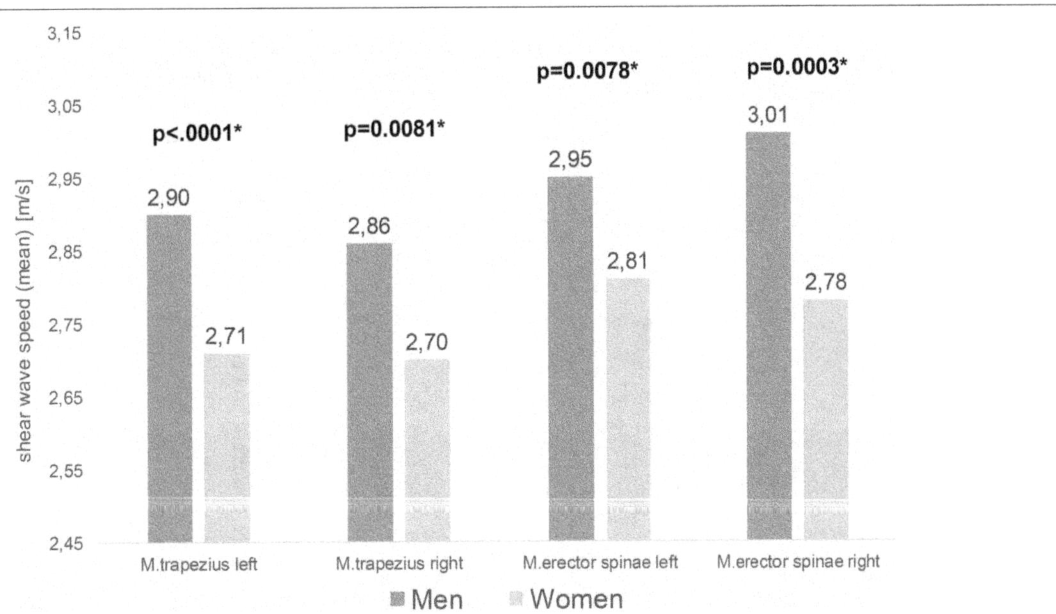

Fig. 2 Shear wave velocities in males and females. Difference between the shear wave velocities of the trapezius and erector spinae muscles in male subjects (n = 110) and female subjects (n = 168); * = statistically significant (Ulm University Hospital, 2013)

Table 2 Shear wave velocities in subjects aged ≤60 and >60 years

N = 278	Mean ± SD ≤ 60 years	Mean ± SD > 60 years	z-value	*p*-value
Left trapezius	2.78 ± 0.38	2.81 ± 0.38	0.3953	0.3463
Right trapezius	2.74 ± 0.41	2.91 ± 0.23	2.05613	*0.0052**
Left erector spinae	2.85 ± 0.52	3.11 ± 0.75	1.7048	*0.0441**
Right erector spinae	2.84 ± 0.58	3.07 ± 0.49	1.9641	*0.0248**

Data not normally distributed: Wilcoxon Two-Sample Test (z-values); * = significant

significant correlations in the comparison of healthy subjects and subjects with frequent backache (n = 65), headache (n = 56) or scoliosis (n = 44). Nor were there any significant results in the comparison between right hand-dominant (n = 242) and left hand-dominant individuals (n = 22). The calculation of differences in shear wave velocities of the trapazius and spinae regarding adipose people (BMI > 25 and <25) adjusted for right and left handed probands showed no significant results and differences ($p > 0.05$).

Discussion

According to our present state of knowledge, this is the first study to perform measurements of the trapezius and erector spinae muscles using virtual touch imaging quantification (VTIQ) technology and the Siemens Acuson S3000 (Siemens Healthcare, Erlangen, Germany). A significant advantage of this study is its large patient population consisting of 278 subjects, as there are currently no studies available with a comparably large study population. Using the Acuson S2000 and virtual touch tissue imaging quantification (VTTQ) technology, Kuo et al. calculated a mean value of 2.0865 ± 0.4480 m/s with their measurements of the trapezius muscle of 20 subjects, a value that is lower than the mean values calculated by the present study for the trapezius [24]. Since Kuo et al. examined their subjects seated, and therefore in a different position from that used in the present study, and also used different Siemens software applications, a comparison between the two studies does not provide very meaningful information.

There are differences between the muscles of males and females, with females, for example, having less muscle strength, a smaller muscle cross-section area and a slower muscle contraction compared to males [4]. With their measurements of the masseter and gastrocnemius muscles of 127 subjects (Supersonic Shear Imaging), Arda et al. demonstrated significantly higher shear wave velocities for males compared to females [1]. Akagi et al. also reached this result with their measurement of the rectus femoris, gastrocnemius and soleus muscles of 80 subjects (Acuson S2000, Siemens Healthcare, Erlangen, Germany) [3]. Akagi et al. assume that the difference in muscle thickness of males and females is the reason for the gender-specific differences in shear wave velocities found in several studies [3]. Kuo et al. examined the trapezius, anterior scalene, levator scapulae and sternocleidomastoid muscles and found no significant difference between males and females (Acuson S2000, Siemens Healthcare Erlangen) [24]. However, the study population was comparatively small with 20 subjects, nine of which were male and 11 female, which rather restricted the informative value of this study. The present study demonstrated that male subjects had significantly higher shear wave velocities in their trapezius and erector spinae muscles and a significantly thicker

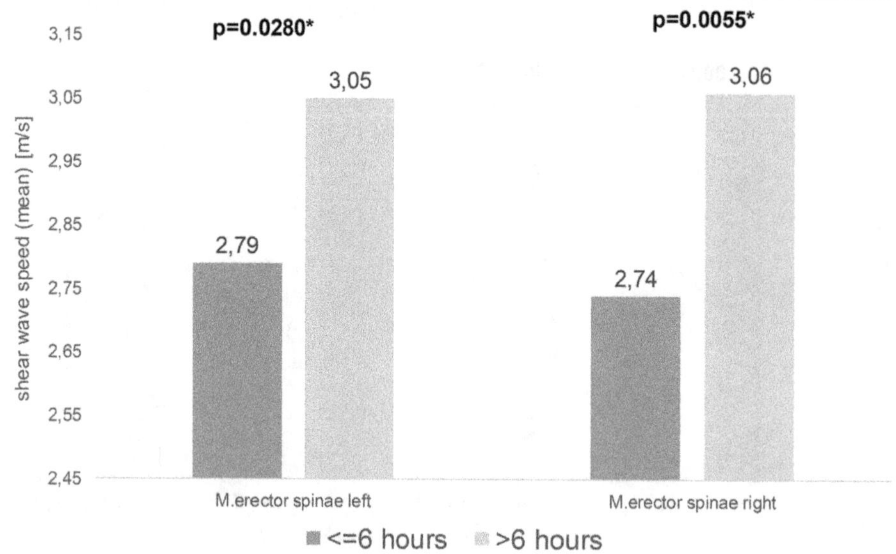

Fig. 3 Physical activity. Difference in shear wave velocity of the erector spinae muscle, depending on the physical activity of the 18- to 30-year-old subjects, specified in hours per week (subdivided into ≤ 6 h per week (n = 131) and >6 h per week (n = 24); * = significant (Ulm University Hospital, 2013)

Table 3 Correlation between the thickness of the trapezius and muscle elasticity

N = 278		Left trapezius	Right trapezius	Left erector spinae	Right erector spinae
Thickness left trapezius	Correlation coefficient r	0.10468	0.11260	0.25657	0.18751
	p-value	0.0826	0.0617	*<.0001**	*0.0018**
Thickness right trapezius	Correlation coefficient r	0.04784	0.14225	0.26859	0.16656
	p-value	0.4286	*0.0180**	*<.0001**	*0.0055**

* = significant

trapezius compared to female subjects. This result supports the assumption of Akagi et al. that the higher shear wave velocities in the muscle tissue of males are related to the greater muscle thickness compared to females [3]. Since the majority of the studies demonstrated a significant difference in muscle elasticity and/ or stiffness, these results are important with regard to use of shear wave elastography in patients with musculoskeletal symptoms and disorders and show that a sex-specific differentiation is necessary when determining reference values.

The ageing process of muscles already sets in at about the age of 25, although this does not result in any significant morphological changes until about the sixth decade of life. Only after about the sixth decade does this process start to accelerate, the number, quality and strength of the muscle fibres decrease, while collagen content on the other hand increases [3, 4]. According to our state of knowledge, these alterations of the muscles with increasing age, known as sarcopoenia, result in increased stiffness of the muscle [3, 4]. After creating two age groups (≤ 60 and >60 years), the present study revealed a significant difference between these two entities with regard to the right and left erector spinae muscles and the right trapezius. No significant difference was demonstrated for the left trapezius, which could be due to the fact that the sub-group of over-sixty-year-olds only comprised 24 subjects, while the group of under-sixty-year-olds consisted of 254. Further studies with approximately the same number of subjects in each group would be helpful in confirming this age-related difference in muscle elasticity. Eby et al. confirmed the results of the present study with their measurements of the biceps brachii muscle in 133 subjects between the ages of 21 and 94 years (Supersonic Shear Imaging) in as much as they also demonstrated higher shear wave velocities in subjects over 60 years of age [4]. Akagi et al., on the other hand, did not discover any greater shear wave velocities in the over-sixty-year-olds [3]. Since Akagi et al. examined muscles of the lower limbs, while the present study and that of Eby et al. measured muscles of the upper limbs and back muscles, it is difficult to make any comparison between the studies and to attempt to explain their discrepancies [3]. It may be worth considering in this respect whether muscles of the lower limbs are more affected by the living circumstances and everyday activities of older people than the muscles of the upper limbs. Furthermore, the issue should be clarified as to whether during the process of sarcopoenia the above alterations affect and alter the properties of muscles of the upper and lower limbs to the same degree.

The results regarding the relationship between shear wave velocities and physical activity show that regular sport does have an effect on stiffness and elasticity of the erector spinae muscle and on the thickness of the trapezius. It should be noted that for the trapezius no significant difference and no significant correlation of the shear wave velocities were evident in relation to physical activity, although the thickness of the trapezius muscle was significantly influenced by a physical activity of more than six hours sport per week. In this regard, it is noticeable that on calculating the correlation between the thickness of the trapezius muscle and the shear wave velocities of the trapezius and erector spinae, significant correlations were evident between the thickness of the trapezius muscle and the shear wave velocities of the erector spinae muscle. It should also be noted that the thickness of the trapezius muscle did not correlate with the shear wave velocities of the trapezius. There is therefore an association between the shear wave velocities of the erector spinae and the thickness of the trapezius, which is related to the results of calculations of the dependency of shear wave velocities on physical activity. There are practically no studies available which have examined the relation between physical activity and muscle elasticity in a similar fashion. Eby et al. also enquired about the degree of physical activity in their 133 subjects, but found no significant connection between the shear wave velocity of the biceps brachii and the physical activity of the subjects [4]. Therefore, the results of the present study indicate that increased regular physical activity changes the elasticity of muscle tissue. This relationship should be examined more exactly and be reassessed in further studies. It would also be important to take into account the type and intensity of the various physical activities, e.g. whether they mainly involve strength or endurance and which muscle groups are being trained.

The results of the measurements did not reveal any significant difference between subjects with backache and headache and those without these symptoms. Although the questionnaire did ask about frequent headache and backache, this was a yes/no question, and the subjects were not asked about the quality, duration, location and frequency of occurrence of the symptoms. Since the results of the subjects with backache and headache did not show any significant difference from those without symptoms, these subjects remained in the study population. The fact that headache and backache are very common symptoms only serves to support this approach. An aim of further studies would be to compare the values obtained in healthy subjects with those of patients with specifically ascertained, examined and located muscle-related backache and headache. In their study using the VTTQ technique, Kuo et al. examined the relationship between neck pain and shear wave velocities of the trapezius muscle. They asked their subjects about neck pain which had lasted longer than six months. They found a significant difference in shear wave velocities between subjects with and without pain involving the trapezius muscle; however, only three of 20 subjects reported neck pain [24]. The small number of participants and the very low number of subjects with symptoms did, however, somewhat restrict the informative value of this study.

Conclusions

The essential results regarding the clinical use of shear wave elastography in muscle tissue are the significantly different values obtained between male and female subjects and between subjects under and over the age of 60, making it clear that normal value ranges need to be adapted to sex and age.

These results obtained in the present study provide a basis for further studies examining the relation between muscle pain/stiffness and the shear wave velocity of muscle tissue or, following on, the significance of various influencing factors for muscle tissue and thus reassessing the clinical application of shear wave elastography in muscles.

Abbreviations

BMI: Body-Mass-Index; m/s: Meters per second; Mean: Average; mm: Milimeter; ROI: region of interest; SAS: Statistical Analysis System; SD: standard deviation; VTIQ: virtual touch imaging quantification; VTTQ: virtual touch tissue imaging quantification

Funding

Not applicable.

Authors' contributions

AH, WK and BG wrote the manuscript. WK and ST was involved in designing and conducting the study. JS and ST collected and analysed the data. TG, BG, JS, TG and AH were involved in interpreting the data and writing the manuscript. All authors read and approved the final manuscript.

Consent for publication

Not applicable.

Competing interests

The authors declare that they have no competing interests.

Author details

[1]Department of Internal Medicine I, Ulm University Hospital, Albert-Einstein-Allee, 23 89081 Ulm, Germany. [2]Department of Diagnostic and Interventional Radiology, Ulm University Hospital, Albert-Einstein-Allee 23, Ulm 89081, Germany. [3]Department of Internal Medicine III, Ulm University Hospital, Albert-Einstein-Allee 23, Ulm 89081, Germany.

References

1. Arda K, Ciledag N, Aktas E, Aribas BK, Kose K. Quantitative assessment of normal soft-tissue elasticity using shear-wave ultrasound elastography. AJR Am J Roentgenol. 2011;197:532–6.
2. Drakonaki EE, Allen GM, Wilson DJ. Ultrasound elastography for musculoskeletal applications. Br J Radiol. 2012;85:1435–45.
3. Akagi R, Yamashita Y, Ueyasu Y. Age-related differences in muscle shear moduli in the lower extremity. Ultrasound Med Biol. 2014;41:2906–12.
4. Eby SF, Cloud BA, Brandenburg JE, Giambini H, Song P, Chen S, et al. Shear wave elastography of passive skeletal muscle stiffness: influences of sex and age throughout adulthood. Clin Biomech (Bristol, Avon). 2015;30:22–7.
5. Eby SF, Song P, Chen S, Chen Q, Greenleaf JF, An KN. Validation of shear wave elastography in skeletal muscle. J Biomech. 2013;46:2381–7.
6. Klauser AS, Miyamoto H, Bellmann-Weiler R, Feuchtner GM, Wick MC, Jaschke WR. Sonoelastography: musculoskeletal applications. Radiology. 2014;272:622–33.
7. Ballyns JJ, Turo D, Otto P, Shah JP, Hammond J, Gebreab T, et al. Office-based elastographic technique for quantifying mechanical properties of skeletal muscle. J Ultrasound Med. 2012;31:1209–19.
8. Ballyns JJ, Shah JP, Hammond J, Gebreab T, Gerber LH, Sikdar S. Objective sonographic measures for characterizing myofascial trigger points associated with cervical pain. J Ultrasound Med. 2011;30:1331–40.
9. Botar-Jid C, Damian L, Dudea SM, Vasilescu D, Rednic S, Badea R. The contribution of ultrasonography and sonoelastography in assessment of myositis. Med Ultrason. 2010;12:120–6.
10. Lacourpaille L, Hug F, Bouillard K, Hogrel JY, Nordez A. Supersonic shear imaging provides a reliable measurement of resting muscle shear elastic modulus. Physiol Meas. 2012;33:N19–28.
11. Brandenburg JE, Eby SF, Song P, Zhao H, Brault JS, Chen S, et al. Ultrasound elastography: the new frontier in direct measurement of muscle stiffness. Arch Phys Med Rehabil. 2014;95:2207–19.
12. Turo D, Otto P, Shah JP, Heimur J, Gebreab T, Zaazhoa M, et al. Ultrasonic characterization of the upper trapezius muscle in patients with chronic neck pain. Ultrason Imaging. 2013;35:173–87.
13. Garra BS. Elastography: current status, future prospects, and making it work for you. Ultrasound Q. 2011;27:177–86.
14. Benson J, Fan L. Tissue strain analytics - a complete ultrasound solution for Elastography. Inc: Siemens Medical Solutions USA; 2012. p. 1–20.
15. Akamatsu FE, Ayres BR, Saleh SO, Hojaij F, Andrade M, Hsing WT, et al. Trigger points: an anatomical substratum. Biomed Res Int. 2015;2015:623287.
16. Shah JP, Thaker N, Heimur J, Aredo JV, Sikdar S, Gerber L. Myofascial trigger points then and now: a historical and scientific perspective. PM R. 2015;7:746–61.
17. Schilder A, Hoheisel U, Magerl W, Benrath J, Klein T, Treede RD. Sensory findings after stimulation of the thoracolumbar fascia with hypertonic saline suggest its contribution to low back pain. Pain. 2014;155:222–31.
18. Thiese MS, Hegmann KT, Wood EM, Garg A, Moore JS, Kapellusch J, et al. Prevalence of low back pain by anatomic location and intensity in an occupational population. BMC Musculoskelet Disord. 2014;15:283–93.
19. Suri P, Fry AL, Gellhorn AC. Do muscle characteristics on lumbar spine magnetic resonance imaging or computed tomography predict future low back pain, physical function, or performance? A systematic review. PM R. 2015;7:1269–81.
20. Fortin M, Gibbons LE, Videman T, Battie MC. Do variations in paraspinal muscle morphology and composition predict low back pain in men? Scand J Med Sci Sports. 2015;25:880–7.

21. Teichtahl AJ, Urquhart DM, Wang Y, Wluka AE, O'Sullivan R, Jones G, et al. Physical inactivity is associated with narrower lumbar intervertebral discs, high fat content of paraspinal muscles and low back pain and disability. Arthritis Res Ther. 2015;17:114.
22. Teichtahl AJ, Urquhart DM, Wang Y, Wluka AE, Wijethilake P, O'Sullivan R, et al. Fat infiltration of paraspinal muscles is associated with low back pain, disability, and structural abnormalities in community-based adults. Spine J. 2015;15:1593–601.
23. Wan Q, Lin C, Li X, Zeng W, Ma C. MRI assessment of paraspinal muscles in patients with acute and chronic unilateral low back pain. Br J Radiol. 2015;88:20140546.
24. Kuo WH, Jian DW, Wang TG, Wang YC. Neck muscle stiffness quantified by sonoelastography is correlated with body mass index and chronic neck pain symptoms. Ultrasound Med Biol. 2013;39:1356–61.

11

Magnetic resonance imaging evaluation of the distal oblique bundle in the distal interosseous membrane of the forearm

Yeon Ho Kim[1], Hyun Sik Gong[1,4*], Jin Woo Park[1], Hyun Kyung Yang[2], Kahyun Kim[1] and Goo Hyun Baek[3]

Abstract

Background: Some cadaveric studies have reported the role of the distal oblique bundle (DOB) in the distal radioulnar joint stability. We aimed to determine whether the presence of the DOB can be identified and its thickness can be measured in magnetic resonance imaging (MRI) examinations.

Methods: We retrospectively reviewed 468 wrist and forearm MRIs. Inclusion criteria were wrist or forearm MRIs taken in patients older than 18 years of age, and exclusion criteria were patients with acute wrist or forearm fractures, infections, or malignant tumors. We selected 80 MRIs that provided adequate coverage of the distal interosseous membrane (DIOM). The thickness of the DIOM in the T2-weighted transverse plane was measured on the picture archiving and communicating system. We used a model-based clustering method to determine whether some individuals have thicker DIOMs that can be considered as the DOB.

Results: The thickness of the DIOM demonstrated a bimodal distribution, indicating the presence of patients with a thick DIOM (DOB). The model-based clustering method indicated that the optimal cutoff point was 1.0 mm. Twenty-six individuals (32.5%) had thick DIOMs with a mean thickness of 1.4 mm (standard deviation, 0.2 mm), while 54 individuals (67.5%) had thin DIOMs with a mean thickness of 0.6 mm (standard deviation, 0.2 mm).

Conclusion: Our study demonstrates that it is possible to identify the DOB and measure its thickness using MRI. Future in-vivo studies of the DOB using MRI in patients with distal radioulnar joint pathologies may reveal its role in the distal radioulnar joint stability.

Keywords: Distal interosseous membrane, Distal oblique bundle, Distal radioulnar joint, Magnetic resonance imaging

Background

The interosseous membrane of the forearm is a ligamentous complex connecting the radius to the ulna, and it consists of distal membranous, middle ligamentous, and proximal membranous portions. The distal interosseous membrane (DIOM) acts as a secondary stabilizer of the distal radioulnar joint (DRUJ) when the dorsal and palmar radioulnar ligaments of the triangular fibrocartilage complex (TFCC) are cut [1, 2]. Noda et al. reported that the thickness of the DIOM varied widely among the specimens and identified the distal oblique bundle (DOB), which is a thick fiber running within the DIOM that originates from the distal one-sixth of the ulnar shaft and runs distally to insert on the inferior rim of the sigmoid notch of the radius [3]. A biomechanical study found that the DOB had little changes in length during forearm rotation, suggesting that it is an isometric stabilizer of the forearm [4].

Recently, studies have reported the role of the DOB in the DRUJ stability. Kitamura et al. reported in a cadaveric study that DRUJ laxity was greater in the group without a DOB than in the group with a DOB [5]. Arimitsu et al. found in another cadaveric study that ulnar shortening with the osteotomy carried out proximal to

* Correspondence: hsgong@snu.ac.kr
[1]Department of Orthopedic Surgery, Seoul National University Bundang Hospital, Seongnam, South Korea
[4]Department of Orthopedic Surgery, Seoul National University Bundang Hospital, Seoul National University College of Medicine, 300 Gumi-dong, Bundang-gu, Seongnam-si, Gyeonggi-do 463-707, South Korea
Full list of author information is available at the end of the article

the attachment of the DIOM had a more favorable effect on DRUJ stability compared with distal osteotomy, especially when there was a DOB [6]. In addition, Dy et al. demonstrated that in the setting of an ulnar styloid fracture, coronal shift of the distal radius fracture is associated with increased DRUJ instability in specimens with a distinct DOB, but not in specimens without a distinct DOB [7]. Furthermore, Moritomo suggests that a thick DIOM (or DOB) has an important role in stabilizing the ulnar stump after the Sauvé-Kapandji procedure [8]. However, these studies are done in cadavers, and it is still unknown whether the presence or absence of the DOB affects clinical outcomes. Therefore, identifying the DOB clinically would be important for future clinical studies exploring the role of this structure in DRUJ stability.

Several studies reported that magnetic resonance imaging (MRI) could evaluate an intact or disrupted interosseous membrane in its central or proximal part in the setting of longitudinal forearm instability (Essex-Lopresti lesion) [9–11]. We hypothesized that MRI might also evaluate the interosseous membrane at its distal part. The purpose of this study was to determine whether the presence of the DOB can be identified and its thickness can be measured in MRI examinations.

Methods

Subjects

We obtained an approval for this study from our institutional review board. Using the electronic medical data record program, we retrieved the list of all patients who had undergone MRI examinations between March 2003 and March 2015 at our hospital, which is an urban tertiary referral hospital. Inclusion criteria were wrist or forearm MRIs taken in patients older than 18 years of age, and exclusion criteria were patients with acute wrist or forearm fractures, infections, or malignant tumors. Thus, 468 wrist and forearm MRIs were retrieved from the data and reviewed.

In these 468 MRIs, we examined whether the MRI provided sufficient coverage of the length of the DIOM that originates from the distal one-sixth of the ulnar shaft and runs toward dorsal and distal direction to insert on the dorsal inferior rim of the sigmoid notch of the radius. A previous anatomical study reported that the mean proximal edge of the DIOM was 59 mm (range, 53–63 mm) proximal to the ulnar head [5]. Therefore, we selected MRIs that covered the forearm from the wrist to at least 60 mm proximal to the ulnar head. Finally, 80 MRIs (17%) that provided adequate resolution and coverage of the DIOM were included in the study. The mean age of the patients was 46. 9 years (range, 22–86 years). There were 38 men (47.5%) and 42 women (52.5%). The diagnoses of the patients included benign soft tissue mass in 38 patients (47.5%), TFCC lesions in 16 patients (20%), peripheral neuropathy in 7 patients (8.8%), Kienböck disease in 5 patients (6.3%), scaphoid nonunion in 4 patients (5%), and other conditions with wrist pain in 10 patients (13%).

MRI protocol and measurement

All MR examinations were performed on a 3.0T unit (Achieva & Ingenia; Philips Healthcare, Best, the Netherlands) with the subject in the supine position. Images were taken according to the standard MR protocol for wrist and forearm imaging in our hospital. The DIOM was identified on T2-weighted Turbo Spin-echo (TSE) imaging in a transverse plane (2–6 mm thickness sections; repetition time (TR) / echo time (TE), 2694-5011/80-100 msec; field of view of 80-150 × 80-150 or 160-320 × 160-320 matrix). The DIOM was seen as a linear low signal intensity band between the radius and the ulna. As the DOB runs obliquely from the ulna proximally to the radius distally, no single transverse cut can show the thick part in the entire length of the DIOM. An anatomic study reports that the DOB showed variations; the DOB can be linear, can spread in a fan shape distally, or can occupy the whole DIOM [5]. Therefore, we traced the thick part from proximal, ulnar side to the distal, radial side, and measured the maximum thickness by using the picture archiving and communicating system in every transverse cut from proximally (6cm proximal to the ulnar styloid) to distally (sigmoid notch of the radius) within the range of the DIOM. The data of the thickest part of the DIOM were collected and analyzed (Fig. 1).

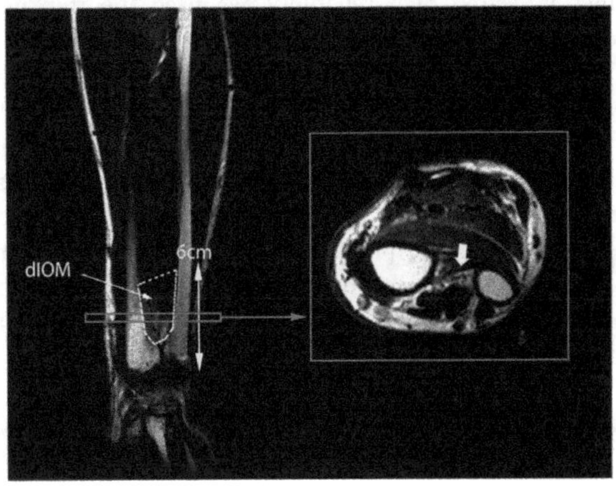

Fig. 1 The distal interosseous membrane (DIOM), which is schematically represented in the coronal image of the forearm (*white dotted area*), was traced in the transverse images of the forearm from proximally to distally within the range of the DIOM (*yellow arrow*). The thickest part of the DIOM was chosen from the transverse images and the thickness was measured (*white arrow*)

Two authors (one orthopedic surgeon and one radiologist), who were blinded to patient information, measured the DIOM thickness. We evaluated the intra-rater reliability by repeating all measurements after 2 weeks, and inter-rater reliability by the independent assessment by 2 examiners. The intra- and inter-rater reliabilities of the thickness measurement were tested using intraclass correlation coefficients (ICCs).

Statistical analysis

Model-based clustering method (Mclust package in R) was used to determine the optimal number of Gaussian mixtures and the cutoff value based on the Bayesian information criterion (BIC). This statistical method demonstrates the number of clusters in the distribution [12], and is often used for medical statistical analysis [13, 14]. We compared the thickness of the DIOM between groups using the *t*-test, and frequency of the DOB between groups using the chi-square test. A power analysis indicated that a sample size of 18 patients to each of the group would provide 90% statistical power ($\alpha = 0.05$; $\beta = 0.10$) with use of *t*-test for an effect size of 1.0 (0.2mm difference between the groups with a standard deviation of 0.2mm).

We used two types of MRI scanners (Achieva and Ingenia), and the section thickness varied from 2 to 6mm. Therefore, we compared the DOB thickness between the two scanners and between sections of 3mm or thinner and sections of more than 3mm.

Results

Reliability of measurements

The ICC value of intra-rater reliability was 0.833, and that of inter-rater reliability was 0.748. As these ICC values indicated high reliability, we used the thickness measured by one of the authors.

Identification of the DOB

The thickness of the DIOM demonstrated a bimodal distribution, indicating the presence of two groups that had a normal distribution. The two groups were divided on the basis of a cutoff point which was established by the model-based clustering method and the optimal cutoff point was suggested as 1.0 mm (Fig. 2). The group with a thick DIOM was considered to have the DOB.

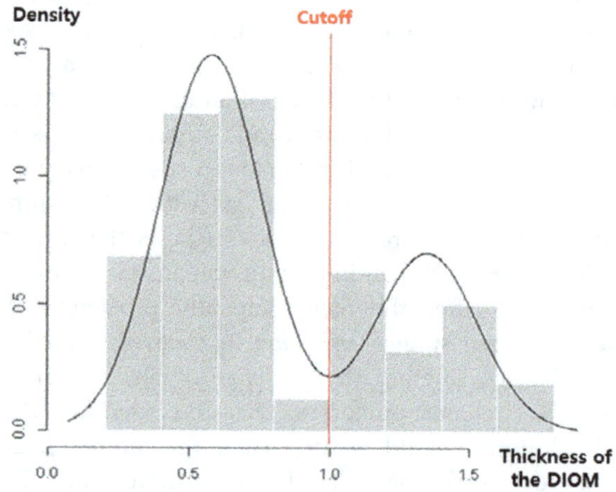

Fig. 2 The density plot of the thickness of the distal interosseous membrane (DIOM) and the cutoff value based on the Model-based clustering method. The optimal cutoff point was suggested as 1.0 mm

Frequency and thickness of the DOB

The number of patients who had a thicker DIOM (DOB Group) was 26 (32.5%) and that of patients who had a thinner DIOM (no-DOB Group) was 54 (67.5%). The mean thickness of the DIOMs in the DOB group was 1.4 mm (standard deviation, 0.2 mm; range, 1.1–1.7 mm), and that in the no-DOB group was 0.6 mm (standard deviation, 0.2 mm; range, 0.2–0.9 mm) (Fig. 3). The mean thickness was significantly different between the two groups ($p = 0.044$).

There were no significant differences in the frequency of the DOB ($p = 0.549$), or in the thickness of the DIOM ($p = 0.716$) between men and women. In addition, there were no significant differences in the frequency and thickness according to the scanner type (Achieva and Ingenia) or section thickness (equal to or less than 3mm vs. more than 3mm) (Table 1).

Discussion

Cadaveric studies have reported the presence of the DOB within the DIOM and its potential role in stabilizing the DRUJ. Identification of the DOB by an imaging modality in clinical studies may further clarify its role in the DRUJ stability, and may allow better prediction of the prognosis or planning of the surgery. Our study demonstrates that the presence of the DOB can be identified and its thickness can be measured in the T2-weighted transverse plane of MRI that provides adequate coverage of the wrist and the distal forearm.

In our study, the frequency of the DOB was 32.5% (26 out of the 80 patients), which is comparable to previous findings in cadaveric studies [3, 5]. Noda et al. reported an frequency of 40% (12/30) in a study using 30 forearms from 15 embalmed cadavers (9 females and 6 males, mean age 85 years), [3] and Kitamura et al. found that 4 out of the 10 fresh-frozen cadavers (5 females and 5 males, mean age 79 years) had the DOB [5]. Our study found that the mean thickness of the DIOM in the DOB group was 1.4 mm and that in the no-DOB group was 0.6 mm, which were comparable to the study by Kitamura et al, where these values were 1.2 mm and 0.4

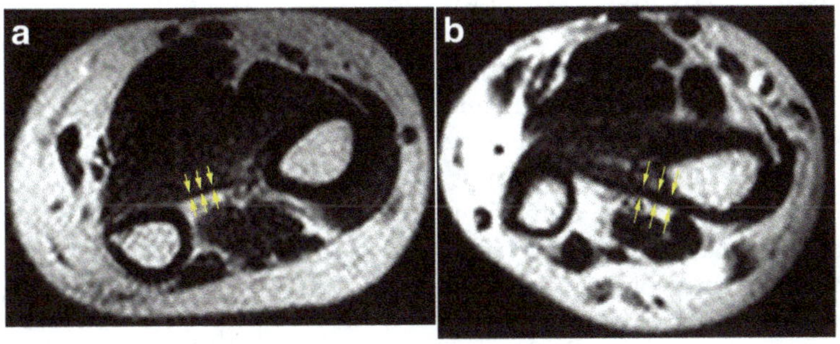

Fig. 3 Two representative cases of the patients with a thin DIOM (**a**, no-DOB Group, 54-year-old female) and with a thick DIOM (**b**, DOB Group, 25-year-old female). The DIOMs were measured 0.67 mm thick (**a**) and 1.32 mm thick (**b**) respectively

mm, respectively [5]. The mean thickness of the DOB was 1.5 mm in the study by Noda et al. [3].

Studies suggest that identifying the presence or absence of the DOB by MRI preoperatively may be helpful in decision-making for patients with ulnar-sided wrist pain or DRUJ problems. Arimitsu et al. found that the DRUJ stability is improved when ulnar shortening osteotomy is performed proximal to the ulnar attachment of the DIOM [6]. They suggest that an enhanced DRUJ stabilizing effect can be expected in patients having a DOB, and an additional or alternative procedure may be considered when the DRUJ instability remains a concern in patients without a DOB [6]. On the other hand, they found significant differences in the longitudinal closure difficulty for proximal compared with distal osteotomy sites, depending on the DOB thickness. Accordingly, they suggest that for patients with a stable DRUJ, an osteotomy performed distal to the ulnar attachment of the DOB may allow better healing of the osteotomy site. A few studies report the advantages of distal metaphyseal ulnar shortening osteotomy [15, 16]. However, the study by Arimitsu is a cadaveric study based on 10 cases. Future clinical studies might determine the clinical relevance of the DOB in ulnar shortening osteotomy, by identifying the presence of the DOB and correlating the outcomes.

Table 1 Comparison according to scanner type, sex, and section thickness

		Mean Thickness of the DIOM	Frequency of the DOB
Scanner type	Achieva ($n = 32$)	0.89mm	15
	Ingenia ($n = 48$)	0.77mm	11
P value		0.772	0.604
Sex	Men ($n = 38$)	0.80mm	13
	Women ($n = 42$)	0.84mm	13
P value		0.716	0.549
Section thickness	>3mm ($n = 51$)	0.86 mm	18
	≤3mm ($n = 29$)	0.74 mm	8
P value		0.157	0.479

The DIOM originates from the distal ulna on average 59 mm (range, 53–63 mm) proximal to the ulnar head [5]. We selected MRIs that covered the forearm from the wrist to at least 60 mm proximal to the ulnar head, and it was possible to see the DIOM in all of the selected MRIs. Previous studies on the IOM also demonstrated that IOM injury was detected using the T2-weighted sequence with a reduced slice thickness [10, 11]. In addition, Fast Spin-echo (FSE) technique, which is similar to the TSE technique used in our study, was reported to yield clearer images by limiting distortion and to allow the images to be produced more quickly [9]. Our study suggests that changing the MRI protocol to include at least 60 mm proximal to the ulnar head and T2-weighted TSE (or FSE) imaging may be necessary to check the status of the DOB in patients presenting with DRUJ problems. Okada et al. evaluated the DIOM in 14 patients using ultrasound, and the sensitivity of ultrasound evaluation in confirming presence of the DOB was 80% [17]. Although ultrasound can be a useful and relatively inexpensive tool in detecting the presence of DOB, MRI can evaluate most of the cartilage and ligament lesions and does not depend on the competence of examiners.

There are a few limitations to this study. First, we evaluated patients who underwent the MRI examination for wrist or forearm problems. The prevalence of the DOB in the general population needs to be investigated further. Furthermore, Most of the wrist MRIs were excluded because they did not cover the distal forearm proximally long enough, which could be a selection bias. Second, our study identified the DOB on imaging only. Studies using both the MRI and surgical findings should confirm the accuracy of the MRI findings. However, evaluation of the DIOM involves elevation of the deep forearm muscles, thus it could be difficult to examine the DIOM for study purposes in patients with common wrist conditions. Third, we collected cases from 12 years period and therefore there must have been lots of variability in the MRI pulse sequence parameters. Forth, although the thickness of the DIOM and the frequency of the DOB were not different between sections of thin and thick sections, thin sections less than 3mm would be ideal for accurate measurement of the DIOM thickness. Finally, we could not stadiardise the position of the forearm in relation to supination/pronation, which may have affected the thickness measurement. However, the DOB was shown to be isometric during forearm rotation, [4] and we did not observe any wavy deformity of the DOB in the transverse planes.

Conclusions

This study demonstrates that it is possible to identify the DOB and measure its thickness using MRI. The frequency and thickness of the DOB in our study support the findings of previous cadaveric studies on its morphology. Future in-vivo studies of the DOB using MRI in patients with distal radioulnar joint pathologies may reveal its role in the distal radioulnar joint stability.

Abbreviations

DIOM: Distal interosseous membrane; DOB: distal oblique bundle; DRUJ: distal radioulnar joint; ICCs: intraclass correlation coefficients

Acknowledgement

The authors thank the Medical Research Collaboration Center at our institution for statistical analyses.

Funding

This study was in part supported by a research fund (2015R1D1A1A01058562) from National Research Foundation of Korea.

Authors' contributions

YHK, HSG, GHB participated in the design of the study. YHK and HKY measured the data. JWP and KK were responsible for the statistical analysis of the study. All authors read and approved the final manuscript

Competing interests

The authors declare that they have no competing interests.

Consent for publication

Not applicable.

Author details

Department of Orthopedic Surgery, Seoul National University Bundang Hospital, Seongnam, South Korea. [2]Department of Radiology, Seoul National University Bundang Hospital, Seongnam, South Korea. [3]Department of Orthopedic Surgery, Seoul National University Hospital, Seoul, South Korea. [4]Department of Orthopedic Surgery, Seoul National University Bundang Hospital, Seoul National University College of Medicine, 300 Gumi-dong, Bundang-gu, Seongnam-si, Gyeonggi-do 463-707, South Korea.

References

1. Watanabe H, Berger RA, Berglund LJ, Zobitz ME, An KN. Contribution of the interosseous membrane to distal radioulnar joint constraint. J Hand Surg. 2005;30:1164–71.
2. Kihara H, Short WH, Werner FW, Fortino MD, Palmer AK. The stabilizing mechanism of the distal radioulnar joint during pronation and supination. J Hand Surg. 1995;20:930–6.
3. Noda K, Goto A, Murase T, Sugamoto K, Yoshikawa H, Moritomo H. Interosseous membrane of the forearm: an anatomical study of ligament attachment locations. J Hand Surg Am. 2009;34(3):415–22.
4. Moritomo H, Noda K, Goto A, Murase T, Yoshikawa H, Sugamoto K. Interosseous membrane of the forearm: length change of ligaments during forearm rotation. J Hand Surg Am. 2009;34A:685–91.
5. Kitamura T, Moritomo H, Arimitsu S, Berglund LJ, Zhao KD, An KN, Rizzo M. The biomechanical effect of the distal interosseous membrane on distal radioulnar joint stability: a preliminary anatomic study. J Hand Surg Am. 2011;36(10):1626–30.
6. Arimitsu S, Moritomo H, Kitamura T, Berglund LJ, Zhao KD, An KN, Rizzo M. The stabilizing effect of the distal interosseous membrane on the distal radioulnar joint in an ulnar shortening procedure: a biomechanical study. J Bone Joint Surg Am. 2011;93(21):2022–30.
7. Dy CJ, Jang E, Taylor SA, Meyers KN, Wolfe SW. The impact of coronal alignment on distal radioulnar joint stability following distal radius fracture. J Hand Surg Am. 2014;39(7):1264–72.
8. Moritomo H. The distal interosseous membrane: current concepts in wrist anatomy and biomechanics. J Hand Surg Am. 2012;37(7):1501–7.
9. Starch DWD, Eugene J. Magnetic resonance imaging of the interosseous membrane of the forearm. J Bone Joint Surg Am. 2001;83(2):235–8.
10. Fester EWMP, Sanders TG, Ingari JV, Leyendecker J, Leis HL. The efficacy of magnetic resonance imaging and ultrasound in detecting disruptions of the forearm interosseous membrane: a cadaver study. J Hand Surg Am. 2002; 27(3):418–24.
11. McGinley JC, Roach N, Hopgood BC, Limmer K, Kozin SH. Forearm interosseous membrane trauma: MRI diagnostic criteria and injury patterns. Skeletal Radiology. 2006;35(5):275–81.
12. Fraley CR, Adrian E. Model-based clustering, discriminant analysis, and density estimation. J Am Stat Assoc. 2002;97(458):611.
13. Pflueger M, Seppänen-Laakso T, Suortti T, Hyötyläinen T, Achenbach P, Bonifacio E, Orešič M, Ziegler AG. Age- and islet autoimmunity-associated differences in amino acid and lipid metabolites in children at risk for type I diabetes. Diabetes. 2011;60(11):2740–7.
14. Tang WH, Hartiala J, Fan Y, Wu Y, Stewart AF, Erdmann J, Kathiresan S, Roberts R, McPherson R, Allayee H, Hazen SL. Clinical and genetic association of serum paraoxonase and arylesterase activities with cardiovascular risk. Arterioscler Thromb Vasc Biol. 2012;32(11):2803–12.
15. Slade 3rd JF, Gillon TJ. Osteochondral shortening osteotomy for the treatment of ulnar impaction syndrome: a new technique. Tech Hand Up Extrem Surg. 2007;11:74–82.
16. Hammert WC, Williams RB, Greenberg JA. Distal metaphyseal ulnar-shortening osteotomy: surgical technique. J Hand Surg Am. 2012;37:1071–7.
17. Okada K, Moritomo H, Miyake J, Kataoka T, Tanaka H, Murase T, Yoshikawa H. Morphological evaluation of the distal interosseous membrane using ultrasound. Eur J Orthop Surg Traumatol. 2014;24(7):1095–100.

12

Comparative study of the paraspinal muscles after OVF between the insufficient union and sufficient union using MRI

Marina Katsu, Tetsuro Ohba*, Shigeto Ebata and Hirotaka Haro

Abstract

Background: Identification of poor prognostic factors for OVF is important but has not yet been clearly established. Despite paraspinal muscles could play an important role in the etiology of OVF, what influence time-dependent changes in paraspinal muscles have after OVF, and the impact on conservative treatments for patients who have an OVF remain largely unknown. The purposes of this study were to (1) evaluate time-dependent changes of the paraspinal musculature using MRI after injury in patients with osteoporotic vertebral fractures (OVFs), and (2) compare paraspinal muscles between conservatively treated patients with OVF who have successful union and those failed to conservative treatment.

Methods: A total of 115 consecutive patients who had sustained a recent OVF injury in the thoracolumbar region were assessed for eligibility using medical records and all required data were available from 90 patients who had been followed up for at least 6 months. Patients who needed to undergo surgery and patients who were diagnosed as having insufficient union after 6 months of follow-up were assigned to a group with insufficient union. Lumbar trunk parameters, relative cross-sectional area (rCSA) and proportion of fat infiltration (FI%) were calculated from MRI. To evaluate the time-dependent changes in the paraspinal muscle in patients after OVF injury, correlations between the timing of MRI and rCSA, FI% were determined. To clarify the impact of paraspinal muscles on the outcome of conservative treatments of patients with OVF, we compared rCSA between the groups.

Results: Sixty-five patients were assigned to a group with insufficient union and 25 patients were assigned to a group with successful union. FI% of the multifidus and erector spinae in the group with insufficient union were significantly greater than in the group with union. The timing of MRI in relation to initial injury was significantly correlated with FI% of the multifidus and erector spinae. rCSA of the erector spinae was significantly larger in the group with successful union than in the group with insufficient union.

Conclusions: These findings indicated a time-dependent increase of fatty degeneration of the multifidus and erector muscles, but no change in the rCSA and larger rCSAs of spinal erectors may play a role in successful union in patients with OVF.

Keywords: Osteoporotic vertebral fractures, Magnetic resonance imaging, Cross sectional area, Insufficient bone union, Fat infiltration rate, Paraspinal muscles

* Correspondence: tooba@yamanashi.ac.jp
Department of Orthopaedic Surgery, University of Yamanashi, 1110, Shimokato, Chuo, Yamanashi 409-3898, Japan

Background

Osteoporotic vertebral fractures (OVFs) increase overall mortality [1, 2], and are becoming increasingly common as the proportion of the population that is older continues to increase [3]. Described as stable spinal injuries, OVF are treated with conservative methods such as rest, immobilization, drug treatment and brace therapy [4]. However, these vertebral fractures sometimes fail to union, resulting in progressive collapse or pseudarthrosis and these patients often suffered from persistent back pain or neurological deficits [5]. The prevalence of insufficient union in elderly patients with OVFs ranges from 10 to 13.5% after conventional conservative treatments, resulting in marked reductions in the quality of life and activities of daily living of these patients [6–8]. Therefore, identification of risk factors associated with a poor prognosis for OVF is important but has not yet been clearly established.

Magnetic resonance imaging (MRI) plays crucial role in evaluation of spinal pathologies [9]. Recent studies have indicated the clinical importance of measuring the cross-sectional area (CSA) and proportion of fat infiltration (FI%) of paraspinal muscles using MRI to evaluate OVF or lumbar degenerative disease [10–15]. The CSA and FI% of paraspinal muscles correlate with spinal stability and alignment [11]. Additionally, trunk muscles could play an important role in the etiology of OVF based on how they affect spinal stability and vertebral strength via muscle–bone interactions [16]. However, what influence time-dependent changes in paraspinal muscles have after OVF, and the outcomes of conservative treatments for patients who have an OVF remain largely unknown.

The purpose of the present study was to (1) evaluate time-dependent changes of the paraspinal musculature after injury in patients with OVFs using MRI, and (2) compare paraspinal muscles between conservatively treated patients with OVF with successful union and insufficient union after conservative treatment.

Methods

Patient population

A total of 115 consecutive patients older than 65 years who had sustained a recent OVF injury in the thoracolumbar region were assessed for eligibility using their medical records between 2010 and 2016 in this retrospective single-center cohort study. During their initial visit to our institute, a new vertebral fracture was diagnosed if the following were present: onset of back pain within 3 weeks before presentation, a deformed vertebral body visible on radiographs, and an abnormal intensity within the vertebral bodies visible with MRI had on the initial visit. Patients with multiple fracture, pathological fractures associated with a tumor, high-energy injury, or those with neurological deficits, or who had not undergone MRI of thoracolumbar spine were not eligible to participate in the present study. Initially, patients underwent conservative treatment determined by three board-certified spinal surgeons at a single institution and were followed-up for a minimum of 6 months. Treatment options, including the use of a brace or drug therapy, or both, were selected by the individual physicians based on their experience. All of the required data were available from 90 patients who had been followed up for at least 6 months (Fig. 1).

Insufficient union was diagnosed when patients underwent surgery within 6 months or were diagnosed based on intravertebral vacuum clefts on plain radiography or CT, or had apparent segmental motion on plain X-ray dynamic images (≥5° between supine and weight-bearing positions) after 6 months of follow-up, as assessed by two spine surgeons independently [17]. Surgical treatment was indicated for patients with progressive neurological deficits or continuous severe lower back pain

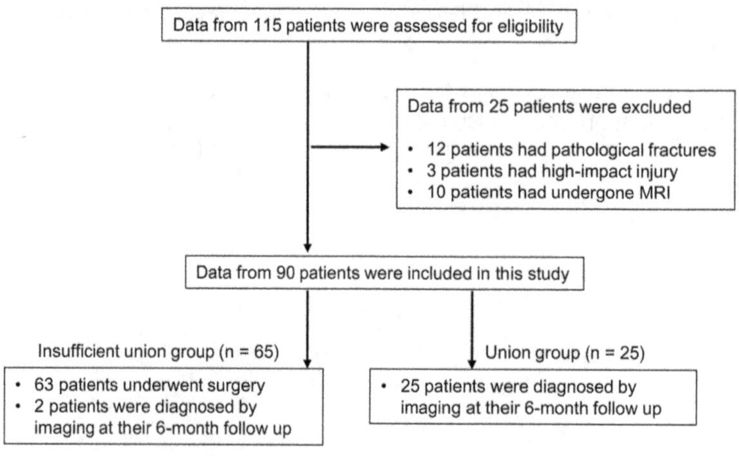

Fig. 1 Flow diagram showing the enrollment and assignment of patients

(visual analog scale > 80/100 points) caused by insufficient vertebral bone union, or both. Sixty-three patients required surgical treatment because of insufficient bone union of their OVF for the present study.

Patient groups

Patients who needed to undergo surgery and patients who were diagnosed as having insufficient union after 6 months of follow-up were assigned to a group with insufficient union (Fig. 1). Average time from original injury to surgery was 4.2 ± 1.5 months. After 6 months of follow-up, based on radiographs of satisfactory bony union without associated severe pain, we assigned 25 patients to a group with successful union (Fig. 1).

MRI protocol

The patients were placed in a supine position with the spine in a neutral position and a pillow was placed under their knees. Imaging was performed using a 3.0 T dual gradient superconducting MRI system (Discovery 750; GE Medical Systems, Milwaukee, WI, USA) with an 8-channel NeuroVascular-full neck coil, at a gradient strength of 40 mT/m, and a slew rate of 150 mT/m/ms. Sagittal and axial T1-weighted and T2-weighted MRI was performed routinely.

Measurement of the CSA and FI% of paraspinal muscles as visualized by MRI

All MRI measurements were made by an experienced orthopedic surgeon blinded to the clinical information and study hypothesis. Following a previously used method [18], the regions of interest (ROI) were defined by manual tracing of the fascial boundary of the following muscles on both sides of the spinal column to the superior endplate of the L3 vertebral body on T1 axial images: psoas major, multifidus (including rotatores lumborum spinae), spinal erectors (encompassing both the longissimus and iliocostalis), and quadratus lumborum muscles (Fig. 2A). The ROIs were analyzed, and histograms showing the signal intensity were generated using digitalized image processing software (Image J, National Institutes of Health, Bethesda, MD, USA). The FI% in the total CSA of both muscles was evaluated using a threshold technique. Briefly, the number of pixels representing intramuscular fatty tissue were distinguished using a threshold grayscale value of 120 [15]. Relative CSA (rCSA) was defined as the CSA of each of the muscles divided by the CSA of the L3 vertebral body [12, 18]. The investigator evaluated and re-evaluated MRI, 2 weeks apart, blinded to MRI identifiers, to assess the intraobserver reliability of the rCSA and FI% of paraspinal muscle measurement. The intraobserver error of FI% of all patients is shown in a Additional file 1.

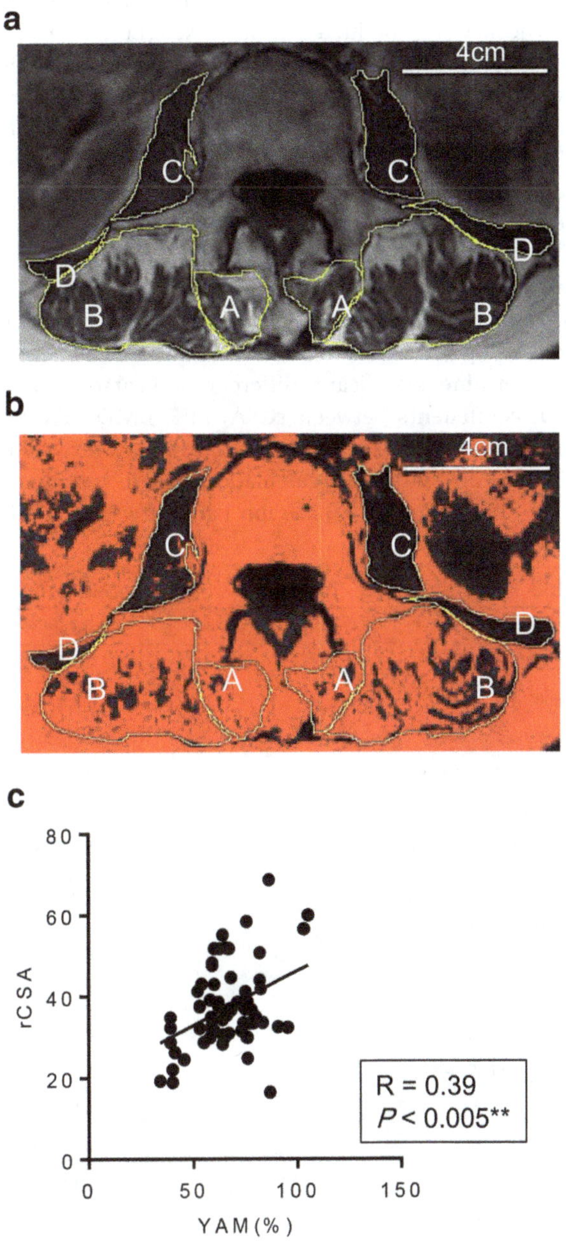

Fig. 2 Measurement of the cross-sectional area on T1 axial image (**a**) and fatty infiltration of paraspinal muscles using Image J (**b**). A = multifidi; B = erector spinaeC = psoas; D = quadratus lumborum. **c** Correlation between rCSA of total paraspinal muscles and BMD (YAM%)

Data collection

For each patient who was treated for OVF, we searched the clinical records and laboratory database to record their basic characteristics, such as age, sex, body mass index (BMI), vertebral levels of injury, and which type of brace was used initially. Standardized bone mass density (BMD) measurements at the femoral neck were conducted using DXA (Lunar Prodigy; GE Medical Systems) within 4 weeks from the first visit. OVF were classified according to Genant's semi-quantitative criteria using plain X-ray images at the initial visit [19]. The severity of lumbar spinal stenosis seen on MRI was graded qualitatively according to the classification reported previously [20].

Statistical analysis

All data are reported as mean ± SD. Data were analyzed using an unpaired t test and a Fisher exact test to determine significant differences. Pearson correlation coefficients between rCSA, FI%, BMD (YAM%), and timing of MRI after the initial injury were determined. All statistical calculations were conducted using Prism, version 6.0 (Graph Pad Software, La Jolla, CA). For all tests, $P < 0.05$ was considered significant ($^{*}P < 0.05$, $^{**}P < 0.005$, $^{***}P < 0.0005$, $^{****}P < 0.0001$).

Results

We included 90 patients (58 women and 22 men) with an average age of 75.4 (65–88) years in the present study. Table 1 summarizes the characteristics of the patients, type of brace that was used initially and drug treatment for osteoporosis at their initial visit to our institute. There was no significant difference in the mean age, sex, BMD, and grading of LSS severity between the groups. The patients in the group with insufficient bony union had a more severe Genant grade of OVF than patients in the group with successful union. Overall, there were no significant differences in conservative management with hard braces or elastic braces between the groups. The

Table 1 Summary of the characteristics of each group

Characteristic	Insufficient union ($n = 65$)	Union ($n = 25$)	p
Age[a] y, mean ± SD	75.9 ± 7.9	74.1 ± 11.2	0.41
BMI, kg/m^2, mean ± SD	22.3 ± 2.9	22.4 ± 3.1	0.87
Sex, female/male	42/23	16/9	0.27
BMD (%YAM), mean ± SD	66.9 ± 16.3	69.2 ± 10.4	0.58
Level of injury			
Thoracolumbar junction level (T11–L2)	60 (92%)	22 (88%)	
Other level	5 (8%)	3 (12%)	
Genant's classification			
Minimal fracture	9 (14%)	15 (60%)	< 0.0001****
Moderate fracture	15 (23%)	5 (20%)	1.00
Severe fracture	41 (63%)	5 (20%)	< 0.005***
Grading of LSS severity			
A	33 (50%)	11 (44%)	0.64
B	12 (19%)	5 (20%)	1.00
C	20 (31%)	8 (32%)	0.44
D	0	1 (4%)	0.27
Type of braces			
Custom-made hard braces	17 (26%)	6 (24%)	1.00
Elastic braces	31 (48%)	15 (60%)	0.35
No brace	17 (26%)	4 (16%)	0.41
Drug treatment			
Teriparatide	8 (12%)	4 (16%)	0.73
Bisphosphonate	11 (17%)	5 (20%)	0.76
Denosumab	5 (8%)	2 (8%)	1.00
SERMs	8 (12%)	3 (12%)	1.00
No treatment	30 (46%)	11 (44%)	1.00

BMI Body Mass Index, *BMD* bone mass density, *YAM* Young Adult Mean, *LSS* lumbar spinal stenosis, *n* number in group, *SERMs* selective estrogen receptor modulators

$^{*}P < 0.05$, $^{**}P < 0.005$, $^{***}P < 0.0005$, $^{****}P < 0.0001$

[a]Mean ± standard deviation (SD)

rCSAs of total paraspinal muscles were positively correlated with BMD (YAM%) of all patients (Fig. 2c).

Despite that only patients who had undergone MRI were enrolled in this study, the timing of MRI after injury was indefinite and was assessed by three board certified spinal surgeons independently. The average time to obtain MRI in all cases was 64.1 ± 13.71 days after the initial injury. To evaluate the time-dependent changes in the paraspinal muscle in patients after OVF injury, correlations between the timing of MRI and rCSA, FI% were determined (Figs. 3 and 4). Timing of MRI after the initial injury was correlated with the FI% seen in the multifidus and erector spinae (Fig. 3a and b). By contrast, there was no correlation between the timing of MRI after the initial injury and the FI% of the psoas and quadratus, or rCSA of any paraspinal muscles (Fig. 3c and d, Fig. 4a–d). These findings indicated a time-dependent increase in FI% of the multifidus and erector muscles after injury, but no change in the rCSA of any paraspinal muscles (the paraspinal muscles of representative cases are shown in Fig. 4e).

To clarify the impact of paraspinal muscles on the outcome of conservative treatments of patients with OVF, we compared rCSA between the groups. rCSA of the erector spinae of patients in the group with sufficient union was significantly larger than the rCSA in patients in the group with insufficient union (Fig. 5b). No significant difference between the groups was found in the rCSA of multifidus, psoas, or quadratus muscles (Fig. 5a, c, and d). These results indicate that the rCSA of the erector spinae in patients with OVF who were treated successfully with conservative treatment is larger than in patients with OVF who had insufficient union (the paraspinal muscles of representative cases of both groups are shown in Fig. 5e).

Discussion

The present study showed that rCSAs of total paraspinal muscles were positively correlated with BMD (YAM%) of patients with OVF (Fig. 2c). The timing of MRI after injury was not controlled because of the retrospective nature of the present study, but the average timing of MRI was 64.1 ± 13.71 days after the initial injury. We found a correlation between rCSA and FI% of paraspinal muscles and the timing of MRI after injury, and found FI% of the multifidus and erector muscles was positively correlated with the timing of MRI after initial injury. Interestingly, the rCSA of paraspinal muscles was not correlated with the timing of MRI after the initial injury. Based on this finding, we compared rCSA, but not FI, of paraspinal muscles in patients with insufficient union to the rCSA of patients with successful union. We found

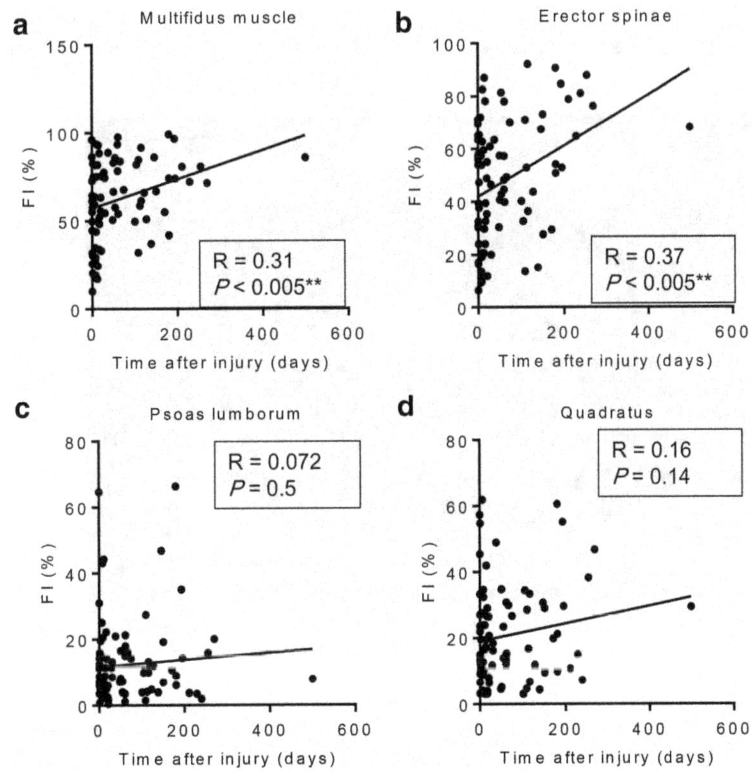

Fig. 3 a Correlation between the timing of MRI after the initial OVF injury and the FI% of the (**a**) multifidus muscle, (**b**) erector spinae, (**c**) psoas lumborum, and (**d**) quadratus

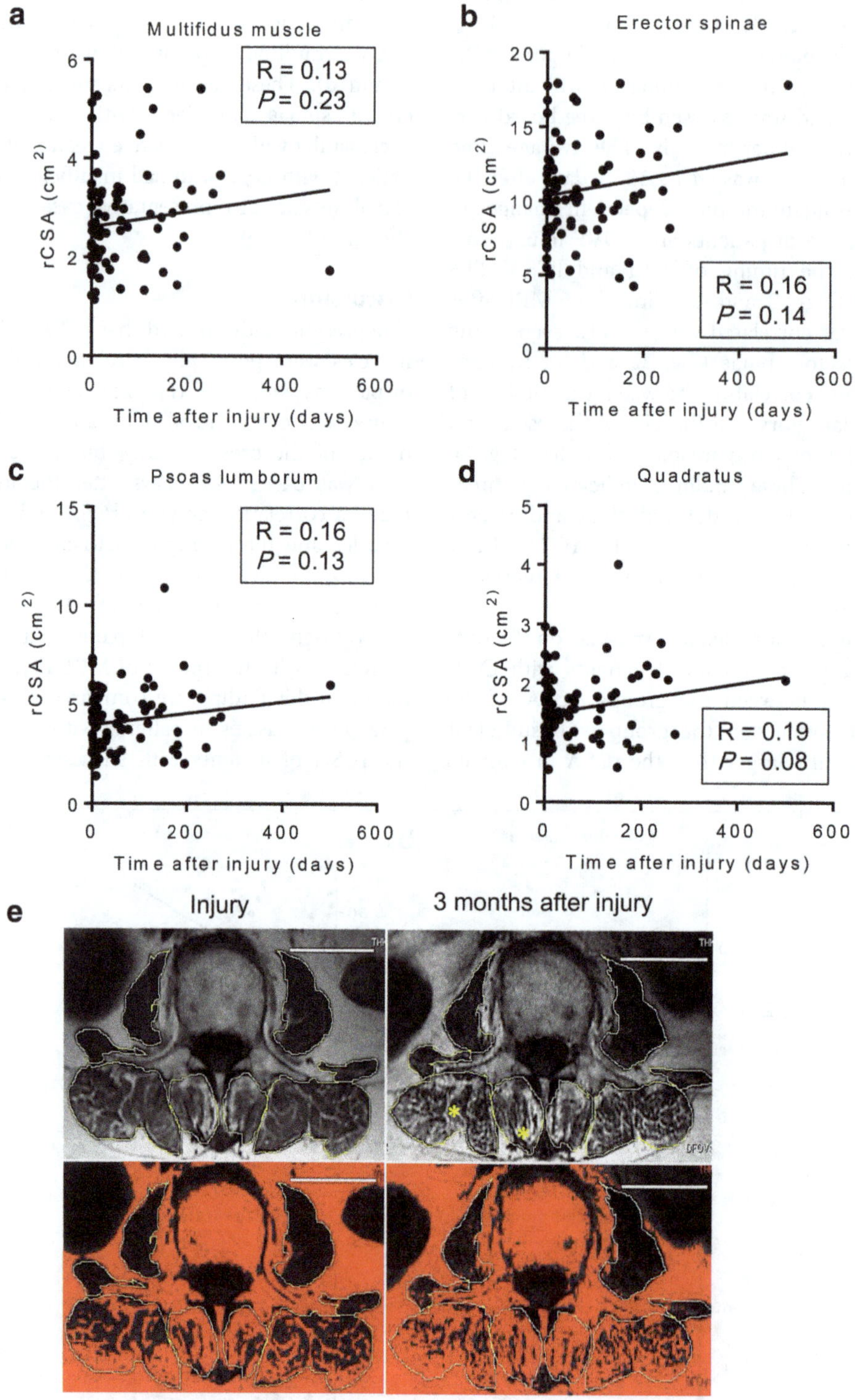

Fig. 4 a Correlation between the timing of MRI after the initial OVF injury and the rCSA of the (**a**) multifidus muscle, (**b**) erector spinae, (**c**) psoas lumborum, and (**d**) quadratus. **e** Representative images of the time-dependent increase in FI%, but no change in rCSA of the multifidus and erector muscles

that the rCSA of the erector spinae of patients in the group with successful union was significantly larger than that in patients in the group with insufficient union.

MRI plays crucial role in evaluation of spinal pathologies [9]. Numerous studies have found an association linking morphological changes in paraspinal

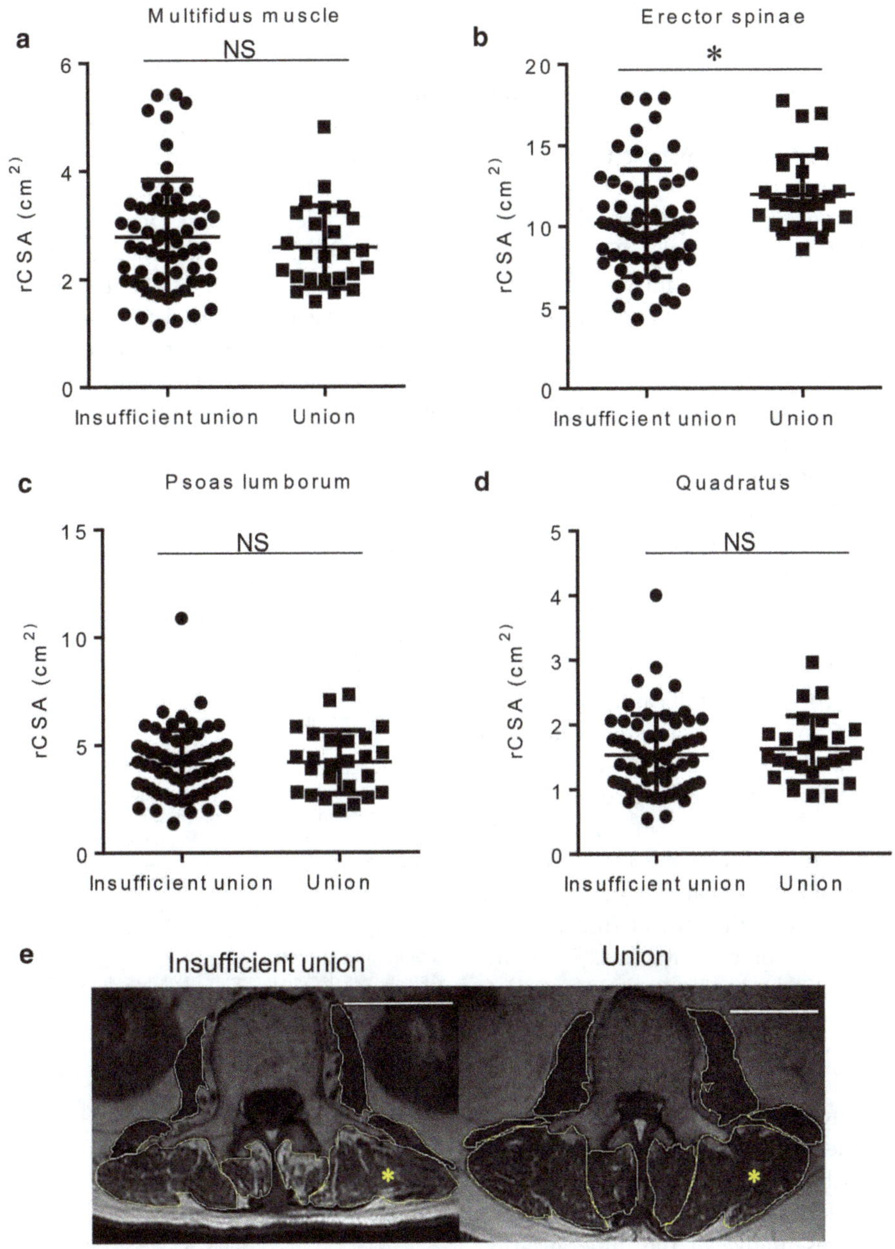

Fig. 5 Graph comparing rCSA of the multifidus (**a**), erector spinae (**b**), psoas lumborum (**c**), and quadratus (**d**) between the groups (*$P < 0.05$, **$P < 0.005$, ****$P < 0.0001$, NS denotes no significant difference). **e** Representative images of paraspinal muscles of patients in both groups

muscles with low back pain (LBP), lumbar spinal stenosis and spinal pathology using MRI [10, 12, 21]. Advancing age is associated with profound changes in the spine and its surrounding musculature, such as atrophied lumbar paraspinal muscles, with a reduction in their CSA and increased intramuscular FI [22]. Despite current study showed there was no significant difference LSS severity between groups, influence of morphometric change of paraspinal muscle by reduced innervation in LSS patients has been focused [12]. However, whether muscle control problems contribute to cause LBP, or whether LBP is a trigger for morphological changes in musculature, such as disuse muscle atrophy, remains largely unknown [21]. A recent report stated that profound changes in lumbar paraspinal muscles, a reduction in the CSA, and increased intramuscular FI occur in patients with osteoporotic spinal compression fractures [23]. However, this report lacked detailed information on the timing of the MRI assessments that were performed after injury. Therefore, we first examined the time-dependent changes of the paraspinal muscles of patients with OVFs to determine the influence of persistent back pain on paraspinal muscle morphology. We found a time-dependent increase in FI% of the multifidus and spinal erectors, but found no change in the rCSA of the paraspinal muscles of patients with OVF. These findings might suggest the mechanism underlying changes in muscle morphology in which fatty degeneration of the paraspinal muscles has occurred ahead of muscle atrophy (Fig. 4e). Further study using muscle biopsy during surgery is needed to elucidate the mechanism, which is likely related to the relationship between fatty degeneration and pathological muscle atrophy.

Despite the numerous studies in which efforts have been made to screen patients with an OVF who are at high risk of a poor prognosis [8, 24, 20], images of fresh vertebral fractures remain difficult to interpret. Recent studies have indicated the roles paraspinal muscles can play in OVFs, fracture prevention, interventions for management, rehabilitation after fracture, and modification of kyphotic changes after fracture [16, 25, 26]. We believe the present study has clinical importance because it shows that rCSAs correlate significantly with bone union; that is, larger rCSAs of spinal erectors can play a crucial role in reducing the risk of an insufficient union in patients with an OVF by contributing to spinal column stability in a protective way (Fig. 5e). Future mechanical study is needed to elucidate the reason for the significant contribution of the spinal erectors among all paraspinal muscles as found in the present study.

The present study has some limitations. First, because of the comparatively small sample size, data from men and women were analyzed together. Differences in the quality and size of paraspinal muscles by sex should be considered in future studies. Second, the retrospective study design was not conducive to obtaining control patients (no fracture) and MRI data from patients according to a structured routine. Third, measuring BMD at the femoral neck using DXA may not be representative of the mineralization of the axial skeleton, because osteoporosis in the peripheral and axial skeleton often develops disparately; thus, quantitative computed tomography of the lumbar spine should be used for further study. Last, conservative treatment was not fully standardized according to drug treatment including calcium/vitaminD, physiotherapy, brace type or the time the brace was worn as these items were selected by 3 physicians independently. The mechanism of fatty degeneration in the paraspinal muscles is presumed to be influenced by brace immobilization, the influence of persistent back pain, or degeneration as a result of muscle disuse, so these possibilities limit identification of the specific mechanism. In current study, 63% of the patients in insufficient group had severe fracture in Genant's classification as compared to 20% in successful union group. This might be one factors the difference of fatty degeneration between groups. Further prospective studies, in which the timing of MRI after injury is controlled and conservative treatment is standardized, are needed to clarify the mechanism of fatty degeneration in the paraspinal muscles. Nevertheless, to our knowledge, this is the first report to determine that (1) fatty degeneration of the paraspinal muscles has occurred ahead of muscle atrophy in patients after OVF injury, and (2) larger rCSAs of spinal erectors can play a crucial role in in successful union in patients with OVF.

Conclusions

These findings indicated a time-dependent increase of fatty degeneration of the multifidus and erector muscles, but no change in the rCSA and larger rCSAs of spinal erectors may play a role in successful union in patients with OVF.

Authors' contributions

MK substantially contributed to the study design and analyzed the patient data. TO substantially analyzed and interpreted the patient data and was a major contributor in drafting the manuscript. SE substantially contributed to the conception and design of the study and contributed to drafting the manuscript. HH substantially contributed to the study design and critically revised the manuscript. All authors read, approved, and take responsibility for the final manuscript.

Competing interests

The authors declare that they have no competing interests.

References

1. Center JR, Nguyen TV, Schneider D, Sambrook PN, Eisman JA. Mortality after all major types of osteoporotic fracture in men and women: an observational study. Lancet. 1999;353(9156):878–82.
2. Lau E, Ong K, Kurtz S, Schmier J, Edidin A. Mortality following the diagnosis of a vertebral compression fracture in the Medicare population. J Bone Joint Surg Am. 2008;90(7):1479–86.
3. Lee YL, Yip KM. The osteoporotic spine. Clin Orthop Relat Res. 1996;323:91–7.
4. Francis RM, Aspray TJ, Hide G, Sutcliffe AM, Wilkinson P. Back pain in osteoporotic vertebral fractures. Osteoporos Int. 2008;19(7):895–903.
5. Hasegawa K, Homma T, Uchiyama S, Takahashi H. Vertebral pseudarthrosis in the osteoporotic spine. Spine (Phila Pa 1976). 1998;23(20):2201–6.
6. Cook DJ, Guyatt GH, Adachi JD, Clifton J, Griffith LE, Epstein RS, Juniper EF. Quality of life issues in women with vertebral fractures due to osteoporosis. Arthritis Rheum. 1993;36(6):750–6.
7. Kim DY, Lee SH, Jang JS, Chung SK, Lee HY. Intravertebral vacuum phenomenon in osteoporotic compression fracture: report of 67 cases with quantitative evaluation of intravertebral instability. J Neurosurg. 2004;100(1 Suppl Spine):24–31.
8. Tsujio T, Nakamura H, Terai H, Hoshino M, Namikawa T, Matsumura A, Kato M, Suzuki A, Takayama K, Fukushima W, et al. Characteristic radiographic or magnetic resonance images of fresh osteoporotic vertebral fractures predicting potential risk for nonunion: a prospective multicenter study. Spine (Phila Pa 1976). 2011;36(15):1229–35.
9. Kumar Y, Gupta N, Chhabra A, Fukuda T, Soni N, Hayashi D. Magnetic resonance imaging of bacterial and tuberculous spondylodiscitis with

associated complications and non-infectious spinal pathology mimicking infections: a pictorial review. BMC Musculoskelet Disord. 2017;18(1):244.

10. Singh R, Yadav SK, Sood S, Yadav RK, Rohilla R. Magnetic resonance imaging of lumbar trunk parameters in chronic low backache patients and healthy population: a comparative study. Eur Spine J. 2016;25(9):2864–72.
11. Choi MK, Kim SB, Park CK, Malla HP, Kim SM. Cross-sectional area of the lumbar spine trunk muscle and posterior lumbar interbody fusion rate: a retrospective study. Clin Spine Surg. 2017;30(6):E798–E803.
12. Chen YY, Pao JL, Liaw CK, Hsu WL, Yang RS. Image changes of paraspinal muscles and clinical correlations in patients with unilateral lumbar spinal stenosis. Eur Spine J. 2014;23(5):999–1006.
13. Kim H, Lee CK, Yeom JS, Lee JH, Cho JH, Shin SI, Lee HJ, Chang BS. Asymmetry of the cross-sectional area of paravertebral and psoas muscle in patients with degenerative scoliosis. Eur Spine J. 2013;22(6):1332–8.
14. Arbanas J, Pavlovic I, Marijancic V, Vlahovic H, Starcevic-Klasan G, Peharec S, Bajek S, Miletic D, Malnar D. MRI features of the psoas major muscle in patients with low back pain. Eur Spine J. 2013;22(9):1965–71.
15. Ranson CA, Burnett AF, Kerslake R, Batt ME, O'Sullivan PB. An investigation into the use of MR imaging to determine the functional cross sectional area of lumbar paraspinal muscles. Eur Spine J. 2006;15(6):764–73.
16. Mokhtarzadeh H, Anderson DE. The role of trunk musculature in osteoporotic vertebral fractures: implications for prediction, prevention, and management. Curr Osteoporos Rep. 2016;14(3):67–76.
17. Takahashi S, Hoshino M, Takayama K, Iseki K, Sasaoka R, Tsujio T, Yasuda H, Sasaki T, Kanematsu F, Kono H, et al. Predicting delayed union in osteoporotic vertebral fractures with consecutive magnetic resonance imaging in the acute phase: a multicenter cohort study. Osteoporos Int. 2016;27:3567–75.
18. Sions JM, Smith AC, Hicks GE, Elliott JM. Trunk muscle size and composition assessment in older adults with chronic low back pain: an intra-examiner and inter-examiner reliability study. Pain Med. 2016;17(8):1436–46.
19. Genant HK, Wu CY, van Kuijk C, Nevitt MC. Vertebral fracture assessment using a semiquantitative technique. J Bone Miner Res. 1993;8(9):1137–48.
20. Schizas C, Theumann N, Burn A, Tansey R, Wardlaw D, Smith FW, Kulik G. Qualitative grading of severity of lumbar spinal stenosis based on the morphology of the dural sac on magnetic resonance images. Spine (Phila Pa 1976). 2010;35(21):1919–24.
21. Barker KL, Shamley DR, Jackson D. Changes in the cross-sectional area of multifidus and psoas in patients with unilateral back pain: the relationship to pain and disability. Spine (Phila Pa 1976). 2004;29(22):E515–9.
22. Mengiardi B, Schmid MR, Boos N, Pfirrmann CW, Brunner F, Elfering A, Hodler J. Fat content of lumbar paraspinal muscles in patients with chronic low back pain and in asymptomatic volunteers: quantification with MR spectroscopy. Radiology. 2006;240(3):786–92.
23. Kim JY, Chae SU, Kim GD, Cha MS. Changes of paraspinal muscles in postmenopausal osteoporotic spinal compression fractures: magnetic resonance imaging study. J Bone Metab. 2013;20(2):75–81.
24. Hoshino M, Nakamura H, Terai H, Tsujio T, Nabeta M, Namikawa T, Matsumura A, Suzuki A, Takayama K, Takaoka K. Factors affecting neurological deficits and intractable back pain in patients with insufficient bone union following osteoporotic vertebral fracture. Eur Spine J. 2009;18(9):1279–86.
25. Greig AM, Briggs AM, Bennell KL, Hodges PW. Trunk muscle activity is modified in osteoporotic vertebral fracture and thoracic kyphosis with potential consequences for vertebral health. PLoS One. 2014;9(10):e109515.
26. Katzman WB, Miller-Martinez D, Marshall LM, Lane NE, Kado DM. Kyphosis and paraspinal muscle composition in older men: a cross-sectional study for the osteoporotic fractures in men (MrOS) research group. BMC Musculoskelet Disord. 2014;15:19.

13

The added value of musculoskeletal ultrasound to clinical evaluation in the treatment decision of rheumatoid arthritis outpatients: physician experience matters

C. Sifuentes-Cantú[1], I. Contreras-Yáñez[1], L. Saldarriaga[2], A.C. Lozada[2], M. Gutiérrez[2] and V. Pascual-Ramos[1*]

Abstract

Background: Musculoskeletal ultrasound improves the accuracy of detecting the level of disease activity (DA) in RA patients, although its impact on the final treatment decision in a real clinical setting is uncertain. The objectives were to define the percentage of clinical scenarios from an ongoing cohort of RA outpatients in which the German Ultrasound Score on 7 joints (GUS-7) impacted the treatment and to explore if the impact differed between a senior rheumatologist (SR) vs. a trainee (TR).

Methods: Eighty-five consecutive and randomly selected RA outpatients underwent 170 assessments, 85 each by the SR and the TR. Initially, both physicians (blinded to each other) performed a rheumatic assessment and recommended a preliminary treatment. Then, the patients underwent the GUS-7 evaluation by an experienced rheumatologist blinded to clinical evaluations; selected joints of the clinically dominant hand were assessed by gray-scale and power Doppler (PD). In the final step, the TR and the SR integrated the GUS-7 findings with their previous evaluation and reviewed their recommendations. The patients received the final recommendation from the SR to avoid patient confusion. The study was approved by the Internal Review Board and all the patients signed informed consent. GUS-7 usefulness was separately evaluated by the SR and the TR according to a visual analogue scale (0 = not useful at all, 10 = very useful). Descriptive statistics were used.

Results: The patients were primarily middle-aged females (91.4%) with (mean ± SD) disease duration of 7.5 ± 3.9 years. The majority of them (69.2% according to TR and 71.8% to SR) were in DAS28-ESR-remission. In 34 of 170 clinical scenarios (20%), the GUS-7 findings modified the final treatment proposal; 24 of these scenarios were determined by the TR vs. 10 by the SR: 70.5% vs. 29.5%, $p = 0.01$. Treatment changes (increase, decrease and joint injection) were similar between both specialists. As expected, the TR rated the GUS-7 usefulness higher than the SR, particularly in the clinical scenarios where the GUS-7 findings impacted treatment.

Conclusions: Musculoskeletal ultrasound added to standard rheumatic assessments impacted the treatment proposal in a limited number of patients; the impact was greater in the TR.

Keywords: Ultrasound impact, Ultrasound value in Rheumatoid Arthritis treatment decisions

* Correspondence: virtichu@gmail.com
[1]Department of Immunology and Rheumatology. Instituto Nacional de Ciencias Médicas y Nutrición Salvador Zubirán, Vasco de Quiroga 15, colonia sección XVI, Tlalpan, 14000 México City, Mexico
Full list of author information is available at the end of the article

Background

Disease activity is a central aspect in the evaluation of patients with rheumatoid arthritis (RA) because it comprises signs and symptoms of the disease, impacts patient reported outcomes and is responsible for the progression of joint damage [1, 2]. Disease activity is reversible, and its abolishment or reduction to desirable levels is the major target of any therapeutic intervention. In clinical practice, it is advisable to regularly evaluate disease activity; a core set of clinical measures [3–5] and pooled indices that combine a variable number of disease activity measures [6] are available and have shown to be beneficial in following RA patients.

In 2013, the EULAR task force on imaging in RA clinical practice [7] developed 10 recommendations on various aspects of imaging in RA using research-based evidence, expert opinions and recommendations aimed to address clinical questions relevant to current practice and stated that ultrasound was a valuable candidate to detect clinical joint inflammation (superior to clinical examination), monitor disease activity, predict progression and therapeutic response and detect damage and persistent inflammation even when clinical remission was achieved. These recommendations summarized the experience gained in routine clinical practice over more than two decades, in which ultrasound was efficiently incorporated as a bedside method to enable clinical evaluation and therapy monitoring with high patient acceptability; novel scores that evaluated a reduced number of joints had been tested and were found to effectively reflect overall joint inflammation in RA, in addition to being less time consuming [8–12]. In this clinical context, the German Ultrasound 7 Score (GUS-7) combines soft tissue changes as well as erosive bone lesions in a single ultrasound scoring system [12]; the score concentrates on a small number of joint regions and examination time is reduced to approximately 10–20 min, making it a suitable candidate to integrate into daily rheumatologic practice.

It is generally accepted that disease activity is the most important factor that determines treatment consideration during routine evaluation of an outpatient with RA, although additional factors, such as comorbidities [13], costs/availability of DMARDs [14] and treatment related adverse/events, are increasingly recognized [15]. In addition, although maintained disease activity or remission status might prompt the clinician to suggest a medication change, patient's willingness to change treatment might affect the final proposal [16]. In a study designed to capture patients with moderate to high disease activity that would prompt a discussion of medications, only in 39% of the study visits did the clinician report a medication change [17].

Ultrasound assessment has certainly improved our accuracy to detect (the level of) disease activity in RA patients, although its real impact on the final treatment proposal in real world practice has not been assessed. The primary objective of this study was to define the percentage of routine clinical scenarios in which GUS-7 findings impacted the treatment indicated by the rheumatologist in an ongoing cohort of early (at cohort inclusion) RA outpatients; we were particularly interested in exploring if the impact differed among rheumatologists categorized by experience, senior (SR) vs. trainee (TR). Additional objectives were to describe GUS-7 findings in our cohort of patients, compare GUS-7 usefulness and factors that impact treatment among physicians and explore GUS-7 patient acceptance.

Methods

Study population

Patients invited to participate belonged to the early arthritis clinic (EAC) of the Instituto Nacional de Ciencias Médicas y Nutrición Salvador Zubirán, a referral center for Rheumatic Diseases in México City. When first evaluated in the EAC, patients had a disease duration of < 1 year and no specific rheumatic diagnosis except for RA. Patients were evaluated every two months during the first two years of follow-up and every two, four or six months (fixed for all patients from the baseline evaluation) thereafter, depending on the patient and the disease characteristics. Treatment was prescribed by the rheumatologist in charge of the clinic and was treat-to-target oriented (T2 T). Traditional DMARDs were used in 99% of the patients with/without corticosteroids (50% of the patients received low doses of oral corticosteroids during their follow-up). In November 2015, when the study was initiated, the cohort comprised 180 RA patients with variable follow-up recruited from 2004 onward. From November 2015 to May 2016, 87 randomly selected patients from the EAC were invited to participate; 2 of these patients denied because they had time constraints. Finally, 85 patients agreed to have study evaluations and were informed about the whole process of the study.

Study evaluations

Patients included had 2 clinical assessments; one assessment was performed by the SR in charge of the EAC and the other assessment was performed by a TR, and both were blinded to each other's evaluation. Completed clinical assessments included 66/68 swollen/tender joint counts, acute reactant-phase determination (both erythrocyte sedimentation rate [ESR] and C reactive protein [CRP]) and a patient visual analogue scale for overall disease activity; the DAS 28 was obtained [18]. After the clinical assessments, each physician was directed to write a treatment proposal on a standardized format. Clinical charts with information regarding comorbidities, previous treatment and serious adverse events were available for both the TR and the SR.

Then, each patient had GUS-7 performed by an experienced rheumatologist trained in musculoskeletal ultrasound and blinded to the clinical evaluations. The findings were immediately recorded on standardized formats and shared with both clinicians, who were instructed to review their previous treatment proposal and confirm/change the proposal on the standardized format (blinded to each other's proposal). In addition, both physicians were instructed to rate on a 0 to 100 mm scale, the GUS-7 usefulness for the final treatment proposal (were 100 indicates the maximum usefulness) and to select (and rate) which of the following factors was/were determinant in the final treatment proposal: clinical assessments, GUS-7, comorbidities, treatment related adverse events, costs/availability, patient's preference and DMARD maximum dose.

Finally, only the SR met with each patient and gave him/her the final treatment recommendation.

GUS-7 assessments

Ultrasound assessments were performed using a General Electric Logiq E ultrasound machine equipped with a high-frequency (8–18 MHz) linear transducer. All joints were scanned using a multiplanar technique, adopting the European League Against Rheumatism (EULAR) guidelines [19]. Ultrasounds were performed by a senior rheumatologist experienced in musculoskeletal ultrasound (at least 10 years of experience) who was blinded to the clinical evaluations performed by the SR and the TR, with the patient seated with hands lying in prone position (for wrist, metacarpophalangeal and proximal interphalangeal joints examination) and the patients in supine position with the legs bent at the knee (for metatarsophalangeal joints examination). All joint regions were assessed by gray-scale and power Doppler (PD), as previously published.

The following joints were assessed during the GUS-7: the wrist, second and third metacarpophalangeal (MCP2 and MCP3), second and third proximal interphalangeal joints (PIP2 and PIP3), and the second and fifth metatarsophalangeal joints (MTP2 and MTP5) of the clinically dominant side. During the GUS-7, the wrist was examined for synovitis and tenosynovitis from the dorsal, palmar and ulnar aspects; the MCP2 and MCP3 joints were evaluated for synovitis and tenosynovitis from the palmar view. Erosions were detected from the dorsal, palmar and radial (for MCP2 joint) aspects or from the dorsal and palmar aspects (for MCP3 joint). The PIP2 and PIP3 joints were assessed for synovitis from the palmar aspect and for erosions from the dorsal and palmar aspects [12]. The MTP2 and MTP5 joints were examined for synovitis from the dorsal aspect, and erosions were detected from the dorsal and palmar aspects for MTP2 joint and from the dorsal, plantar and lateral aspects for MTP5 joint. Synovitis by GUS-7 was described semiquantitatively as absence (=0), mild (=1), moderate (=2) and severe (=3) (see definitions below). Tenosynovitis and erosions were registered as being absent or present (see definitions below).

PD was performed for synovitis and tenosynovitis from the palmar and dorsal aspects in each region evaluated except for the MTP joints, which were evaluated from the plantar aspect. PD activity for synovitis and tenosynovitis were semi-quantitatively scored from grade 0 to grade 3 (see definitions below).

All the documentation was obtained on standardized formats. The GUS-7 examination of each patient took 10 to 20 min. Immediately after the GUS-7 was performed, the patients were instructed to complete a questionnaire that evaluated the following items according to a Likert scale: pain (new or increase) related to GUS-7, convenience of GUS-7 duration, patient satisfaction with GUS-7, patient preference for disease activity assessments (GUS-7 vs. clinical assessment) and patient disposition to have GUS-7 included in their routine evaluations.

Definitions

Clinical disease activity was graded by the following classification criteria: DAS28 ≤ 2.6 as clinical remission, DAS28 ≤ 3.2 as mild disease activity, DAS28 ≤ 5.2 as moderate disease activity and DAS28 > 5.2 as high disease activity [20].

Erosion: bone surface interruption in 2 perpendicular planes [21].

Tenosynovitis: hypoechoic/anechoic thickened tissue with or without fluid within the tendon sheath [21].

Grade 1 synovitis: small hypoechoic/anechoic line beneath the joint capsule; *grade 2 synovitis:* joint capsule elevated, parallel to the joint area; *synovitis grade 3:* strong distention of the joint capsule [21].

PD ultrasound activity: grade 0 = no intra-articular color signal, grade 1 = up to 3 color signals or 2 single and 1 confluent signal in the intraarticular area, grade 2 = greater than grade 1 to < 50% of the intraarticular area filled with color signals, and grade 3 = ≥50% of the intraarticular area filled with color signals [21, 22].

GUS-7 disease activity was defined as present if ≥grade 1 PD activity was detected in at least one joint/area examined.

Statistics

A sample size of 84 pairs of evaluations was calculated, assuming a difference between both physicians of at least

40% in the proportion of evaluations where GUS-7 impacted the treatment, with a 95% two-side confidence level and 80% power [23–26].

We performed a descriptive statistical analysis, presenting frequencies for categorical variables and measures of position and dispersion for numerical variables. The Mann-Whitney test was used to compare continuous variables, and Chi-squared and Fisher's exact test were used to compare proportions. The weighted kappa coefficient was used to establish the agreement between the SR and the TR for level of disease activity.

The statistical analysis was performed using SPSS IBM V.21.

Results

Characteristics of the patients evaluated

The patients included had 170 clinical assessments performed, 85 each by the TR and the SR. At study inclusion, the patients were primarily middle-aged females with substantial follow-up, although they had short disease duration at cohort inclusion ([mean ± SD] disease duration of 5.7 ± 2.5 months); the majority of the patients had disease-specific autoantibodies as summarized in Table 1 and up to 49% had at least one comorbid condition.

Patients level of disease activity at study entry (Table 2)

The majority of the patients were classified as in remission according to the DAS28-ESR, although all 4 levels of disease activity (remission, low, moderate and high disease activity) were represented. There was a good correlation between the SR and the TR in patient disease activity level, with kappa = 0.822, $p \leq 0.0001$.

GUS-7 findings

Table 3 summarizes the relevant findings. All the patients but one had at least some degree of synovitis on gray-scale US in at least one joint; the MTP2 joint was the most frequently involved, in 84.7% of the patients; the (mean ± SD) number of joints/patient with gray-scale synovitis was 3.2 ± 1.5, almost half of the patients had grade 2 synovitis, and 19 (23%) showed PD activity (Fig. 1-a); the most frequently affected joint was the MTP2 in 94.7% of the patients showing PD activity. In addition, one-third of the patients had tenosynovitis, although few (12%) had PD activity (Fig. 1-b). Finally, 33 patients (38.8%) had erosions detected by the GUS-7, and the most frequently affected bones were the MC2 and MT5 heads, each in 18.1% of the patients (Fig. 1-c).

Twenty patients were classified with GUS-7 active disease, 19 of them based on PD activity on at least one joint and the other patient based on the presence of tenosynovitis with PD activity.

Table 1 Population characteristics at study inclusion

N° (%) of female	77 (90.6)
Age, (mean ± SD), years	44.9 ± 12.2
Formal education, (mean ± SD), years	11.9 ± 4.2
N° (%) of patients RF+	78 (91.8)
N° (%) of patients ACCP+	76 (89.4)
Follow-up at the EAC, (mean ± SD), years	7.5 ± 4.1
N° (%) of patients with disease duration <5 years	31 (36.5)
N° (%) of patients with disease duration within 5 to 10 years	28 (32.9)
N° (%) of patients with disease duration >10 years	26 (30.6)

N° number, *SD* standard deviation, *RF* rheumatoid factor, *APCC* antibodies to cyclic citrullinated peptides, *EAC* early arthritis clinic

GUS-7 impact on treatment

In 34 (20%) clinical scenarios (among 170 assessments), the GUS-7 findings impacted treatment; treatment changes (after GUS-7 findings were incorporated to clinical findings) consisted of an increase in 24 (70.6%) scenarios, a decrease in 8 (23.5%) and joint injection with corticosteroids in 2 (5.9%).

A total of 24 of the 34 clinical scenarios with GUS-7 treatment impact were determined by the TR vs. 10 determined by the SR: 70.5% vs. 29.5%, $p = 0.01$. In 18 clinical scenarios (52.8%) the TR and the SR agree in their decision to modify the treatment after GUS-7. Treatment changes (increase, decrease and joint injection) were similar among both physicians (data not shown). There was a good correlation between the SR and the TR in the treatment indicated (kappa = 0.645, $p \leq 0.0001$) although the incorporation of GUS-7 findings did not improve it (kappa = 0.474, $p \leq 0.0001$).

Finally, we compared demographic characteristics (gender, age, education), disease characteristics (rheumatoid factor, antibodies to cyclic citrullinated proteins, disease duration, DAS28, ESR, CRP, disease activity status), comorbidities and treatment (corticosteroids use and DMARDs/patient) between patients in whom the GUS-7 findings modified the treatment and their counterpart; no differences were found in the variables examined (data not shown).

Comparison of GUS-7 usefulness between the SR and the TR

Table 4 summarizes the VAS scores from the SR and the TR. As expected, the TR rated the GUS-7 usefulness higher than the SR, particularly in the clinical scenarios where the GUS-7 findings impacted treatment. This finding was replicated within the SR GUS-7 usefulness scores.

The GUS-7 was rated as a determinant in the final treatment proposal in 84.7% of the clinical scenarios after clinical assessment, which was rated as determinant

Table 2 DAS28-ESR disease activity level according to the SR and the TR

	SR assessments (*N* = 85)	TR assessments (N = 85)	Agreement (%)
N° (%) of patients with remission	59 (69.4)	61 (71.8)	98.3
N° (%) of patients with low disease activity	8 (9.4)	7 (8.2)	71.4
N° (%) of patients with moderate disease activity	15 (17.6)	15 (17.6)	86.7
N° (%) of patients with high disease activity	2 (2.4)	2 (2.4)	66.7

DAS28-ESR disease activity score (28 joints evaluated)-erythrocyte sedimentation rate, *N* number, *SR* senior rheumatologist, *TR* trainee in rheumatology

in all of the clinical scenarios; the DMARD maximum dose was rated in 41.2%, comorbidities in 23.5%, DMARD cost/availability in 21.2%, DMARD-related adverse events in 20% and patient preference was rated as determinant in 14.1% of the clinical scenarios. The SR and the TR differed in the selection of the factors they considered determinant for the treatment proposal, as shown in Fig. 2; GUS-7 and DMARD-related adverse events were more frequently considered determinant in the treatment proposal by the TR, and the opposite trend was true for the SR regarding DMARD cost/availability and DMARD maximum doses.

Table 3 Description of GUS-7 findings

Synovitis	
N° (%) of patients with synovitis in ≥ 1 joint (grey scale)	84 (98.8)
(Mean ± SD) N° of joints/patient with synovitis (grey scale)[a]	3.2 ± 1.5
N° (%) of patients with grade 1 synovitis[a]	24 (28.6)
N° (%) of patients with grade 2 synovitis[a]	43 (51.2)
N° (%) of patients with grade 3 synovitis[a]	19 (22.6)
N° (%) of patients with synovitis (greys scale) and PD activity[a]	19 (22.6)
(Mean ± SD) N° of joints/patient with synovitis and PD activity[a]	1.6 ± 1
Tenosynovitis	
N° (%) of patients with tenosynovitis	25 (29.4)
(Mean ± SD) N° of tendons/patient with tenosynovitis (grey scale)[b]	1.5 ± 0.7
N° (%) of patients with tenosynovitis and PD activity[b]	3 (12.2)
(Mean ± SD) N° of tendons/patient with tenosynovitis and PD activity[b]	2 ± 1
Erosions	
N° (%) of patients with erosions (in ≥ 1 joint)	33 (33.8)
(Mean ± SD) N° of joints/patient with erosions[c]	1.6 ± 1

GUS-7 German ultrasound score on 7 joints, *N°* Number, *SD* Standard deviation, *PD* Power Doppler
[a]Among 84 patients with synovitis in at least 1 joint
[b]Among 25 patients with synovitis in at least 1 joint
[c]Among 33 patients with at least one erosion in at least 1 joint

Patient satisfaction with GUS-7

The majority of the patients reported that the GUS-7 was painless (97.6%), the duration of the assessment was appropriate (84.7%), they were satisfied with the ultrasound assessment (95.3%), they agreed that the GUS-7 should be part of routine clinical assessments (76.5%) and they confirmed their willingness to have future ultrasound assessments (100%).

Discussion

In the present study, we assessed the impact of adding musculoskeletal ultrasound information to the treatment decisions in an ongoing cohort of early RA outpatients and evaluated if the impact differed according to the experience of the rheumatologist involved in the treatment decision, SR vs. TR; we also compared how both physicians rated additional factors that might impact treatment decisions; finally, we explored patient satisfaction with the radiological assessment.

The study was performed in a real clinical setting of an ongoing cohort of early (at cohort inclusion) RA patients who had been treated since the beginning of their enrollment according to a T2 T strategy with traditional DMARDs (with/without corticosteroids) following current recommendations [27]; in addition, up to 49% of the patients had comorbidities. The simultaneous presence of multiple pathological conditions is more a rule than an exception in RA patients and has important academic issues and implications in daily practice [13]. We consider our results contribute to define the impact of ultrasound in RA patients' clinical care. Additional strengths of the study were the blinding for ultrasound evaluations and for clinical assessments (between the TR and the SR).

Four years ago, the Targeted Ultrasound Initiative (TUI) group stated that targeting therapy to PD activity provided superior outcomes in RA patients compared with treating to clinical targets alone [28] and undertook an international study in 8 countries to determine the added value of musculoskeletal ultrasound to the state-of-the-art management of RA, the Targeted Ultrasound in RA (TURA) study; the results of the TURA study have not been published yet. In the present study, we found that musculoskeletal ultrasound impacted the

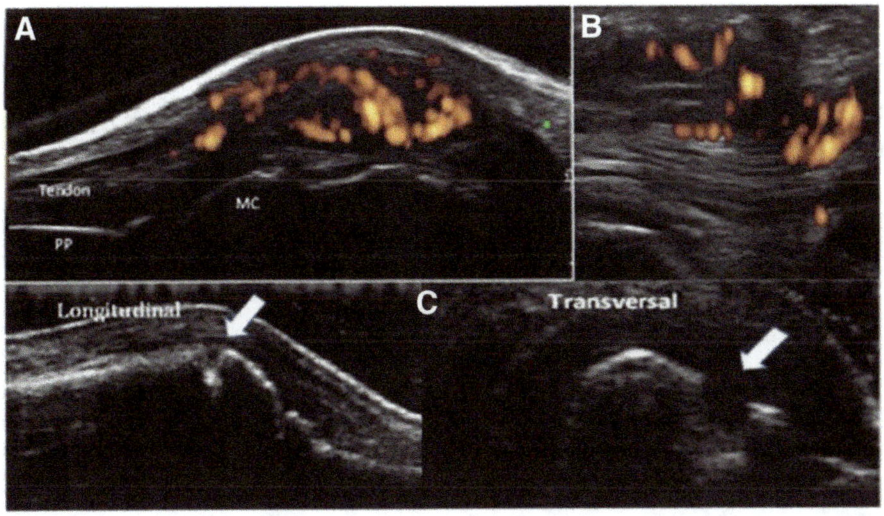

Fig. 1 **a**. Synovitis at the MCP joint of the clinically dominant hand. Dorsal view in a longitudinal scan of the MCP joint. A moderate joint cavity widening with signs of synovial proliferation and PD signal (grade 3) is appreciated. MC = metacarpal head; PP = proximal phalanx; Tendon = common digital extensor tendon. **b**. Tenosynovitis at the first extensor compartment of the clinically dominant hand. Longitudinal scan that shows the image with PD technique, where an inflammatory process of the intra-synovial sheath consistent with tenosynovitis is appreciated along with a correlation with the area in the tendon and the anatomical damage. **c**. Bone erosion at the MC2 head. Longitudinal (*upper image*) and transversal (*bottom image*) planes. There is a bone surface interruption (*arrow*) in 2 perpendicular planes (longitudinal and transversal)

treatment decision in a limited number of the clinical scenarios, 20%, and the impact was greater for the lesser experienced rheumatologist, the TR, compared to the SR. The role of ultrasound in RA management has been recently revisited [29], and the need to counterbalance the expanded scientific literature on the generalized benefits of ultrasound in RA management with appropriate strategy trials has been addressed. Two recent studies performed in early RA populations [30, 31] highlighted discrepancies between the potential benefits of adding ultrasound information to the treatment decisions in early RA patient management and the actual impact on clinical and imaging outcomes. In addition, although musculoskeletal ultrasound provides a more accurate additional (to clinical assessment) method for assessing disease activity, its incorporation to a T2 T strategy in

Table 4 Comparison of GUS-7 usefulness VAS-scores between the SR and the TR

	SR VAS-score[a]	TR VAS-score[a]	*p*
Usefulness score among all the clinical scenarios	4.1 ± 1.9	4.9 ± 2.5	0.023
Usefulness score among clinical scenarios where GUS-7 impacted treatment	7.2 ± 0.9	8.4 ± 1.3	0.011
Usefulness score among clinical scenarios where GUS-7 did not impact treatment	3.7 ± 1.5	3.6 ± 1.3	0.47

GUS-7 German ultrasound score on 7 joints, *SR* Senior rheumatologist, *TR* Trainee in rheumatology, *VAS* Visual analogue scale
[a]Data presented as (mean ± SD)

early RA patients modified only 29% of all DAS-28-based DMARD decisions and did not impact patient outcomes [32]; this percentage is close to that recently reported by Diaz-Torné et al. [33], who assessed RA patients with a longer disease duration (mean follow-up of 15.5 ± 10.7 years), the majority of them treated with conventional DMARDs (68%); in their study, ultrasound information made a change in the therapeutic decision in 32% of the patients. The above mentioned studies are consistent and highlight the complexity of RA patient management that goes far beyond the assessment of disease activity and even in the clinical context of remission; a careful assessment of the risk-benefit of targeting ultrasound remission also needs to be performed. As recently highlighted by van der Heijde D [34], the ultimate target should be better long-term patient-reported outcomes. We also found that the impact was greater in the TR than in the more experienced rheumatologist. This finding could be related to a greater experience of the SR in early RA and a deeper knowledge of the patients from the clinic, so the SR can be more confident in deciding treatment based on a limited number of traditional medical and serological factors. In addition, young rheumatologists have identified training on novel imaging technologies as among the most important educational needs [35]; a more accurate understanding of novel technology might favor a rapid incorporation to routine clinical practice. Nonetheless, it should be emphasized that both clinicians (the TR and the SR) completed a 12-h course of musculoskeletal ultrasound in

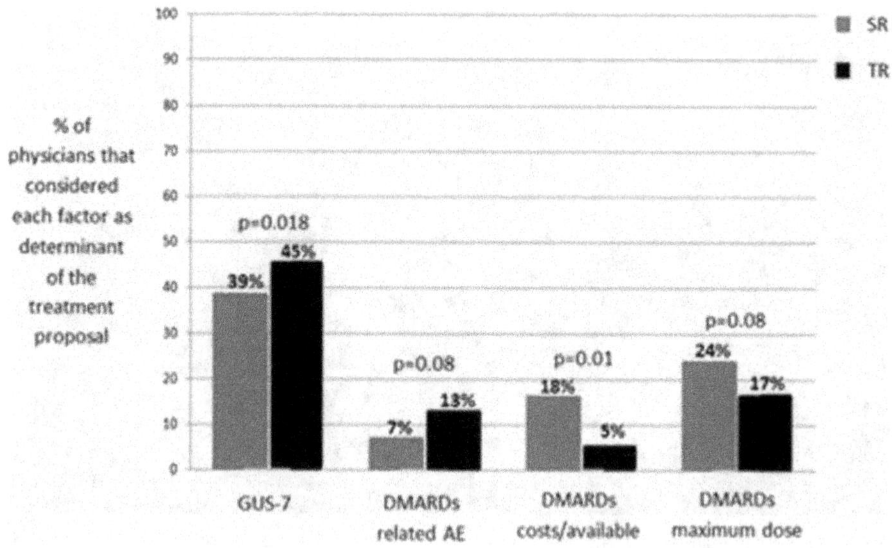

Fig. 2 Comparison of the percentage of SR and TR that considered GUS-7, DMARD related AE, DMARD costs/availability and DMARD maximum doses as determinant in the treatment proposal

rheumatic diseases and that in addition to the GUS-7, 3 other factors among 6 were differently rated by the TR and the SR to impact the treatment decision.

Both physicians agreed on the impact on the treatment proposal in 3 factors (the clinical evaluation of disease activity according to DAS28, the presence and type of comorbidities and the patients' preferences) and disagreed on the other 3 (the DMARD cost/availability, a tendency to see DMARD-related adverse events and DMARD maximum doses), although the physicians had access to the same patient medical information. The management plan for RA might be a relatively simple task if only disease activity is considered but might become more complex when additional factors are considered; in particular, patients from Latin-America share particular sociodemographic and clinical characteristics that impact their access to health care and commitment with treatment that need to be included in the treatment equation during routine clinical practice [36, 37]. In addition, considerable variation has been observed in doctors' decisions, and these variations are known to depend on a physician's medical characteristics and medical experience [38].

In accordance to a greater impact of the ultrasound findings in the TR's treatment decision vs. the SR's decision, the TR rated the GUS-7 usefulness significantly higher than the SR in the totality of the clinical scenarios and in those where the GUS-7 impacted the final recommendation. Additionally, both physicians agreed on a higher GUS-7 usefulness in those scenarios where ultrasound findings did impact the treatment. These results suggest that the SR did not discard a priori the potential benefits of incorporating musculoskeletal ultrasound findings in the treatment decision; they rather confirmed that ultrasound assessments were among the most important factors included in the final management proposal.

In the present study, the GUS-7 findings were similar to those previously described in RA patients in whom gray-scale synovitis is frequently observed, even in patients with clinical remission, as were the majority of our patients [39]; tenosynovitis was less frequently identified and confirmed previous publications [12, 40]; erosions were identified in 34% of our patients, similar to what was observed in RA patients (43%) with disease duration proxy to that of our patients [12]; erosions were frequently located in the clinically dominant MTP5 (in addition to the MCP2) as previously published [41]. Interestingly, we found that the MTP2 was the joint most frequently scored with gray-scale synovitis and PD activity; we are unaware of similar findings, although erosions have been frequently described as located in the MTP2 head [41], and there is an association between PD ultrasound activity [42], anatomical and biomechanical factors [43], and a higher risk of erosive disease; our population had a (mean ± SD) body mass index of 25.9 ± 1.8, and 22% were obese.

Finally, patients were highly satisfied with the ultrasound assessment, with minimum discomfort, adequate time requirements and agreed to have ultrasound incorporated to routine clinical assessments, although they did not pay for the study; previous studies have also shown that musculoskeletal ultrasound favors patients' RA knowledge and their adherence to medication [44, 45].

Limitations of the study need to be addressed. First, a 40% difference between the TR and the SR in the percentage of treatment modification after GUS-7 was estimated; the difference between both physicians was 17%, and the 85 pairs of assessments performed could have been underpowered to test the primary objective. With the sample studied, the study had a 78.2 power to detect the primary objective. Second, the majority of the clinical scenarios described corresponded to remission status, some levels of disease activity (such as high DA level) were underrepresented, and the results might not be generalized to patients with such clinical status; nonetheless, in routine clinical practice, RA outpatients are expected to be in remission or to have low disease activity. Third, an important variable of the GUS-7 evaluation to impact the treatment proposal was the identification of DA; there is no consensus on the optimal scoring system for ultrasound in rheumatoid arthritis [46]. Additionally, DA definition was based on PD activity on at least one area, and low-grade PD signal might not necessarily reflect active synovitis [39]. Fourth, the GUS-7 assessed a limited number of joint sets compared to the clinical evaluation, although the existing literature confirms that they perform as well as extended joint sets [10, 47]. Finally, our study does not assess the adequacy of the final treatment in the ultimate terms of better disease and patient-reported outcomes. We are currently performing a study aimed to address the topic (Ultrasound impact in Rheumatoid Arthritis patient-reported outcomes [ULTRAPRO], ClinicalTrials.gov Identifier: NCT03228342).

Conclusions

Disease activity is important for the treatment decision during RA patient assessment; in routine clinical practice, additional factors also need to be considered. Musculoskeletal ultrasound added to "traditional rheumatic assessments" impacted the treatment proposal in a limited number of RA outpatients, most of them were classified with remission and low disease activity; the impact was greater in the trainee in rheumatology, who also scored better ultrasound usefulness compared to the senior rheumatologist. Both physicians differed in the impact of additional factors in the final treatment proposal.

Significance and innovations:

- Musculoskeletal ultrasound added to "traditional rheumatic assessments" impacts the treatment decision in 20% of RA outpatients.
- The impact of musculoskeletal ultrasound in the treatment decision of RA outpatients is limited for more experienced rheumatologists.
- Additional factors to disease activity determine treatment consideration during routine evaluation of an outpatient with RA. Physician experience impacts how those factors are rated.

Abbreviations

ACCP: Antibodies to cyclic citrullinated peptides; CRP: C reactive protein; DA: Disease activity; DAS 28: Disease activity score of 28 joints; DMARD: Disease-modifying anti-rheumatic drug; EAC: Early arthritis clinic; ESR: Erythrocyte sedimentation rate; EULAR: European League Against Rheumatism; GUS-7: German ultrasound score on 7 joints; MCP: Metacarpophalangeal joint; MTP: Metatarsophalangeal joint; PD: Power doppler; PIP: Proximal interphalangeal joint; RA: Rheumatoid arthritis; RF: Rheumatoid factor; SD: Standard deviation; SR: Senior rheumatologist; T2 T: Treat-to-Target; TR: Trainee in rheumatology; TUI: Targeted ultrasound initiative; TURA: Targeted ultrasound in RA study; VAS: Visual analogue scale

Acknowledgements

None.

Funding

None.

Authors' contributions

CSC: Participated in the conception and design of the study, performed patient's clinical evaluations, and reviewed the manuscript. ICY: Participated in the conception and design of the study, performed the statistical analysis, in charge of databases integrity of the early arthritis clinic. LSR: Participated in the conception of the study and reviewed the manuscript. ACL: Participated in the conception of the study and reviewed the manuscript. MG: Participated in the conception of the study, performed ultrasound evaluations and reviewed the manuscript. VPR: Participated in the conception and design of the study, performed patient's clinical evaluations; performed the statistical analysis and drafted the manuscript. In charge of the early arthritis clinic. All authors read and approved the final manuscript.

Consent for publication

Not applicable.

Competing interests

The authors declare that they have no competing interests.

Author details

[1]Department of Immunology and Rheumatology. Instituto Nacional de Ciencias Médicas y Nutrición Salvador Zubirán, Vasco de Quiroga 15, colonia sección XVI, Tlalpan, 14000 México City, Mexico. [2]Division of Musculoskeletal Ultrasound. Instituto Nacional de Rehabilitación y Ortopedia, Calzada México-Xochimilco 289, Arenal de Guadalupe, 14389 México City, Mexico.

References

1. Smolen JS, Aletaha D, Bijlsma JW, Breedveld FC, Boumpas D, Burmester G, et al. Treatment rheumatoid arthritis to target: recommendations of an international task force. Ann Rheum Dis. 2010;69:631–7.
2. National Institute for Health Care and Excellence (NICE). Nice clinical guideline 79. url: http://guidance.nice.org.uk/CG79. Accessed 11 Aug 2017.
3. Felson DT, Anderson JJ, Boers M, Bombardier C, Chernoff M, Fried B, et al. The American College of Rheumatology preliminary core set of disease

activity measures for rheumatoid arthritis clinical trials: The Committee on Outcome Measures in Rheumatoid Arthritis Clinical Trials. Arthritis Rheum. 1993;36:729–40.

4. Smolen JS. The work of the EULAR Standing Committee on International Clinical Studies including Therapeutic Trials (ESCISIT). Br J Rheumatol. 1992; 31:219–20.
5. Boers M, Tugwell P, Felson DT, van Riel PL, Kirwan JR, Edmonds JP, et al. World Health Organization and International League of Associations for Rheumatology core endpoints for symptom modifying antirheumatic drugs in rheumatoid arthritis clinical trials. J Rheumatol Suppl. 1994;41:86–9.
6. Grigor C, Capell H, Stirling A, McMahon AD, Lock P, Vallance R, et al. Effect of treatment strategy of tight control for rheumatoid arthritis (the TICORA study): A single-blind randomised control trial. Lancet. 2004;364:263–9.
7. Colebatch AN, Edwards CJ, Østergaard M, vasn Der Heidje D, Balint PV, D'Agistino MA, et al. EULAR recommendations for the use of imaging in the clinical management of rheumatoid arthritis. Ann Rheum Dis. 2013;72:804–14.
8. Chary-Valckenaere I, Sommier JP, MicheL-Batot C, Sauliere N, Rat AC, Hoenen-Clavert V, et al. Erosion and joint space narrowing in RA: proposition for a new quantitative score (ScuSST: Scoring by Ultrasound Structural Total) [abstract]. Arthritis Rheum. 2006;54:S 139.
9. Scheel AK, Hermann KG, Kahler E, Pasewaldt D, Fritz J, Hamm B, et al. A novel ultrasound synovitis scoring system suitable for analyzing finger joint inflammation in rheumatoid arthritis. Arthritis Rheum. 2005;52:733–43.
10. Naredo E, Gamero F, Bonilla G, Uson J, Carmona L, Laffon A. Ultrasonographic assessment of inflammatory activity in rheumatoid arthritis: comparison of extended versus reduced joint evaluation. Clin Exp Rheumatol. 2005;23:881–4.
11. Loeuille D, Sommier JP, Michel-Batot C, Sauliere N, Rat AC, Fintinger H, et al. ScUSI, and ultrasound inflammatory score, predicts Sharp progression at 7 months in RA patients [abstract]. Arthritis Rheum. 2006;54:S139.
12. Backhaus M, Ohrndorf S, Kellner H, Strunk J, Backhaus TM, Wartung W, et al. Evaluation of a novel 7-joint ultrasound score in daily rheumatologic practice: a pilot project. Arthritis Rheum. 2009;61(9):1194–201.
13. Dougados M. Comorbidities in rheumatoid arthritis. Curr Opin Rheumatol. 2016;28(3):282–8.
14. Pascual-Ramos V, Contreras-Yáñez I. Motivations for inadequate persistence with disease modifying anti-rheumatic drugs: The patient's perspective. BMC Musculoskelet Disord. 2013;14:336.
15. Neame R, Hammond A. Beliefs about medications: a questionnaire survey of people with rheumatoid arthritis. Rheumatology (Oxford). 2005;44(6):762–7.
16. Wolfe F, Michaud K. Resistance of rheumatoid arthritis patients to changing therapy: discordance between disease activity and patient's treatment choices. Arthritis Rheum. 2007;56:2135–42.
17. Barton JL, Trupin L, Shillinger D, Evans-Young G, Imboden J, Montori VM, et al. Use of low-literacy decision aid to enhance knowledge and reduce decisional conflict among a diverse population of adults with rheumatoid arthritis: results of a pilot study. Arthritis Car Res. 2016;68(7): 889–98.
18. Prevoo ML, van't Hof MA, Kuper HH, van Leeuwen MA, van de Putte LB, van Riel PL. Modified disease activity scores that include twenty-eight-joint counts. Development and validation in a prospective longitudinal study of patients with rheumatoid arthritis. Arthritis Rheum. 1995;38:44–8.
19. Backhaus M, Burmester GR, Gerber T, Grassi W, Machold KP, Swen WA, et al. Guidelines for musculoskeletal ultrasound in rheumatology. Ann RheumDis. 2001;60:641–9.
20. Taylor WJ, Harrison AA, Highton J, Chapman P, Stamp L, Dockerty J, et al. Disease Activity score 28-ESR bears a similar relationship to treatment decisions across different rheumatologists, but misclassification is too frequent to replace physician judgement. Rheumatology (Oxford). 2008;47:514–8.
21. Wakefield JR, Balint PV, Szkudlarek M, Filipucci E, Backhasu M, D'agostino MA, et al. OMERACT 7 special interest group: musculoskeletal ultrasound including definitions for ultrasonographic pathology. J Rheumatol. 2005;32:2485–7.
22. Szkudlarek M, Cpourt-Payen M, Strandberg C, Klarlund M, Klausen T, Ostergaad M. Contrast-enhanced power Doppler ultrasonography of the metacarpophalangeal joints in rheumatoid arthritis. Eur Radiol. 2003;13:163–8.
23. Micu MC, Alcalde M, Sáenz JI, Crespo M, Collado P, Bolboacă SD, et al. Impact of musculoskeletal ultrasound in an outpatient rheumatology clinic. Arthritis Care Res. 2013;65:615–21.
24. Agrawal S, Bhagat SS, Dasgupta B. Improvement in diagnosis and management of musculoskeletal conditions with one-stop clinic-based ultrasonography. Mod Rheumatol. 2009;19:53–6.
25. Mendonça JA, Yazbek MA, Costallat BL, Gutiérrez M, Barros-Bertolo M. The modified US7 score in the assessment of sinovitis in early rheumatoid arthritis. Rev Bras Reumatol. 2014;54(4):287–94.
26. Matsos M, Harish S, Zia P, Ho Y, Chow A, Ioannidis G, Khalidi N. Ultrasound of the hands and feet for rheumatological disorders: influence on clinical diagnostic confidence and patient management. Skelet Radiol. 2009;38: 1049–54.
27. Nam JL. Rheumatoid arthritis management of early disease. Curr Opin Rheumatol. 2016;28:267–74.
28. Wakefield RJ, D'Agostino MA, Naredo E, Buch MH, Iagnocco A, Terslev L, et al. After treat-to-target: can targetd ultrasound initiative improve RA outcomes? Ann Rheum Dis. 2012;71:799–803.
29. D'Agostino MA, Boers M, Wakefield RJ, Émery P, Conaghan PG. It is time to revisit the role of ultrasound in rheumatoid arthritis. Ann Rheum Dis. 2016;0:1–2. doi:10.1136/annrheumdis-2016-210453.
30. Haavarsdsholm EA, Aga AB, Olsen IC, Lillegraven S, Hammer HB, Uhlig T, et al. Ultrasound in management of rheumatoid arthritis: ARTIC randomised controlled strategy trial. BMJ. 2016;354:i42051.
31. Dale J, Stirling A, Zhang R, Purves D, Foley J, Sambrook M, et al. Targeting the ultrasound remission in early rheumatoid arthritis: the results of the TaSER study, a randomised clinical trial. Ann Rheum Dis. 2016;75:1043–50.
32. Dale J, Purves D, McConnachie A, McInnes I, Porter D. Tightening up? Impact of musculoskeletal ultrasound disease activity assessment on early rheumatoid arthritis patients treated using a treat to target strategy. Arthritis Car Res. 2014;66:19–26.
33. Díaz-Torné C, Moragues C, Toniolo E, Geli C, Castellví I, Moya P, Gich I, Llobet JM. Impact of ultrasonography on treatment decision in rheumatoid arthritis: the IMPULSAR study. Rheumatol Int. 2017;37(6): 891–6.
34. van der Heijde D. Remission by imaging in rheumatoid arthritis: should this be the ultimate goal? Ann Rheum Dis. 2012;71(Suppl 2):i89–92.
35. Beyer C, Ramiro S, Sivera F, Mandl P, Machado PM, Ospelt C, et al. Educational needs and preferences of young European clinicians and physician researchers working in the field of rheumatology. RMD Open. 2016;2:e000240.
36. Mody GM, Cardiel MH. Challenges in the management of rheumatoid arthritis in developing countries. Best Pract Res Clin Rheumatol. 2008;22:621–41.
37. Pascual-Ramos V, Contreras-Yáñez I, Villa AR, Cabiedes J, Rull-Gabayet M. Medication persistence over two years of follow-up in a cohort of early rheumatoid arthritis patients: associated factors and relationship with disease activity and disability. Arthritis Res Ther. 2009;11(1):R26.
38. Hinkka H, Kosunen E, Metsänoja R, Lammi U-K, Kellokumpu-Lehtinen P. Factors affecting physicians' decisions to forgo life-sustaining treatments in terminal care. J Med Ethics. 2002;28:109.14.
39. Gärtner M, Mandl P, Radner H, Supp G, Machold KP, Aletaha D, et al. Sonographic joint assessment in rheumatoid arthritis. Associations with clinical joint assessment during a state of remission. Arthritis Rheum. 2013; 65(8):2005–14.
40. Naredo E, D'Agostino MA, Wakefield R, Möller I, Balint PV, Filippucci E, et al. Reliability of a consensus-based ultrasound score for tenosynovitis in rheumatoid arthritis. Ann Rheum Dis. 2013;72:1328–34.
41. Siddle HJ, Hensor EMA, Hodgson RJ, Grainger AJ, Redmond AC, Wakefield RJ, et al. Anatomical location of erosions at the metatarsophalangeal joints in patients with rheumatoid arthritis. Rheumatology. 2014;53:932–6.
42. Brown AK, Quinn MA, Karim Z, Conaghan PG, Peterfy CG, Hensor E, et al. Presence of significant synovitis in rheumatoid arthritis patients with disease-modifying antirheumatic drug-induced clinical remission: evidence from an imaging study may explain structural progression. Arthritis Rheum. 2006;54(12):3761–73.
43. Tuna H, Birtane M, Tastekin N, Kokino S. Pedobarography and its relation to radiologic erosion scores in rheumatoid arthritis. Rheumatollnt. 2005;26:42–7.
44. Joplin SK, van der Zwan R, Bagga H, Joshua F, Wong PK. Pilot study assessing the novel use of musculoskeletal ultrasound in patients with rheumatoid arthritis to improve patient attitudes and adherence to medication. Int J Rheum Dis. 2016;19(7):658–64.

45. Kumar K, Raza K, Gill P, Greenfield S. The impact of using musculoskeletal ultrasound imaging and other influencing factors on medication adherence in patients with rheumatoid arthritis: a qualitative study. Patient Prefer Adherence. 2016;10:1091–10.
46. Mandl P, Naredo E, Wakefield RJ, Conaghan PG, D'Agiatino MA. OMERACT ultrasound task force. A systematic literature review analysis of ultrasound joint count and scoring systems to assess synovitis in rheumatoid arthritis according to the OMERACT filter. J Rheumatol. 2011;38:2055–62.
47. Dougados M, Jousse-Joulin S, Mistretta F, d'Agostino MA, Backhaus M, Bentin J, et al. Evaluation of several ultrasonography scoring systems for synovitis and comparison to clinical examination: results from a prospective multicenter study of rheumatoid arthritis. Ann Rheum Dis. 2010;69:828–33.

14

Arthroscopic findings of a diagnostic dilemma-hip pathology with normal imaging

Joel Glenn Buikstra[1*], Camdon Fary[2] and Phong Tran[2]

Abstract

Background: Patients with groin, hip and pelvic pain but normal findings on MRI and minimal changes on x-ray can be a diagnostic problem. This paper looks at the arthroscopic findings of patients who have had hip pain and a positive response to an intra-articular anaesthetic but have non-contributory imaging. We hypothesized that standard MRI's were missing significant pathology and if there was a response to intra-articular local anaesthesia, pathology found during arthroscopy was likely.

Methods: A retrospective review of all hip arthroscopies performed from March 2011 to January 2015 by two orthopaedic surgeons specializing in hip arthroscopy was conducted to identify patients with clinically suspected intra-articular hip pathology despite a normal MRI report and X-ray. Clinical suspicion of intra-articular hip pathology was confirmed with a positive response to a fluoroscopically guided intra-articular injection of local anaesthetic and corticosteroid. Pathologic findings were collated from the standardised operative notes.

Results: Fifty-three hip arthroscopies performed in 51 patients met the inclusion criteria from a total of 1348 hip arthroscopies performed over a 46-month period. All but one of the 53 (98%) hips had arthroscopically confirmed pathology. Mean patient age was 32.5 years [15 to 67 years] with 40 (78%) females and 11 (22%) males. 92.5% of the hips (49/53) were FADIR (flexion, adduction and internal rotation) positive on clinical examination, giving this test a positive predictive value of 98% (95% CI: 89.31 to 99.67%) for intra-articular pathology.

Conclusions: In patients with a normal MRI without contrast and a positive response (relief of pain) to an intra-articular injection that failed conservative management, there is a 98% chance of intra-articular hip pathology being discovered on hip arthroscopy.

Keywords: Hip arthroscopy, Magnetic resonance imaging, Image-guided injection, Intra-articular hip pathology

Background

This study explores the arthroscopic findings in patients with suspected hip pathology and normal hip X-ray (standing anteroposterior (AP) Pelvis, Lateral hip and Dunn views) and Magnetic Resonance Imaging (MRI) without contrast imaging but a positive response to an intra-articular hip injection of a local anaesthetic and corticosteroid. These patients pose diagnostic dilemmas that can be difficult to manage with little literature addressing how to approach the diagnostic workup in this select group. We hypothesized that standard XR and non-contrast MRI miss clinically significant pathology if there was a positive response to intra-articular local anaesthesia.

The diagnostic accuracy of physical examination tests of the hip are unfortunately poor, although combined with a detailed history can often predict the presence of intra-articular pathology [1–3]. The majority of cases require the use of additional investigative and diagnostic tests. Despite the recent advancements in imaging, hip pathology can be missed resulting in progressive symptoms and pathology. Diagnosis may not be made until sufficient damage has occurred that is irreversible (e.g. cartilage loss). Early diagnosis is therefore crucial for early successful management.

* Correspondence: joelbuikstra@gmail.com
[1]Austin Health, Austin Hospital, PO Box 5555, Heidelberg, VIC 3084, Australia
Full list of author information is available at the end of the article

Although it has been well established that a negative MRI should not preclude hip arthroscopy if there is high clinical suspicion [4], there is very limited literature looking at this population. MR arthrography remains the more sensitive diagnostic test when compared to MRI for intra-articular hip pathology and in particular labral tears, although there are discrepancies in the literature [5–8].

Local anaesthetic injection for diagnostic purposes with or without corticosteroid for therapeutic purposes is a common practice [9]. According to Jacobson et al. [10] and Kivlan et al. [11], pain secondary to chondral damage and femoroacetabular impingement (FAI) respond particularly well to diagnostic intra-articular local anaesthetic injections. Another study has demonstrated the response to injection is 90% accurate for detecting the presence of intra-articular pathology [1].

Methods

Inclusion criteria

We retrospectively reviewed all hip arthroscopies performed from March 2011 to January 2015 by two orthopaedic surgeons specializing in hip arthroscopy. Patients with a normal XR and MRI report, failed conservative management (including activity modification, analgesic medication and physical therapy) and positive response to hip joint preoperative anaesthetic injection were identified from the medical records.

Imaging

All patients had three routine plain XR views taken; standing anteroposterior (AP) Pelvis, Lateral hip and Dunn views to exclude osteoarthritis, hip dysplasia and FAI as a cause for the clinical suspicion of hip pathology. XR and MRI's were performed at a range of radiology departments in Melbourne (Australia), and reporting radiologists had a range of experiences although approximately half (25/53 or 47%) had specialist training in musculoskeletal radiology. Of the MRI's 56% were performed with a 3.0 Tesla (T) scanner, 15% with a 1.5 T scanner and of the remaining 29%, the strength of the magnet was unclear in the clinical database. The surgeons agreed with the reporting radiologist in all cases after reviewing the images themselves during the patient's following consultation.

Intra-articular injection

Those patients with unrevealing imaging went on to have a fluoroscopically guided intra-articular injection of corticosteroid and local anaesthetic. Pain relief following the injection was defined by a substantial improvement of pain as indicated by the numerical rating scale (NRS-11), which is a self-reported pain scale from 0 to 10 [12]. Those with pain less than 6 out of 10 prior to injection were excluded. Patients with pain 0 or 1 out of 10 for up to 48 h after the injection were considered to have had a positive result. Additional file 1 demonstrates the pain diary patients were asked to complete at the time of the injection along with verbal instructions.

Operative findings

Once we identified those that met the inclusion criteria, we looked at the arthroscopic findings by 2 fellowship-trained hip arthroscopists and recorded the details of the pathology found. In particular, we reviewed the operative notes for the presence and details of 3 common intra-articular pathologies- Ligamentum teres (LT) tears, labral tears, and chondral damage. LT anatomy was classified as normal, a partial, complete or degenerative tear [13]. As with Devitt et al. [14], we feel that LT fraying and elongation represent partial tears associated with instability/subluxation and so these two findings were classified as such. Labral tear size and location using a clock-face description [15] were recorded. Chondral damage to the acetabulum or femoral head was graded using the Outerbridge system [16].

The two surgeons independently and blindly assessed each other's arthroscopic images to confirm what pathology was present and agreed in all cases. Statistical analyses were performed using the Statistical Package for the Social Sciences (SPSS) software (version 22.0, IBM SPSS, Chicago, IL, USA).

Results

Fifty-three hip arthroscopies performed in 51 patients met the inclusion criteria from a total of 1348 hip arthroscopies performed over the 46-month period. 52 of the 53 (98%) hips included in this retrospective study had arthroscopically confirmed intra-articular hip pathology. Mean patient age was 32.5 years [15 to 67 years]) with 40 (78%) females and 11 (22%) males. There were 23 left hips and 30 right hips.

Running, Australian Rules football, gym, netball and soccer were the most common sporting activities (see Table 1 below) that patients engaged in. 21 patients did not participate in any regular sport at the time of presentation.

The most common precipitating event was pain during sport/physical activity (17/51 patients, or 33%) followed by a gradual onset of pain without an obvious precipitating event (16/51 patients or 31%)- see Table 2.

92.5% of the hips (49/53) were FADIR (flexion, adduction and internal rotation) positive on clinical examination, giving this test a positive predictive value of 98% (95% CI: 89.31% to 99.67%) for intra-articular pathology as all but one of the patients had arthroscopically confirmed pathology.

The most common pathology found during arthroscopy was a tear of the ligamentum teres (47/53, 89%), followed by chondral damage (35/53, 66%) and a labral tear (20/53, 38%). Damage to both the ligamentum teres and medial femoral head cartilage co-existed in 43% (23/53). Two

Table 1 Patient demographics

Number of patients	51 (53 hips)
Mean age (range)	32.5 (15–67)
Female: male	40:11
Left: right	23:30
Main regular sport	
Running	10
Football	3
'Gym''gymnastics'	5
Netball	3
Soccer	2
Cycling	1
Hockey	1
Ice skating	1
Rowing	1
Basketball	1
Volleyball	1
Dancing	1
None/not specified	21

complete tears of the LT were found during arthroscopy. Chondral damage was seen in 23 cases on the femoral head and 23 cases on the acetabulum (most commonly Outerbridge grade 1 or 2, see Table 3 below and also Additional file 2). Eleven patients had chondral damage on both the femoral head and acetabulum.

Labral tears were found in 20 cases (38%), and 17 of these (85%) were anterosuperior, 1 (5%) was posterosuperior and 2 (10%) extended across both anterosuperior and posterosuperior quadrants. Only 1 subject had no identifiable pathology during hip arthroscopy despite experiencing relief of pain following the intra-articular injection. Figure 1 summarizes the proportions of different combinations of pathology that were definitively diagnosed and treated arthroscopically. Figure 2 illustrates the types and incidences of intra-articular hip pathologies, with LT tears being the most common.

Discussion

There is a very high chance of intra-articular pathology being discovered during hip arthroscopy despite normal

Table 2 Precipitating event of pain

Precipitating event	Number of cases
Sport/physical activity	17
Gradual onset (no precipitating event)	16
Unclear from clinical notes	8
Fall/slipped over	7
Childbirth	3

Table 3 Confirmed pathology

Pathology	No. of cases
No pathology	1
LT tear (partial or complete)	47
Labral tear	20
Femoral head chondral damage[a]	
Grade I	4
Grade II	15
Grade III	3
Grade IV	1
Acetabular chondral damage[a]	
Grade I	13
Grade II	8
Grade III	2
Grade IV	0

LT ligamentum teres
[a]I to IV, Outerbridge classification

imaging investigations in this select group of diagnostic dilemmas. With limited literature suggesting a suitable diagnostic workup for these patients, a diagnostic arthroscopy is very likely to yield pathology that *may* be the cause of a patient's symptoms. To our knowledge, this is the first study looking at the arthroscopic findings in this select group.

The majority (89%) of the hips had a LT tear. Partial LT tears are increasingly being recognised as a source of hip pain although clinical examination and MR imaging play a

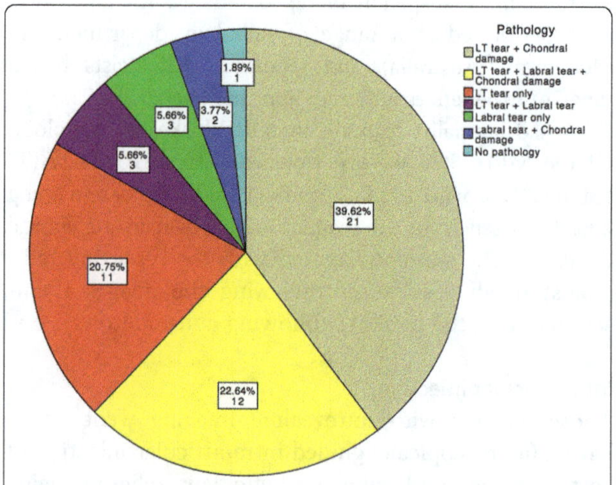

Fig. 1 Combinations of Intra-Articular Pathology Defined at Time of Arthroscopy for Individual Patients. The most frequent pathology combination was a ligamentum teres (LT) tear with associated chondral damage, which was seen as a combination in 21 hips (40%). A combination of all 3 pathologies (LT tear, labral tear and chondral damage) co-existed in 12 hips (23%; also see Table 3 and Additional file 2)

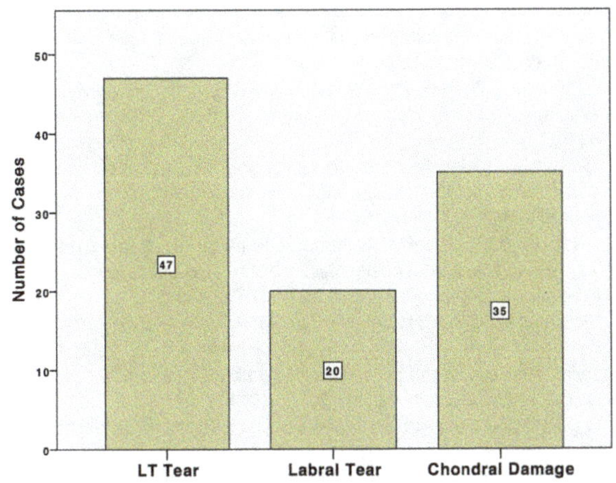

Fig. 2 Total Proportions of Intra-Articular Pathology Identified Arthroscopically. The most common pathology arthroscopically diagnosed in patients with normal imaging was a tear of the ligamentum teres (89% of hips), followed by chondral damage (66%). Labral tears were seen in 20 hips (38%)

limited role in detection. A LT clinical examination test has recently been described by O'Donnell et al. [17], which has been reported to have moderate to high interobserver reliability (κ coefficient 0.80) for detecting the presence of LT tears [17]. LT tears are infrequently reported or described on MRI. The incidence of reported LT tears confirmed with arthroscopy varies in the literature from 4 to 65% [14, 18–21]. The higher prevalence observed in this study may be due to the fact that only subjects with a normal MRI were included. It must also be noted that the diagnosis of LT tears is largely subjective and as previously discussed, we classified fraying and elongation of the LT as a partial tear.

A combination of pathologies were diagnosed and treated arthroscopically in 72% (38/53) of the hips. An LT tear with chondral damage of the femoral head was the most common (21/53) combination and in 9 of these cases, a labral tear was also diagnosed. This is consistent with previous literature on LT biomechanics. LT tears can lead to instability and subluxation of the hip joint with progressive damage to chondral surfaces and the labrum [22]. We observed that the majority of hips that had undergone arthroscopy for hip pain demonstrated chondropathy. Of note, chondral damage wasn't observed as an isolated pathology.

Labral tears were found in 20 (38%) hips and most commonly co-existed with other pathology, which is consistent with previous findings [23–26] The sensitivity and specificity of MRI in the diagnosis of acetabular labral tears is 66 and 79% respectively in the literature [27]. Most labral tears were in the anterior superior quadrant, which is consistent with previous literature [28]. In this group we further postulate that LT tear/ elongation and/or ligamentous instability results in repetitive anterosuperior subluxation of the femoral head in this quadrant during forced external rotation of the hip joint as a cause for this predominant soft tissue damage pattern found.

Limitations

This study is limited by its retrospective nature, lack of control subjects and small sample size. A further limitation of this study is that MR arthrograms were not used, as standard MRIs are routine in clinical practice in this country. There is an argument for an arthrogram with dye and anaesthetic during MRI. However, we feel that a steroid injection does pose a small but significant risk of complication, which is minimised if it is used primarily for this select group after normal investigations or to decrease a large differential diagnosis. We added steroid to local anaesthetic in case there was a therapeutic effect that would limit pain to facilitate the patient's ability to perform physical therapy prior to considering surgery. It should be again noted that the strength of the MRI magnets differed (3.0 T Vs. 1.5 T Vs. unknown) depending on where they were performed, which may have impacted on the findings.

Literature suggests that these intra-articular hip pathologies may be asymptomatic, and associated with increasing age [11, 29, 30]. However, it is important to note that all patients had failed conservative management. Collections of pre and post-operative outcome measurements were not standard practice in our clinic during the first 18 months of data collection. Patients now complete the recently validated 33-item International Hip Outcome Tool (iHOT33) [31] pre and post surgery.

Conclusions

Although MRI is commonly used in imaging hip pathology, fluoroscopic guided injections of local anaesthetic are recommended when there is clinical suspicion, despite otherwise normal imaging. In patients with normal XR and MRI imaging but a positive response to an intra-articular injection that have failed conservative management, our study suggests that there is a 98% chance of intra-articular hip pathology being discovered on hip arthroscopy. In particular, there is a high rate of LT tears in patients with hip pain relieved by local anaesthetic and an MRI reported as normal.

Abbreviations

AP: Anteroposterior; CI: Confidence interval; FADIR: Flexion, adduction and internal rotation; FAI: Femoroacetabular impingement; iHOT33 33-item: International Hip Outcome Tool; LT: Ligamentum teres; NRS: Numerical rating scale; SPSS: Statistical Package for the Social Sciences; T: Tesla

Acknowledgements

We thank Shelley Westgarth-Nugent and Rebecca Cordingly from Western Health for their logistical expertise and help with the ethics approval process. We would also like to extend our appreciation to the staff at the Specialist Orthopaedic Surgery Centre (Melbourne) for help with data acquisition and general matters.

Funding

Not applicable.

Authors' contributions

JB collected and analysed the data and was the major contributor to the writing of the manuscript. PT and CF obtained the clinical history, performed the physical examination and reviewed the MRI films and arthroscopic images. All authors read and approved the final manuscript.

Competing interests

The authors declare that they have no competing interests.

Consent for publication

Not applicable.

Author details

[1]Austin Health, Austin Hospital, PO Box 5555, Heidelberg, VIC 3084, Australia.
[2]Orthopaedic Surgery, Western Health, Footscray, VIC, Australia.

References

1. Byrd JWT, Jones K. Diagnostic accuracy of clinical assessment, magnetic resonance imaging, magnetic resonance arthrography, and intra-articular injection in hip arthroscopy patients. Am J Sports Med. 2004;32(7):1668–74.
2. Martin RL, Irrgang JJ, Sekiya JK. The diagnostic accuracy of a clinical examination in determining intra-articular Hip pain for potential Hip arthroscopy candidates. Arthroscopy. 2008;24(9):1013–8.
3. Reiman MP, Goode AP, Hegedus EJ, Cook CE, Wright AA. Diagnostic accuracy of clinical tests of the hip: a systematic review with meta-analysis. Br J Sports Med. 2012.
4. Mitchell B, McCrory P, Brukner P, O'Donnell J, Colson E, Howells R. Hip joint pathology: clinical presentation and correlation between magnetic resonance arthrography, ultrasound, and arthroscopic findings in 25 consecutive cases. Clin J Sport Med. 2003;13(3):152–6.
5. Botser I, Safran M. MR imaging of the hip: pathologies and morphologies of the hip joint, what the surgeon wants to know. Magn Reson Imaging Clin N Am. 2013;21(1):169–82.
6. Czerny C, Hofmann S, Neuhold A, Tschauner C, Engel A, Recht MP, et al. Lesions of the acetabular labrum: accuracy of MR imaging and MR arthrography in detection and staging. Radiology. 1996;200(1):225–30.
7. Zlatkin M, Pevsner D, Sanders T, Hancock C, Ceballos C, Herrera M. Acetabular labral tears and cartilage lesions of the hip: indirect MR arthrographic correlation with arthroscopy–a preliminary study. AJR Am J Roentgenol. 2010;194(3):709 14.
8. Sutter R, Zubler V, Hoffmann A, Mamisch Saupe N, Dora C, Kalberer F, et al. Hip MRI: how useful is intraarticular contrast material for evaluating surgically proven lesions of the labrum and articular cartilage? AJR. Am J Roentgenol. 2014;202(1):160–9.
9. Singh J, Khan W, Marwah S, Wells G, Tannous D, Sharma H. Do we need radiological guidance for intra-articular hip injections? Open Orthop J. 2014; 8:114–7.
10. Jacobson JA, Bedi A, Sekiya JK, Blankenbaker DG. Evaluation of the painful athletic Hip: imaging options and imaging-guided injections. Am J Roentgenol. 2012;199(3):516–24.
11. Kivlan BR, Martin RL, Sekiya JK. Response to diagnostic injection in patients with femoroacetabular impingement, labral tears, chondral lesions, and extra-articular pathology. Arthroscopy. 2011;27(5):619–27.
12. Hjermstad M, Fayers P, Haugen D, Caraceni A, Hanks G, Loge J, et al. Studies comparing numerical rating scales, verbal rating scales, and visual analogue scales for assessment of pain intensity in adults: a systematic literature review. J Pain Symptom Manage. 2011;41(6):1073–93.
13. Gray AJ, Villar RN. The ligamentum teres of the hip: an arthroscopic classification of its pathology. Arthroscopy. 1997;13(5):575–8.
14. Devitt B, Philippon M, Goljan P, Peixoto L, Briggs K, Ho C. Preoperative diagnosis of pathologic conditions of the ligamentum teres: is MRI a valuable imaging modality? Arthroscopy. 2014;30(5):568–74.
15. Blankenbaker DG, De Smet AA, Keene JS, Fine JP, Blankenbaker DG, De Smet AA, Keene JS, Fine JP. Classification and localization of acetabular labral tears. Skeletal Radiol. 2007;36(5):391–97.
16. Outerbridge RE. The etiology of chondromalacia patellae. J Bone Joint Surg. 1961;43-B:752–7.
17. O'Donnell J, Economopoulos K, Singh P, Bates D, Pritchard M. The ligamentum teres test: a novel and effective test in diagnosing tears of the ligamentum teres. Am J Sports Med. 2014;42(1):138–43.
18. Byrd JWT, Jones K. Traumatic rupture of the ligamentum teres as a source of hip pain. Arthroscopy. 2004;20(4):385–91.
19. Haviv B, O'Donnell J. Arthroscopic debridement of the isolated Ligamentum Teres rupture. Knee Surg Sports Traumatol Arthrosc. 2011;19(9):1510–3.
20. Martin R, Kivlan B, Clemente FR. A cadaveric model for ligamentum teres function: a pilot study. Knee Surg Sports Traumatol Arthrosc. 2013;21(7):1689–93.
21. Botser I, Martin D, Stout C, Domb B. Tears of the ligamentum teres: prevalence in hip arthroscopy using 2 classification systems. Am J Sports Med. 2011;39(Suppl):117S–25.
22. Cerezal L, Kassarjian A, Canga A, Dobado M, Montero J, Llopis E, et al. Anatomy, biomechanics, imaging, and management of ligamentum teres injuries. Radiographics. 2010;30(6):1637–51.
23. McCarthy J, Noble P, Aluisio F, Schuck M, Wright J, Lee JA. Anatomy, pathologic features, and treatment of acetabular labral tears. Clin Orthop Relat Res. 2003;406:38–47.
24. Zaragoza E, Lattanzio P-J, Beaule P. Magnetic resonance imaging with gadolinium arthrography to assess acetabular cartilage delamination. Hip Int. 2009;19(1):18–23.
25. Beaulef P, Zaragoza E, Motamedi K, Copelan N, Dorey F. Three-dimensional computed tomography of the hip in the assessment of femoroacetabular impingement. J Orthop Res. 2005;23(6):1286–92.
26. Wang W-g, Yue D-b, Zhang N-f, Hong W, Li Z-r. Clinical diagnosis and arthroscopic treatment of acetabular labral tears. Orthop Surg. 2011;3(1):28–34.
27. Smith T, Hilton G, Toms A, Donell S, Hing C. The diagnostic accuracy of acetabular labral tears using magnetic resonance imaging and magnetic resonance arthrography: a meta-analysis. Eur Radiol. 2011;21(4):863–74.
28. Reurink G, Jansen SPL, Bisselink J, Vincken PWJ, Weir A, Moen M. Reliability and validity of diagnosing acetabular labral lesions with magnetic resonance arthrography. J Bone Joint Surg Am. 2012;94(18):1643–8.
29. Seldes RM, Tan V, Hunt J, Katz M, Winiarsky R, Fitzgerald RH. Anatomy, histologic features, and vascularity of the adult acetabular labrum. Clin Orthop Relat Res. 2001(382):232–40.
30. McCarthy JC, Noble PC, Schuck MR, Wright J, Lee J. The watershed labral lesion: Its relationship to early arthritis of the hip. J Arthroplasty. 2001;16(8):81–87.
31. Mohtadi NGH, Griffin D, Pedersen ME, Chan D, Safran M, Parsons N, et al. The development and validation of a self-administered quality-of-life outcome measure for young, active patients with symptomatic hip disease: the International Hip Outcome Tool (iHOT-33). Arthroscopy. 2012;28(5):595–605.

15

Quantitative MRI comparison of multifidus muscle degeneration in thoracolumbar fractures treated with open and minimally invasive approach

F. Gilbert[1*], T. M. Heintel[1], M. G. Jakubietz[1], H. Köstler[2], C. Sebald[1], R. H. Meffert[1] and A. M. Weng[2]

Abstract

Background: Minimally invasive pedicle screw fixation has less approach-related morbidity than open screw placement and is allegedly less traumatizing on paravertebral muscles, as there is no requirement to mobilize and retract the adjacent muscle portion. The approach-related long-term effects to the morphology of the paravertebral muscles are unknown. The purpose of this study was to compare the long-term amount of fatty degeneration of the multifidus muscle in patients treated with a classical open or a minimally invasive approach.

Methods: Fourteen Patients meeting inclusion criteria were selected. In all patients a singular fracture of the thoracolumbar spine with a two-level posterior instrumentation was treated, either using an open approach or a minimally invasive approach. All patients underwent quantitative MRI spectroscopy for quantification of the fatty degeneration in the multifidus muscle as a long-term proof for muscle loss after minimum 4-year follow-up. Clinical outcome was assessed using Oswestry Low Back Pain Disability Questionnaire, SF-36 and VA-scale for pain.

Results: The minimally invasive approach group failed to show less muscle degeneration in comparison to the open group. Total amount of fatty degeneration was 14.22% in the MIS group and 12.60% in the open group ($p = 0.64$). In accordance to MRI quantitative results there was no difference in the clinical outcome after a mean follow up of 5.
9 years (±1.8).

Conclusion: As short-term advantages of minimal invasive screw placement have been widely demonstrated, no advantage of the MIS, displaying a significant difference in the amount of fatty degeneration and resulting in a better clinical outcome could be found. Besides the well-known short-term advantage of minimally invasive pedicle screw placement, a long-term advantage, such as less muscle degeneration and thus superior clinical results, compared to the open approach could not be shown.

Keywords: Spine trauma, Muscle degeneration, Minimal invasive surgery, Dorsal instrumentation

Background

Minimally invasive pedicle screw placement is an equally safe and reproducible procedure for treatment of thoracolumbar fractures in comparison to the open approach [9] .Advantages of a minimally invasive approach are less blood loss, lower muscle trauma and a lower rate of surgical site infection than in open approach [2, 6, 18].

Muscle trauma in open approach results from sharp, subperiosteal dissection of the multifidi and rotator muscles, blunt force trough retraction and damage of the posterior branches of the spinal nerves leading to loss of function of the motor unit. The nerve damage has been shown to be solely approach related and unlikely to be caused by the trauma itself [6, 12]. EMG studies have shown that pathological changes in the muscle innervation after open approach are persistent in

* Correspondence: gilbert_f@ukw.de
[1]Department of Trauma, Hand, Plastic and Reconstructive Surgery, Julius-Maximilians-University of Würzburg, Oberdürrbacherstr. 6, D-97080 Würzburg, Germany
Full list of author information is available at the end of the article

midterm follow up and that reduction of the surface EMG signal correlates negatively to the amount of pain. EMG analysis has shown that an open approach leads to pathological innervation patterns of the paravertebral muscles in the long-term [6, 12]. While EMG studies may be a strong predictor of muscle degeneration, the actual true amount of degeneration, visible as fatty degeneration, has not been evaluated quantitatively. Chronic denervation leads to MRI detectable muscle degeneration and fatty infiltration. Whether the amount of fatty degeneration of the paravertebral muscles is further influenced by segmental immobilization is unclear, thus patients, permanently immobilized by implants must not be included in such studies [13]. Apart from an effect in the EMG studies, it remains unclear whether a higher amount of muscle damage in the open approach has long-term effects on the morphology of paravertebral spine muscles, and if there is an approach depended difference in morphology of the paravertebral muscles. Fatty degeneration of the paravertebral muscles has been described even in asymptomatic individuals, thus after surgery an increased degeneration would be expected. The goal of the study was a quantitative evaluation of fatty degeneration in the paravertebral muscles in either an open or a minimal invasive approach in the long term.

Methods

A statistical power analysis was performed using GLMPOWER in SAS 9.3 (SAS Institute Inc., North Carolina, USA), furthermore a 2-way-covariant analysis with ANCOVA for a level of significance of 0.05 was performed. A total number of 6 patients for each group were calculated to detect significant differences related to the type of surgery with a power of 90%. The expectable variation in both groups were based on the findings of Fan et al. with a comparable study design for the investigation of mono-segmental dorsal instrumentation in degenerative spine diseases. The institutional review board approved the study (Etic committee of the Julius-Maximilians-University, Würzburg, Germany approval number 55/15) and written informed consent was obtained from each patient before participation.

The spine register of level 1 Trauma center between 2007 and 2012 included 963 patients who underwent spine surgery for fractures of the thoracolumbar spine. The exclusion criteria were, among others, remaining osteosynthesis material (interference with MRI fat measurement), concomitant neuro trauma (Frankel A-D), osteoporotic fractures, low energy trauma, muscle diseases, Diabetes, use of steroids, obesity (BMI > 30) and claustrophobia.

After application of the inclusion criteria, monosegemental fractures of the thoracolumbar spine from T 11 to L2, treated with a bisegmental dorsal instrumentation, minimal follow up time of 48 months, age 18–65 and Frankel E classification, 34 patients that met inclusion were identified for the retrospective analyzation. Furthermore, two patients had died due to unrelated causes, 6 had moved away and 12 refused participation due to claustrophobia or had contraindications for MRI (pacer, defibrillator). 14 Patients were available for the investigation.

The level of pain was assessed using VAS spine score. For further evaluation of lower back pain the Oswestry Low Back Pain Disability Questionnaire and the SF-36 were surveyed. The fractures were classified according to the AO/Magerl classification [15]. Estimated blood loss and operation time were retrospectively obtained from the anesthesiology protocol of the clinical databank.

A postoperative CT scan was available for all patients, accuracy of pedicles screw placement was analyzed using a pedicle screw scoring system and sagittal alignment was measured [22].

In every patient a MRI with a spectroscopy using the SPLASH technique (spectroscopic fast low angle shot) was performed, which allows an exact quantification of fat in a 2-D MRI layer. The exact technique and the reliability of the spectroscopy was described by our workgroup previously [5, 11]. Borders of the multifidus muscle were delineated manually as custom-made software allows measuring in a random shaped region of interest. The amount of fatty degeneration was measured at the fracture level and in the middle of the adjacent vertebras (Fig. 1). The mean values and standard deviation of the FD were calculated.

Statistical analyses were performed using Excel and SPSS. Level of significance was calculated using the independent samples Mann-Whitney U-test and the Kruskal-Wallis test.

Results

In the open group all patients were treated using a Schanz-screw system (USS fracture Depuy-Synthes) MIS group all patients were treated with a toploader system with polyaxial screws (Longitude Horizon Fa Medtronic). Patients in the open group had a mean age of 46.5 years (±16.3) and in the MIS group an age of 41.3 (±17.6) years ($p = 0.616$). Blood loss was significantly lower in the MIS group and operation time did not show any differences between the two groups. The other baseline characteristics like BMI, follow up time, sex and smoker status did not show any significant difference (table 1). Fracture distribution for the open group revealed five A3 fractures, two B1 and two B3 fractures. In the MIS group four A3 and two B2 fractures were observed. Accuracy of pedicel screw placement revealed a good or excellent position for all screws according to the pedicle screw rating system of Zdichavsky et al. [21].

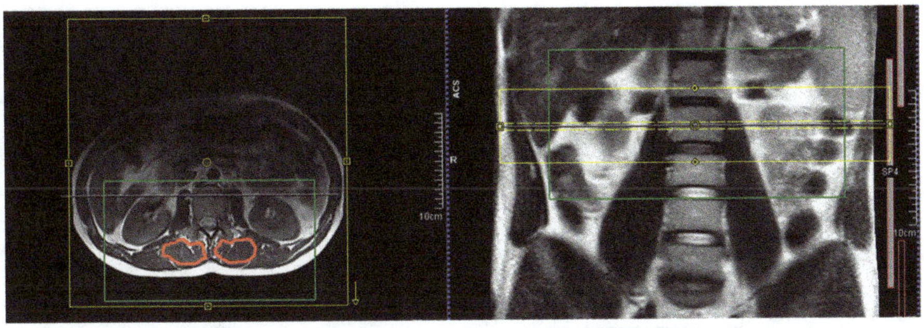

Fig. 1 A quantitative MR-spectroscopy was performed and the fat amount in the multifidus muscle was measured at the fracture level and the adjacent vetebrae

Mean loss of sagittal profile was 7° (±1.7) in the open and 6.8°(±1.7) in the MIS group compared from the initial postoperative lateral x-ray compared to the latest available x ray ($p = 0.73$). Implant removal was performed after a mean of 1.5 (±1.2) years in group A and after 1.3 (±1.4) years in group B ($p = 0.86$).

Functional assessment did not show a significant difference between the two groups. Results of the functional scores are shown in table 2. The result for the Oswestry Low Back Pain Disability Questionnaire for all individuals was 9% which resembles an excellent result. For the open group this score was 6% and for MIS group it was 12% without showing a significant difference $p = 0.13$. For the SF 36 and the VAS spine score no significant differences were detected between the two groups.

Finger floor distance was 5 cm (±4.7) in the MIS and 5.25 cm (±2.4) in the open group.

MR-spectroscopy of the paravertebral muscles revealed a mean fat amount of 13.3% (±6.1%) for all individuals. Patients treated with an open approach ($n = 8$) had a mean fat amount of 12.6% (±6.4%) and Patients with a minimal-invasive approach ($n = 6$) had a mean fat amount of 14.2% (±5.4%) (Fig. 2). Difference did not reach the level of significance ($p = 0.642$).

Table 1 Patients demographic data and results

	All $n = 14$	Open $n = 8$	MIS $n = 6$	p-value
Age [years]	44.3 (±17.1)	46.5 (16.3)	41.3 (±17.6)	0.616
Sex m:f	8:6	5:3	3:3	0.67
BMI	26.9 (±2.3)	27.1 (±2.1)	26.7 (±2.6)	0.75
Smoker	10	5	5	
Follow up Time [years]	5.9 (±1.8)	6.2 (±2.1)	5.43 (±1.1)	0.438
Amount of FD[%]	13.3 (±6.0)	12.6 (±6.8)	14.22 (±5.9)	0.642
Oswestry [%]	9 (±1)	6 (±1)	12 (±1)	0.134
SF 36	84 (±10.7)	86.3 (±8.7)	81 (±12.5)	0.51
VAS	1 (±1.2)	0.95 (±1.3)	1 (±1.1)	0.9
Blood loss [ml]	254 (±46)	110 (±23)	350 (±96)	0.0007
Operation Time [min]	98 (±14)	102 (±17)	97 (±12)	0.82

No implant related complications were observed in the two cohorts.

Discussion

Advantages of MIS

The advantages of minimally-invasive approaches in spine surgery are well investigated and accepted. As a muscle sparing technique, it reduces the approach-related morbidity. In particular use of minimal invasive approaches has less blood loss, lower infection rates, less operation time, faster recovery and a decreased serum concentration of creatinkinase, by providing the same safety and accuracy as open techniques [8, 9]. These effects on muscle have been supported by EMG studies showing a significant reduction of pathological EMG patterns if a minimal invasive approach was used in mid-term investigations [6]. A reduction of muscular disconnection from the bone, a reduction of nerve damage and the reduction of blunt trauma trough retractors are assumed to be beneficial (Fig. 3) [6, 18]. Long term effects of open dorsal approaches have been described, as Kramer et al. found pathological EMG patterns in the muscles of the whole erector spinae after a follow up time of 4 years in a cohort of 32 patients who underwent

Table 2 Inclusion and exclusion criteria for the study

Inclusion criteria
Monosegemental fractures of the thoracolumbar spine from T 11 to L2 which were treated with a bisegmental dorsal instrumentation
Minimal follow up time 48 months
Age 18–65
Frankel E
Exclusion criteria
Metal Implants In the fracture region
Neurological deficits (Frankel A-D)
Osteoporotic fractures, low energy trauma
Muscle diseases
Diabetes, Steroid, Adipositas >BMI 30
Claustrophobia
Contraindications for MRI

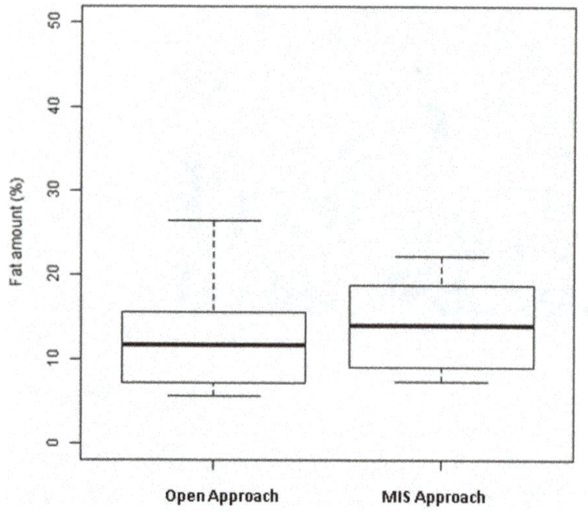

Fig. 2 MR-spectroscopy revealed a fat amount of 12.6% (±6.3) for the open and a amount 14.2% (±5.3) for the MIS group. The upper and the lower whisker of boxplots represent the standard deviation. The heights of box represents the interquartile range (25% and 75% quartile). The line in the middle represents the median

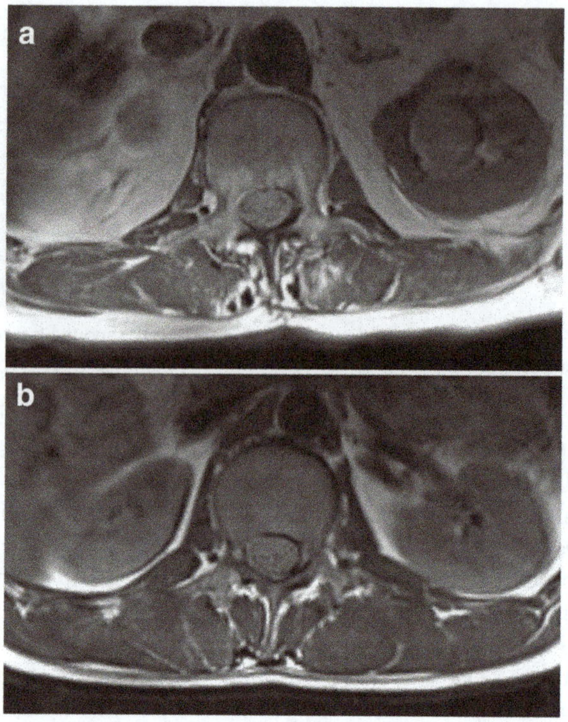

Fig. 4 T1-weighted transversal imagfe of the paravertebral muscles. MR spectroscopy reveald a fat amount of 26.5% for the multifidus muscle in **a** and an amount of 5.6% in **b**

open dorsal pedicle screw placement for fracture stabilization [12]. Patients with minimal invasive approaches were not investigated in this study; so, it remains unclear if these changes persist over a longer period and whether EMG changes translate into quantifiable effects on muscle diameter and ultimately atrophy.

Despite its disadvantages open approaches are still widely used and necessary especially in trauma with concomitant neurological deficit for decompression or if direct reduction of intra-spinal fragments is desired.

Fatty degeneration of paravertebral muscles and influencing factors

As muscular atrophy and degeneration is a promotor of lower back pain, which has been shown trough biopsy and MRI analysis of the lumbar muscles, it is unknown if there is an approach-related impact to FD of the paravertebral muscles in a trauma context [10, 20]. Various quantitative and semi-quantitative MRI methods are employed for analysis of amount of FD, but there is no standardized protocol yet, thus comparison of the different studies is limited. As the relation between the amount of FD and the occurrence of low back pain is well documented, several influencing factors for promoting FD have been described. In detail age, sex, spinal degeneration i.e. lumbar disc herniation, spondylolisthesis and facet joint arthritis influence the amount of FD (Fig. 4). [3, 4, 14, 19]. This is

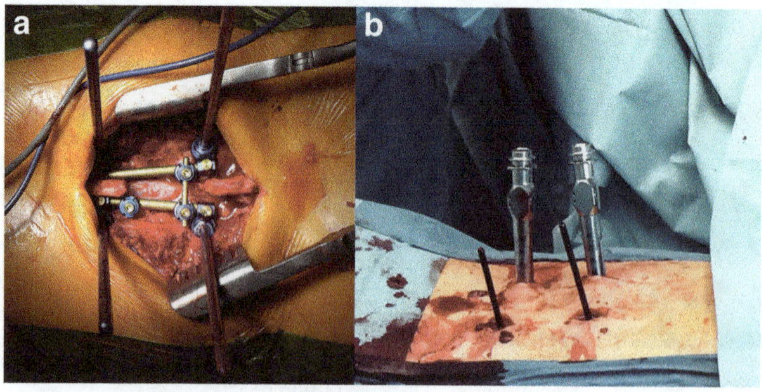

Fig. 3 Open approach (**a**) for pedicle screw placement and Minimal invasive approach (**b**)

supported by histological findings in chronical lumbar spine diseases showing an increase of degenerative changes in the multifidus muscles which occur as decrease of the cross sectional area, reduction of type II fibers, signs of inflammation and decreased vascularity [20]. Thus, an increased amount of fatty degeneration should be expected in patients with fractures that are furthermore treated with an open method in contrast to minimally invasive surgery. Surprisingly the long-term morphological changes in the paravertebral muscles were not approach related in this study and where approximately in the range of healthy individuals found in other spectroscopic MRI and semiquantitative studies [1, 7, 16]. MRI and biopsy studies showed that FD of the paravertebral muscles occurs regularly after spine surgery or with degenerative changes of the spine, even if segmental immobilization is performed trough anterior techniques alone. This suggests that the changes in morphology seem to be mainly triggered by the segmental immobilization, age and degenerative changes than the nerve damage through surgery [1, 3, 17]. Studies using MRI quantification to assess the lumbar spine muscles are rare in trauma situation. In contradiction to our findings Fan et al. found a significant reduction of in the cross-sectional area of the multifidus muscle postoperatively when an open approach was used for dorsal mono-segmental fusion (PLIF) in a cohort of 21 patients after 1 year. The follow up time of 1 year was shorter, the patient cohort was about 10 years older, the focus was on surgery for degenerative changes and a semi-quantitative method for analyzing the amount of FD was used [2]. Therefore, comparison may not be possible. As reinnveration potential has been demonstrated in EMG studies, the effect of the approach may be attenuated in the long term and could lead to a remodeling of the muscle structure [3, 6].

The relatively small number of participants and the retrospective design of the study do not allow conclusions about other influencing factors on the amount of FD. A prospective design would be helpful how FD develops over time, and if FD is a reversible process in the paravertebral muscles.

Conclusion

In this retrospective study setting, we did not find any differences in approach related long-term effects to the morphology of the paravertebral muscles. Studies focusing on the morphology of the paravertebral muscles in a trauma setting are rare, thus this study may serve as an approach to quantitative assessment of muscle morphology after spine trauma surgery. With a prospective design the impact of the surgical approach to the muscle and development of FD over time may be better understood. Nevertheless, we did not find approach-related the long-term effects on muscle morphology in this cohort of trauma patients.

Abbreviations

BMI: Body mass index; EMG: Electromyography; FD: Fatty Degeneration; MIS: Minimally invasive surgery; mm: millimeter; MRI: Magnet Resonance Imaging; SPLASH: Spectroscopic Fast Low Angle Shot; PACS: Picture archiving and communication system; VAS: Visual analog scale

Acknowledgments

None

Funding

This publication was funded by the German Research Foundation (DFG) and the University of Wuerzburg in the funding programme Open Access Publishing.

Authors' contributions

FG: made substantial contribution in design and conception of the study, wrote the manuscript. TH: performed acquisition of data and interpretation of data. JM: made substantial contribution in design an conception of the study, revisited the manuscript. CS: performed acquisition of data and interpretation of data. HK: performed acquisition of data and interpretation of data (spectroscopy), revisited the manuscript critically. RM: made substantial contribution in design an conception of the study. AW: performed acquisition of data and interpretation of data (spectroscopy), revisited the manuscript critically. All authors approved the final version of the manuscript.

Consent for publication

Not applicable

Competing interests

The authors declare that they have no competing interests.

Author details

[1]Department of Trauma, Hand, Plastic and Reconstructive Surgery, Julius-Maximilians-University of Würzburg, Oberdürrbacherstr. 6, D-97080 Würzburg, Germany. [2]Department of Radiology Julius-Maximilians-University of Würzburg, Oberdürrbacherstr. 6, D-97080 Würzburg, Germany.

References

1. Crawford RJ, Elliott JM, Volken T. Change in fatty infiltration of lumbar multifidus, erector spinae, and psoas muscles in asymptomatic adults of Asian or Caucasian ethnicities. Eur Spine J. 2017;1–9. Available from: https://link.springer.com/article/10.1007%2Fs00586-017-5212-6. [cited 2017 Nov 6].
2. Fan S, Hu Z, Zhao F, Zhao X, Huang Y, Fang X. Multifidus muscle changes and clinical effects of one-level posterior lumbar interbody fusion: minimally invasive procedure versus conventional open approach. Eur Spine J. 2010; 19(2):316–24. Available from: https://link.springer.com/article/10.1007%2Fs00586-009-1191-6. [cited 2015 Jan 16].
3. Fischer MA, Nanz D, Shimakawa A, Schirmer T, Guggenberger R, Chhabra A, et al. Quantification of muscle fat in patients with low back pain: comparison of multi-Echo MRI imaging with single voxel MR spectroscopy. Radiology. 2013;266:555–63. Available from: http://pubs.rsna.org/doi/10.1148/radiol.12120399?url_ver=Z39.88-2003&rfr_id=ori%3Arid%3Acrossref.org&rfr_dat=cr_pub%3Dpubmed&.
4. Fortin M, Lazáry À, Varga PP, McCall I, Battié MC. Paraspinal muscle asymmetry and fat infiltration in patients with symptomatic disc herniation.

Eur Spine J. 2016;25:1452–9. https://doi.org/10.1007/s00586-016-4503-7.
5. Gilbert F, Böhm D, Eden L, Schmalzl J, Meffert RH, Köstler H, et al. Comparing the MRI-based Goutallier classification to an experimental quantitative MR spectroscopic fat measurement of the supraspinatus muscle. BMC Musculoskelet Disord. 2016:1–7. Available from: https://doi.org/10.1186/s12891-016-1216-3doi:10.1186/s12891-016-1216-3
6. Grass R, Biewener A, Dickopf A, Rammelt S, Heineck J, Zwipp H. Percutaneous dorsal versus open instrumentation for fractures of the thoracolumbar border. A comparative, prospective study. Unfallchirurg. 2006;109(4):297–305. Available from: https://link.springer.com/article/10.1007%2Fs00113-005-1037-6. [cited 2015 Jan 15].
7. Hebert JJ, Kjaer P, Fritz JM, Walker BF. The relationship of lumbar multifidus muscle morphology to previous, current, and future low back pain: a 9-year population-based prospective cohort study. Spine (Phila Pa 1976). 2014; 39(17):1417–25. Available from: https://insights.ovid.com/pubmed?pmid=24859576. [cited 2017 Dec 14].
8. Heintel TM, Berglehner A, Meffert R. Accuracy of percutaneous pedicle screws for thoracic and lumbar spine fractures: a prospective trial. Eur Spine J. 2013;22(3):495–502. Available from: https://link.springer.com/article/10.1007%2Fs00586-012-2476-8. [cited 2017 Dec 14].
9. Heintel TM, Dannigkeit S, Fenwick A, Jordan MC, Jansen H, Gilbert F, et al. How safe is minimally invasive pedicle screw placement for treatment of thoracolumbar spine fractures? 2017;26, 5:1515–24. Available from: https://link.springer.com/article/10.1007%2Fs00586-016-4908-3. [cited 2017 Nov 6].
10. Kalichman L, Carmeli E, Been E. The association between imaging parameters of the Paraspinal muscles, spinal degeneration, and low back pain. Biomed Res Int. 2017;2017:1–14. Available from: https://www.hindawi.com/journals/bmri/2017/2562957/. [cited 2017 Nov 8].
11. Köstler H, Kenn W, Hümmer C, Böhm D, Hahn D. 2D-SPLASH spectroscopy to determine the fat/water ratio in the muscle of the rotator cuff. Rofo. 2002;174(8):991–5. Available from: https://link.springer.com/article/10.1007%2Fs00330-004-2410-5. [cited 2015 Jan 14].
12. Kramer M, Katzmaier P, Eisele R, Ebert V, Kinzl L, Hartwig E. Surface electromyography-verified muscular damage associated with the open dorsal approach to the lumbar spine. Eur Spine J. 2001;10(5):414–20. Available from: https://www.ncbi.nlm.nih.gov/pmc/articles/PMC3611527/. [cited 2017 Nov 6].
13. Kumar Y, Wadhwa V, Phillips L, Pezeshk P, Chhabra A. MR imaging of skeletal muscle signal alterations: systematic approach to evaluation. Eur J Radiol. 2016; 85(5):922–35. Available from: http://linkinghub.elsevier.com/retrieve/pii/S0720-048X(16)30034-1. [cited 2018 Feb 17].
14. Lerer A, Nykamp SG, Harriss AB, Gibson TWG, Koch TG, SHM B. MRI-based relationships between spine pathology, intervertebral disc degeneration, and muscle fatty infiltration in chondrodystrophic and non-chondrodystrophic dogs. Spine J. 2015;15(11):2433–9. Available from: https://www.sciencedirect.com/science/article/pii/S1529943015012243?via%3Dihub. [cited 2017 Nov 8].
15. Magerl F, Aeb F, Gertzbein SD, Harms JNS. A comprehensive classification of thoracic and lumbar injuries. Eur. Spine J. 1994;3:184–201.
16. Mengiardi B, Schmid MR, Boos N, Pfirrmann CWA, Brunner F, Elfering A, et al. Fat content of lumbar Paraspinal muscles in patients with chronic low back pain and in asymptomatic volunteers: quantification with MR spectroscopy. Radiology. 2006;240(3):786–92. Available from: http://pubs.rsna.org/doi/10.1148/radiol.2403050820?url_ver=Z39.88-2003&rfr_id=ori:rid:crossref.org&rfr_dat=cr_pub%3dpubmed. [cited 2017 Dec 14].
17. Motosuneya T, Asazuma T, Tsuji T, Watanabe H, Nakayama Y, Nemoto K. Postoperative change of the cross-sectional area of back musculature after 5 surgical procedures as assessed by magnetic resonance imaging. J Spinal Disord Tech. 2006;19:318–22. Available from: https://insights.ovid.com/pubmed?pmid=16826001. [cited 2017 Nov 6].
18. O'Toole JE, Eichholz KM, Fessler RG. Surgical site infection rates after minimally invasive spinal surgery. J Neurosurg Spine. 2009;11(December 2007):471–6. https://doi.org/10.3171/2009.5.SPINE08633.
19. Schilling AM, Heidenreich JO, Schulte T, Gräßmann A, Stendel R, Brock M, et al. Veränderugnen des Fett/wasser-Quotienten im Musculus Erector Trunci bei Patienten mit Lumbalem Bandscheibenvorfall: Eine Vergleichende 1H-MRS Studie. RoFo Fortschritte auf dem Gebiet der Rontgenstrahlen und der Bildgeb. Verfahren. 2004;176:229–33. https://doi.org/10.1055/s-2004-817632.
20. Shahidi B, Hubbard JC, Gibbons MC, Ruoss S, Zlomislic V, Allen RT, et al. Lumbar multifidus muscle degenerates in individuals with chronic degenerative lumbar spine pathology. J Orthop Res. 2017; Available from: http://onlinelibrary.wiley.com/doi/10.1002/jor.23597/abstract;jsessionid=A1625AB29133A0BBF1C79B8F4ADFB39A.f02t04. [cited 2017 Nov 8].
21. Zdichavsky M, Blauth M, Knop C, Graessner M, Herrmann H, Krettek C, et al. Accuracy of pedicle screw placement in thoracic spine fractures - part I: inter- and intraobserver reliability of the scoring system. Eur J Trauma. 2004; 30(4):234–40. https://doi.org/10.1007/s00068-004-1422-9.
22. Zdichavsky M, Blauth M, Knop C, Lotz J, Krettek C, Bastian L. Accuracy of pedicle screw placement in thoracic spine fractures. Eur J Trauma. 2004; 30(4):241–7. https://doi.org/10.1007/s00068-004-1423-8.

16

Magnetic resonance imaging of bacterial and tuberculous spondylodiscitis with associated complications and non-infectious spinal pathology mimicking infections

Yogesh Kumar[1], Nishant Gupta[2], Avneesh Chhabra[3], Takeshi Fukuda[4], Neetu Soni[5] and Daichi Hayashi[1,6*]

Abstract

Magnetic resonance (MR) imaging plays an important role in the evaluation of bacterial and tuberculous spondylodiscitis and associated complications. Owing to its high sensitivity and specificity, it is a powerful diagnostic tool in the early diagnosis of ongoing infections, and thus provides help in prompt initiation of appropriate, therapy which may be medical or surgical, by defining the extent of involvement and detection of complications such as epidural and paraspinal abscesses. More specifically, MR imaging helps in differentiating bacterial from tuberculous infections and enables follow up of progression or resolution after appropriate treatment. However, other non-infectious pathology can demonstrate similar MR imaging appearances and one should be aware of these potential mimickers when interpreting MR images. Radiologists and other clinicians need to be aware of these potential mimics, which include such pathologies as Modic type I degenerative changes, trauma, metastatic disease and amyloidosis. In this pictorial review, we will describe and illustrate imaging findings of bacterial and tuberculous spondylodiscitis, their complications and non-infectious pathologies that mimic these spinal infections.

Keywords: Spine, Infection, Abscess, MRI, Spondylitis, Discitis

Background

Magnetic resonance (MR) imaging plays an important role in the evaluation of bacterial and tuberculous spondylodiscitis. Owing to its high sensitivity and specificity of up to 90% or greater [1–5], it is a powerful diagnostic tool in the early diagnosis of spondylodiscitis. MR imaging thus provides help in prompt initiation of appropriate therapy which may be medical or surgical, by defining the extent of involvement and detection of complications such as epidural and paraspinal abscesses. However, other non-infectious pathology can demonstrate similar MR imaging appearances and one should be aware of these potential mimickers when interpreting MR images [6–10]. Radiologists and referring clinicians need to be aware of these potential mimics, which include such pathologies as Modic type I degenerative changes, trauma, metastatic disease and amyloidosis. In this pictorial review, we describe and illustrate imaging findings of bacterial and tuberculous spondylodiscitis, their complications and non-infectious pathologies that mimic these infections.

Epidemiology of bacterial and tuberculous spondylodiscitis

In bacterial spondylodiscitis, *Staphylococcus aureus* is the most commonly responsible organism, accounting for up to >75% of cases [11–13]. Other organisms that may cause bacterial spondylodiscitis include *Escherichia coli* in patients with concurrent urinary tract infections, *Pseudomonas aeruginosa* in patients with a history of

* Correspondence: dhayashi@bu.edu
[1]Department of Radiology, Yale New Haven Health System at Bridgeport Hospital, 267 Grant Street, Bridgeport 06610, CT, USA
[6]Department of Radiology, Boston University School of Medicine, 820 Harrison Avenue, FGH Building 3rd Floor, Boston 02118, MA, USA
Full list of author information is available at the end of the article

intravenous drug abuse, *Streptococcus pneumoniae* in patients with diabetes, and *Salmonella* species in patients with sickle cell disease or asplenia [14, 15].

Tuberculosis (TB) is one of the major causes of morbidity and mortality in developing countries with a rising trend in the United States and other developed countries with a reported worldwide incidence of 10.4 million cases in 2015 according to the World Health Organization global report [16]. Spinal TB is a destructive form of TB affecting the spinal column in less than 1% of all TB cases, causing neurological deficits, spinal deformities and paraplegia which mandates early diagnosis and treatment to avoid permanent damages [17]. According to an epidemiological study in the United States with a 10-year observation period (2002–2011), the incidence of spinal TB is actually decreasing from 0.07 cases per 100,000 persons in 2002 to 0.05 cases per 100,000 in 2011 ($p < 0.001$), corresponding to 1 case per 2 million persons in the latter year [18]. The same study identified men aged approximately 50 years were most commonly affected [18].

Pathogenesis of bacterial and tuberculous spondylodiscitis

Bacterial spondylodiscitis usually occurs due to hematogenous spread from a distant site, particularly from the lung or urinary tract. Bacterial spondylodiscitis can also occur via direct extension, for instance from spinal surgery, myelography, penetrating trauma, and from adjacent infections in the thorax or abdomen. Due to differences in vascular anatomy at different stages of life, discs are usually the first site of infection in pediatric patients followed by metaphyseal involvement, while in adult patients endplates are usually the first site of infection followed by disc involvement [19, 20].

Tuberculous spondylodiscitis, also known as Pott disease, is caused by *Mycobacterium tuberculosis*, a slow-growing gram positive acid fast bacillus which becomes lodged in the bone via Batson's venous plexus and lymphatic from primarily infected lung, lymph nodes, mediastinum and viscera, forming granulomatous inflammation and caseation necrosis [17]. Primary or secondary involvement of the posterior appendicular and articular element along with paraspinal soft tissue can also be seen [17, 21]. Thoracolumbar region is the most commonly affected site while the cervical and sacrum regions are less commonly involved. Usually more than one vertebra is affected because of its segmental arterial distribution and subligamentous spread of the disease. The bacilli reach the disc space causing disc destruction, spreads to adjacent vertebral bodies leading to vertebral collapse, anterior wedging, characteristic kyphotic angulation (Gibbus deformity), which may compress the spinal cord and nerve roots producing functional impairment [17, 22, 23].

Clinical presentation and diagnostic work-up

Bacterial spondylodiscitis most commonly presents with acute to subacute onset of back pain and fever. In many cases, fever of unknown origin is the main presenting complaint. Progressively increasing pain at the surgical site is usually the first symptom of postsurgical infection. For tuberculous spondylitis, patients present with constitutional symptoms such as malaise, loss of weight and night sweats while in chronic healed stage patients present with back stiffness, deformity and neural deficits.

Laboratory evaluation includes elevated inflammatory markers such as erythrocyte sedimentation rate (ESR) and C-reactive protein (CRP). These are very sensitive but non-specific markers of active bacterial spondylodiscitis, and thus can only be used to exclude active infection. Moreover, normal levels can also be seen in chronic infections. Leukocytosis and positive blood cultures are seen in most cases, especially before the initiation of medical treatment. Diagnosis of TB infection is usually based on clinical features, cerebrospinal fluid (CSF) analysis, histology and culture. However, combined use of MR imaging and GeneXpert, a test which detects DNA sequences specific for *Mycobacterium tuberculosis* increases the sensitivity to 97.9% for detection [17]. In doubtful cases, tissue biopsy is required to reach the diagnosis.

The diagnosis is often made by a combination of clinical features and imaging findings in some cases of spinal infection to initiate early empirical treatment in order to reduce the risk of complications, such as vertebral collapse and cord compression. However, a definitive diagnosis of the causative micro-organism is very difficult to establish based on clinical features and imaging alone. Therefore, image-guided percutaneous spinal biopsies are being increasingly performed to get sufficient tissue for culture and sensitivity of the causative organism [24]. However, the biopsy diagnostic yield of percutaneous spinal biopsy for detecting infection ranges from 30 to 40% and aspiration of > or = 2 mL of purulent fluid reported increases the rate of positive cultures [24].

Technical considerations for MR imaging

Usually, MR imaging of the spine is performed with basic sequences including T1 and T2 weighted sagittal and axial images. Additionally, fat-suppressed T2-weighted sequence or Short tau Inversion Recovery (STIR) sequence is used to increase the conspicuity of bone marrow edema and thus increasing the sensitivity [6]. If there is no bone marrow edema on fat suppressed T2-weighted or STIR images, gadolinium contrast administration does not add any value and is not required [25]. However, in many institutions, intravenous gadolinium contrast is usually administered in all suspected cases of vertebral infection. Its main role lies in differentiating phlegmon from epidural abscesses (this latter

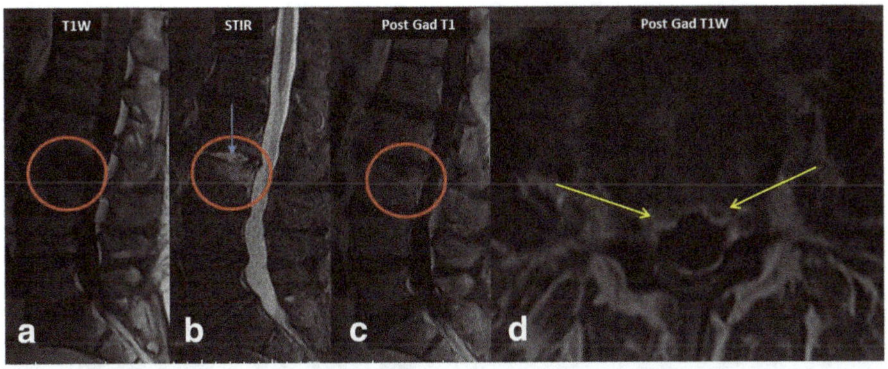

Fig. 1 42-year-old-diabetic-male patient presented with low back pain for 2 weeks. MR imaging showed L2–3 vertebral endplate marrow edema (*red circle* in **a**, **b** and **c**) and increased fluid signal in the L2–3 intervertebral disc on STIR sequence (*blue arrow* in image **b**). Post contrast images (**c** & **d**) show enhancing soft tissue in the epidural space (*yellow arrows*), consistent with phlegmon, which is a very early complication. Post contrast imaging can help in differentiating between phlegmon, which does not contain non-enhancing or liquefied components, from an abscess which does have those components. *Streptococcus pneumoniae* was the causative organism

demonstrates peripheral enhancement with central non-enhancing component), which is very important in deciding the appropriate treatment as epidural abscesses require surgical treatment in many cases, while phlegmon is usually treated with medical treatment [26]. In patients who cannot undergo contrast-enhanced MRI due to contraindications such as poor renal function or allergic reactions, usefulness of diffusion weighted imaging (DWI) for detection of abscesses has been demonstrated in the literature [21, 27, 28]. Some authors advocate its routine use in clinical practice because DWI may help differentiate between abscess and other pathologies such as non-infected cystic lesions (postoperative seroma, hematoma), cerebrospinal fluid leak, cystic/necrotic tumor and unusual patterns of degenerative disc and facet joint changes [21]. For assessment of spinal and paraspinal abscesses, DWI is performed with b values of 50 and 1000 s mm^{-2} and the apparent diffusion coefficient (ADC) map [21]. Image distortion can be reduced by deploying the parallel imaging factor 2. A spin-echo-type echo planar DWI sequence which allows fast imaging is commonly used to reduce motion artifacts [21].

MR imaging features of bacterial and tuberculous spondylodiscitis and associated complications

Bacterial infection

Early bacterial infection within bone marrow typically results in minor ischemia due to septic embolism to the

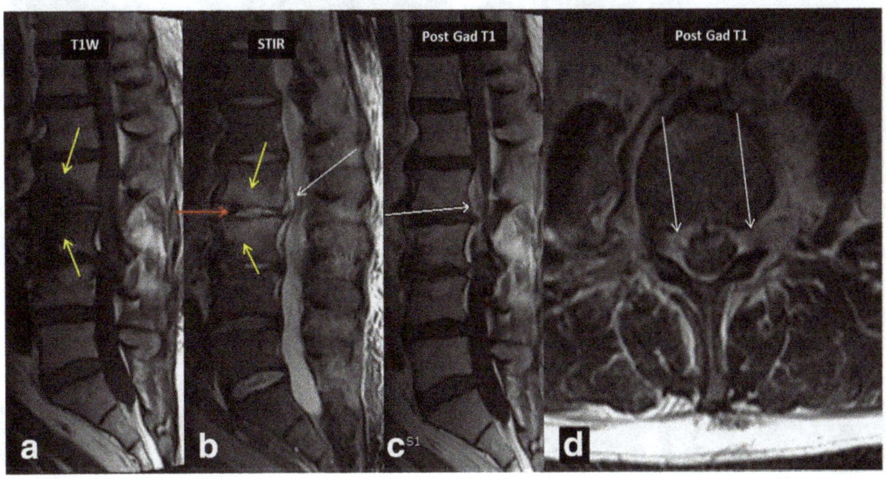

Fig. 2 MR imaging in a 36-year-old intravenous drug abuser female shows marrow edema involving L2–3 vertebra reaching up to the endplates (*yellow arrows* in **a** and **b**), with minimal enhancement on post contrast imaging consistent with osteomyelitis. Note increased amount of fluid signal in L2–3 intervertebral disc suggesting discitis-osteomyelitis complex. Post contrast imaging shows enhancing epidural soft tissue (*white arrows* in **b**, **c** and **d**) without areas of liquefaction, consistent with epidural phlegmon. Once again post contrast imaging can differentiate epidural abscess from phlegmon and thus alter management. Also note the presence of left psoas muscle involvement. Responsible bacteria in this case were *Staphylococcus epidermidis*

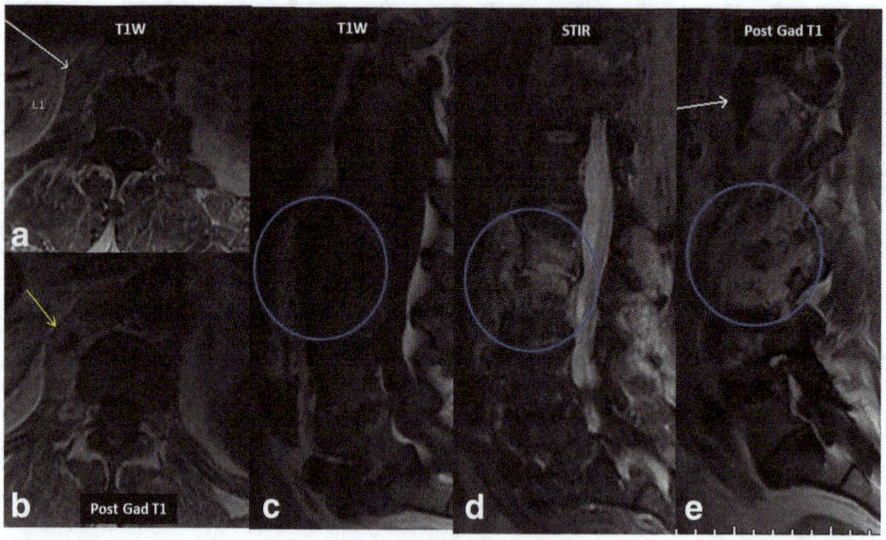

Fig. 3 This is a companion case to the case shown in Fig. 2. 24-year-old male from India presented with low back pain. MR imaging showed involvement of the left diaphragmatic crura (*white arrow* in image **a**) and showing enhancement in post contrast imaging (*yellow arrow* in image **b**). Note the extensive prevertebral tubercular involvement (*blue circles* in **c**, **d** and **e**) on T1 W, STIR and post contrast imaging. *Staphylococcus aureus* was the causative organism

end arteries and the presence of inflammatory exudate. These changes result in low T1 and high T2 signal abnormalities in the bone marrow. High T2 signal intensity abnormalities within the bone marrow are made more conspicuous using fat-suppressed T2 weighted or STIR sequences. In addition, enhancement would be seen in the bone marrow (Fig. 1). The intervertebral disc will also show increased T2 signal with contrast enhancement. With progression of the disease without prompt and appropriate treatment, the end plates will show erosions with subsequent loss of disc and vertebral height. Pre- and paravertebral edema and contrast enhancement is also seen in most of the cases (Fig. 2). Extension into the adjacent soft tissue

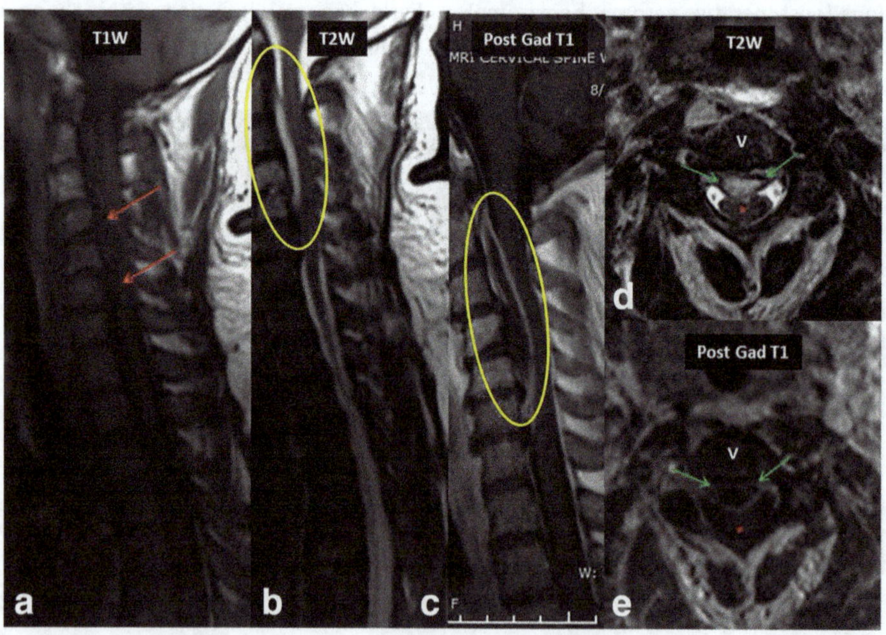

Fig. 4 MR imaging in a 42-year-old female with paraparesis shows heterogeneous signal (*red arrows*) on T1 W image (**a**) and hyperintense epidural collection (*yellow oval*) on T2 W image (**b**) and show rim enhancement (*yellow oval*) on post contrast images (**c**), consistent with an epidural abscess. Axial T2 W (**d**) and post contrast images (**e**) distinctly show the epidural abscess (*green arrows*) causing indentation and posterior displacement of the thecal sac and cord (*red asterisk*). *Escherichia coli* was the causative organism. V- Vertebral body

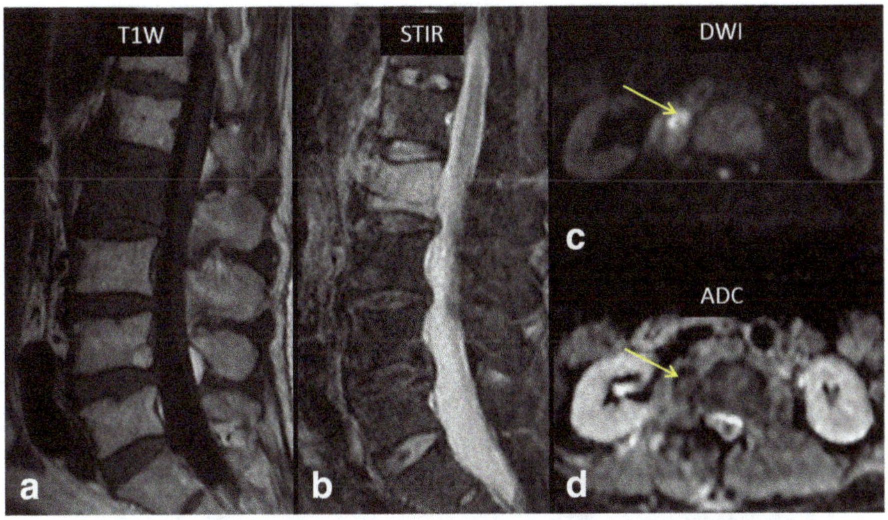

Fig. 5 64-year-old male with fever and low back pain. Sagittal T1 W (**a**) and STIR (**b**) MR images show extensive bone marrow edema involving entire L2 vertebral body and anterior portion of L1 vertebral body. High b-value (1000) axial diffusion weighted image (**c**) shows a right paraspinal soft tissue lesion with restricted diffusion (*arrow*) with associated decreased ADC values on ADC map (**d**, *arrow*). Biopsy of the lesion confirmed bacterial spondylodiscitis at L1/2 with a paraspinal abscess. *Staphylococcus aureus* was the causative organism

structures such as psoas muscle and diaphragmatic crura with phlegmon and abscess formation can also occur (Fig. 3). One of the major roles of MR imaging in evaluation of spinal infections is to look for spread of the infection in the epidural space and spinal canal with any effects on the cord and cauda equina nerve roots (Fig. 4). Contrast administration is necessary to differentiate phlegmon from the abscess in the epidural space (Figs. 2 and 4) as medical treatment may be sufficient in the former, while surgical drainage of abscess combined with medical treatment is necessary in cases of epidural abscesses. In patients who cannot receive gadolinium contrast or in cases where contrast enhanced MRI was not clearly diagnostic, DWI can be used to diagnose epidural abscess, as described earlier (Fig. 5).

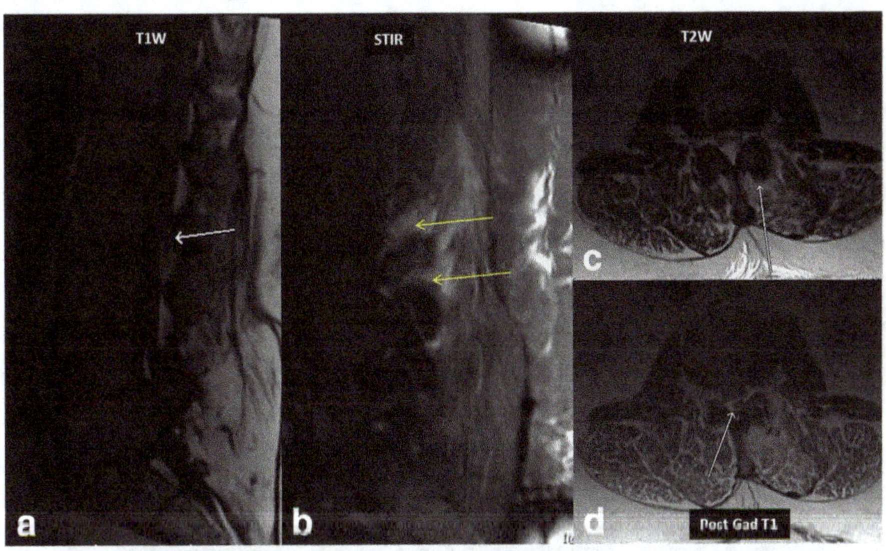

Fig. 6 46-year-old-cashier presented with left lower back pain, especially with bending to the left for picking up shopping bags for customers. Physical exam showed left lower back point tenderness. T1 W images (**a**) showed a left sided hypointense posterior epidural lesion (*white arrow* in image **a**). STIR image (**b**) shows extensive edema in the region of left L2–3 lumbar facet joint (*yellow arrows*). T2 W image (**c**) shows fluid signal in left L2–3 facet joint with adjacent edema (*white arrow* in image **c**). Note the associated posterior epidural abscess (*white arrow* in image **d**) causing anterior displacement of the thecal sac. *Staphylococcus aureus* was the causative organism

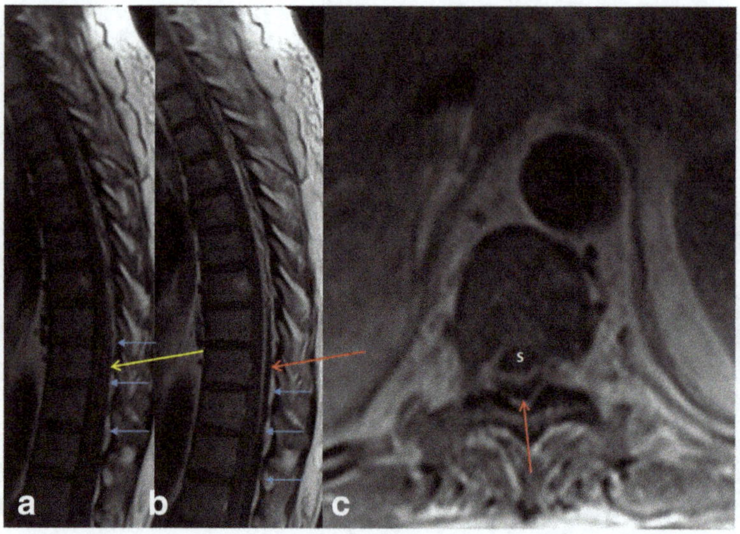

Fig. 7 MR imaging in a 24-year-old intravenous drug abuser male shows heterogeneous signal in the subdural space in the lower thoracic spine (*yellow arrow* in **a**) on T1 W images. There is peripheral rim enhancement on post contrast T1 W images (*red arrows* in **b** and **c**), consistent with subdural abscess causing anterior displacement of the cord (marked as S in **c**). Also note the preserved epidural fat suggesting subdural location of the abscess (*blue* arrows in **a** and **b**). Biopsy of the abscess confirmed *Pseudomonas aeruginosa* infection

In some cases, such as elderly patients, immunocompromised patients and following spinal procedures including facet joint steroid injections, facet joints can be the primary site of infection. This can result in abscesses which tend to be located in the posterior epidural space as compared to anterior epidural space in cases of spondylodiscitis. The MRI findings of facet joint infection includes increased signal in the joint and surrounding edema (Fig. 6). These changes can be very subtle and resemble degenerative joint disease. However, clinical presentation suggesting infective etiology and the presence of an epidural abscess favors infection over degenerative changes. In some cases, subdural abscess may be the main presentation of the spine infections, which is seen as a collection deep to the epidural fat (Fig. 7).

DWI has been shown to be useful in highlighting the extent of bacterial spondylodiscitis and distinguishing it from other pathologies which can mimic it [29]. 'Claw sign', described as a well-marginated, linear region of restricted diffusion at the interface of normal and abnormal marrow within the adjacent vertebral bodies, is seen in Modic type I degenerative changes and can be used to differentiate it from infection. This is due to the fact that a gradual process such as degenerative disc disease is

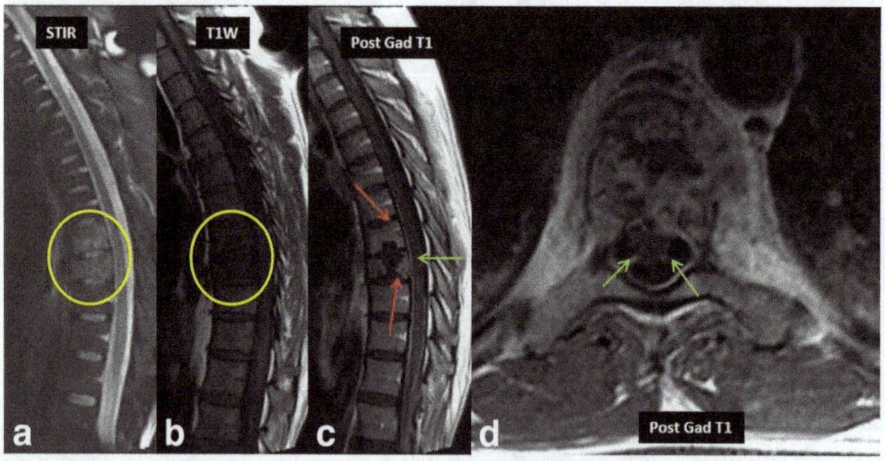

Fig. 8 27-year-old-male patient who was an immigrant from South America presented with back pain. Initial MRI was normal. Follow up MRI of the thoracolumbar spine for persistent back pain revealed marrow edema in the lower thoracic spine (*yellow circle* in **a** and **b**). Post contrast imaging showed discitis-osteomyelitis complex (*red arrows* in **c**). Note the enhancement of nerve roots suggesting extension of infectious process to the nerve roots causing arachnoiditis (*green arrows* in **c** and **d**)

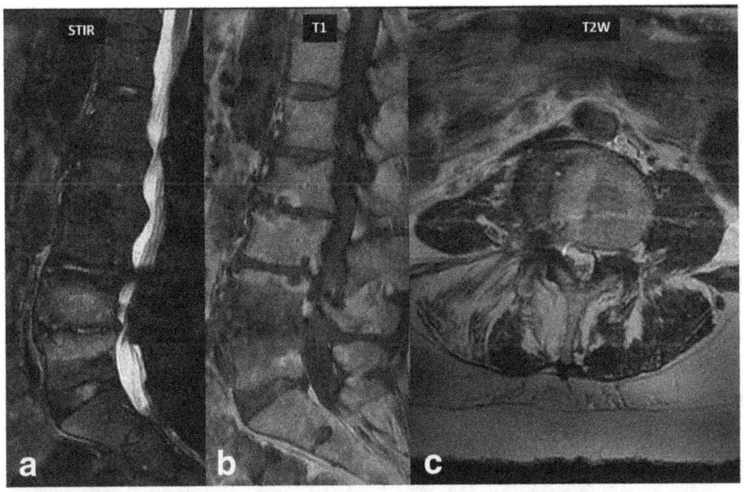

Fig. 9 An example of the Modic changes related to degenerative disease in a 68-year-old farmer. Note the Type I Modic changes at L4–5 endplates showing hyperintense signal on STIR image (**a**) and hypointense signal on T1-weighted image (**b**). Also note the absence of any surrounding paravertebral edema or psoas involvement (**c**), differentiating these Modic changes from vertebral osteomyelitis

expected to produce a well-defined response while infections usually progress quickly and diffusely giving rise to diffuse diffusion abnormalities rather than well-defined linear diffusion changes. DWI is also helpful in differentiating normal postsurgical fluid collections from the infected collections as the latter would show restricted diffusion due to thick viscous pus (Fig. 5) [30].

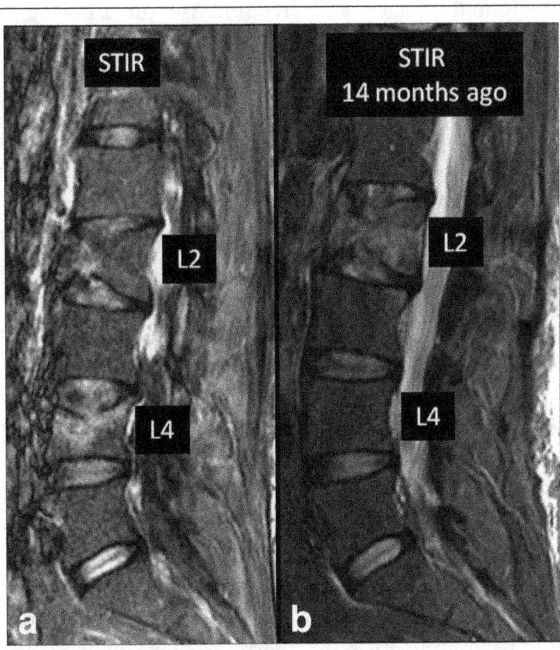

Fig. 10 74-year-old man presenting with acute low back pain following a fall. Sagittal STIR image at the time of presentation (**a**) shows end-plate deformities and bone marrow edema involving L2 and L4 vertebral bodies. When compared to prior study from 14 months ago (**b**), it became clear compression fracture of L2 is actually chronic. Change involving L4 is a new finding consistent with acute Schmorl's node in this patient who had no clinical or laboratory evidence of active infection

Frank bony and disc destruction is usually seen in chronic cases when there is a lack of initiation of prompt and appropriate treatment, either due to delay in presentation or diagnosis. Reactive bony changes, such as new bone formation and sclerosis, normalization of T1 signal intensity within a previously infected vertebral body and resolution of bone marrow edema on T2 weighted images suggest bone healing in a resolving infection.

Tuberculous spondylitis

Radiographs demonstrate reduced disc space, blurred paradiscal margins, increased paravertebral soft tissue opacity with and without calcifications, vertebral body destruction and severe kyphotic angulation in advanced progressive cases. CT is considered superior to MR imaging for visualization of small bony fragments and demonstrates more fine bony details of lytic lesions, endplate destruction and sclerotic margins, while MR imaging is considered superior for accurately defining the epidural extension of the disease and neural structure involvement. Findings of loss of vertebral body cortical definition and the presence of a calcified paraspinal mass with thick irregular rim enhancement favor tubercular over bacterial spondylodiscitis [23, 31]. Because of its superior ability to detect marrow changes before any bony destruction, MR imaging plays an important role in early diagnosis even in patients with normal radiographs. In majority of cases, tubercular spondylitis appears hyperintense on T2-weighted images and hypointense on T1-weighted images with contrast enhancement indicating marrow edema in the infected area (Fig. 8). An important imaging feature that characterizes tuberculous infection

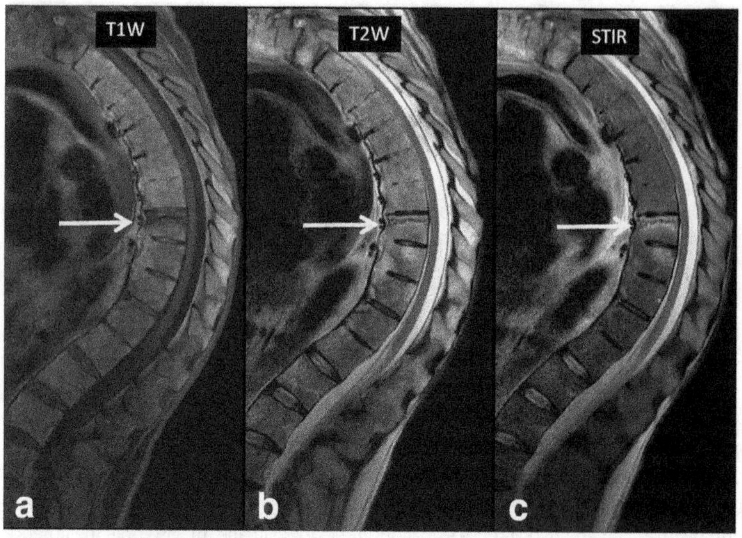

Fig. 11 52-year-old man with known history of ankylosing spondylitis presented with acute back pain following a fall. **a** T1-weighted, **b** T2-weighted and **c** STIR images in the sagittal plane shows a horizontal fracture *line* with associated bone marrow edema involving the superior endplate of T8 vertebral body (*arrows*). The patient showed no clinical evidence of active infection

compared to bacterial infection is sparing of the intervertebral disc in the early stage of infection. Conversely, early spread to discs with loss of disc height and disc herniation favor bacterial infection [4]. Other characteristic involvement of the anterior vertebral body corner, subligamentous spread, multiple vertebral bodies, extensive paraspinal abscess formation, abscess calcification,

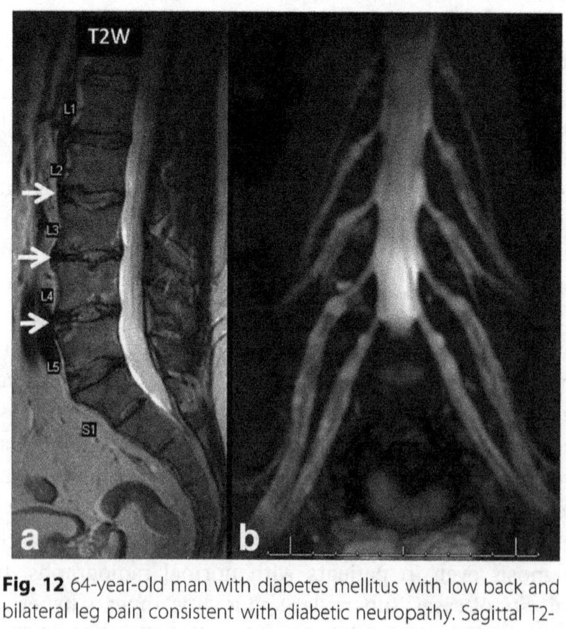

Fig. 12 64-year-old man with diabetes mellitus with low back and bilateral leg pain consistent with diabetic neuropathy. Sagittal T2-weighted image (**a**) shows end plate fragmentation at multiple lumbar levels (L2/3, L3/4, L4/5, *arrows*). MR neurography image (**b**) shows diffuse lumbosacral plexopathy with patchy thickening of all nerves. The patient showed no clinical evidence of active infection

and vertebral destruction differentiates tubercular from bacterial spondylodiscitis [17, 23, 32].

With progression of the disease classic discovertebral involvement can be seen which appear hyperintense on T2-weighted images and hypointense on T1-weighted images. In the chronic stage due to delayed diagnosis, low signal intensity on T1 and T2-weighted images indicates vertebral collapse with endplate sclerosis. During treatment, progressive increase in vertebral signal intensity on T1-weighted images suggests fatty replacement and indicates healing [23, 31, 32]. The infective process can extend into the epidural space causing cord compression, which is associated with a high mortality [23]. Extension into the spinal canal can lead to arachnoiditis (Fig. 8) and tuberculomas in the brain parenchyma in some cases.

Imaging features of pathologies mimicking spinal infections

Many degenerative and inflammatory spinal disorders may mimic spinal infections and it is necessary to be able to differentiate them from infectious spondylitis. In patients with overlapping clinical presentations, Modic type I degenerative changes can mimic infectious spondylitis as it can have endplate bone marrow edema with areas of contrast enhancement (Fig. 9). However, lack of abnormally increased signal in the disc on T2 weighted images and lack of soft tissue involvement including epidural abscess favors a degenerative disease over an infection [7].

Acute traumatic schmorl's node is the extrusion of a disc into the endplate (Fig. 10). Due to associated vascularization and inflammation, bone marrow edema

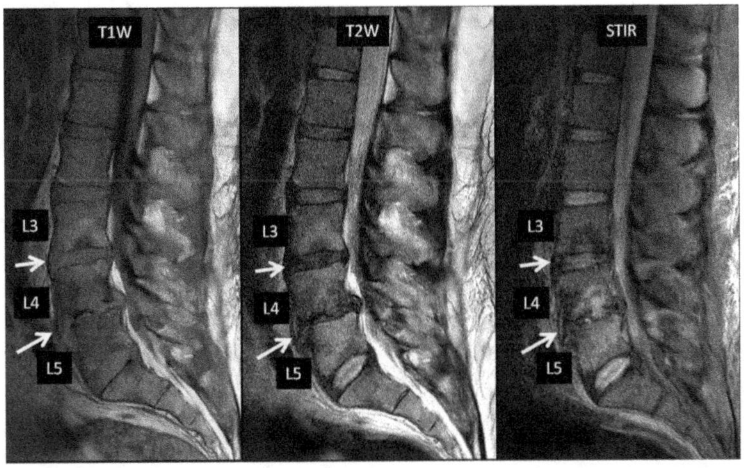

Fig. 13 39-year-old man with chronic renal failure on dialysis, with biopsy-proven amyloid spondyloarthropathy involving the lumbar spine. There are disc space narrowing and end-plate desctruction with associated bone marrow edema at L3/4 and L4/5. There is also grade 1 anterolisthesis of L4 over L5 as well as a disc herniation causing severe central canal stenosis at L4/5. From the imaging findings, initially infectious spondylodiscitis was suspected. However, failure to respond to antibiotic therapy prompted biopsy, which was negative for infectious organism and positive for amyloid stain

and contrast enhancement may be identified, and imaging features may be indistinguishable from those of infectious spondylitis. However, the presence of a high-signal-intensity concentric ring surrounding a cartilaginous node and involvement of only one endplate without disc signal abnormality favor acute traumatic schmorl's node over infection [8].

A common complication of advanced ankylosing spondylitis is spinal fractures which can be either spontaneous or following a trauma. These are commonly caused by osteoporosis in a patient with spinal fusion. These fractures typically are three-column fractures involving juxtadiscal endplate or the disk space. Pseudoarthrosis may develop at the site of the fracture resulting in endplate erosion and bone marrow edema mimicking imaging findings of infectious spondylitis (Fig. 11) [9]. A history of ankylosing spondylitis, proper clinical context and extension of the fracture line into the posterior elements help in differentiating ankylosing spondylitis related pseudoarthrosis from infectious spondylitis.

In patients with diabetes mellitus, syringomyelia, syphilis, or other neuropathic disorders, diminished protective sensation to repetitive trauma results in neuropathic arthropathy. In the spine, the thoracolumbar junction and the lumbar regions are most commonly affected. The clinical presentation and imaging appearance of spinal neuropathic arthropathy may resemble those of severe degenerative disease or spinal infection (Fig. 12). In the spinal neuropathic arthropathy, destructive changes in the vertebral bodies lead to a fracture, followed by bone sclerosis, new bone formation, a loss of disc space followed by pseudoarthrosis in the end stage. However, low signal in the disc and surrounding marrow on T2-weighted images are more likely seen in the neuropathic spine than in bacterial spondylitis. Other findings of vacuum phenomenon, facet involvement, osseous joint debris and joint disorganization are also suggestive of spinal neuropathic arthropathy [10].

Destructive spondyloarthropathies can also be seen in patients with long-term hemodialysis and resultant amyloid deposition in the spine (Fig. 13). Although MR imaging appearances can be similar to those of infection, these patients are usually clinically silent and bone marrow edema is not as prominent as infection [33]. Differentiation between infectious spondylodiscitis and amyloid spondylopathy can be achieved by biopsy, with negative culture and positive stain for amyloid.

Conclusions

A better understanding of the clinical features and pathophysiologic basis of bacterial and tuberculous spondylodiscitis contributing to their imaging appearances help the radiologist to make an accurate diagnosis and differentiate infections from other abnormalities which may mimic infections. This may result in early diagnosis and prompt initiation of appropriate treatment to avoid complications such as abscess formation, spinal deformities and neurological deficits.

Abbreviations

CNS: Central nervous system; CRP: C-reactive protein; CSF: Cerebrospinal fluid; CT: Computed tomography; DWI: Diffusion weighted imaging; ESR: Erythrocyte sedimentation rate; MR: Magnetic resonance; STIR: Short tau inversion recovery; T1W: T1 weighted; T2W: T2 weighted; TB: Tuberculosis; TE: Time to echo

Acknowledgements

None.

Funding

None.

Authors' contributions

All authors made the following contribution in preparation of this paper. Made substantial contributions to conception and design, or acquisition of data, or analysis and interpretation of data; Been involved in drafting the manuscript or revising it critically for important intellectual content; Given final approval of the version to be published. Each author should have participated sufficiently in the work to take public responsibility for appropriate portions of the content; and agreed to be accountable for all aspects of the work in ensuring that questions related to the accuracy or integrity of any part of the work are appropriately investigated and resolved. All authors read and approved the final manuscript.

Competing interests

AC is a consultant to ICON Medical and receives royalties from Jaypee and Wolters. YK, AC and DH are members of the Editorial Board of BMC Musculoskeletal Disorders. The authors declare that they have no competing interests.

Consent for publication

Not applicable.

Author details

[1]Department of Radiology, Yale New Haven Health System at Bridgeport Hospital, 267 Grant Street, Bridgeport 06610, CT, USA. [2]Department of Radiology, St. Vincent's Medical Center, 2800 Main Street, Bridgeport 06606, CT, USA. [3]Department of Radiology, University of Texas Southwestern Medical Center, 5323 Harry Hines Blvd, Dallas 75390, TX, USA. [4]Department of Radiology, The Jikei University School of Medicine, 3-25-8 Nishi-shimbashi, Minato-ku, Tokyo 105-8461, Japan. [5]Department of Neuroradiology, Sanjay Gandhi Postgraduate Institute of Medical Sciences, Lucknow, U.P, India. [6]Department of Radiology, Boston University School of Medicine, 820 Harrison Avenue, FGH Building 3rd Floor, Boston 02118, MA, USA.

References

1. Tali ET. Spinal infections. Eur J Radiol. 2004;50:120–33.
2. Kourbeti IS, Tsiodras S, Boumpas DT. Spinal infections: evolving concepts. Curr Opin Rheumatol. 2008;20:471–9.
3. Tins BJ, Cassar-Pullicino VN. MR imaging of spinal infection. Semin Musculoskelet Radiol. 2004;8:215–29.
4. Galhotra RD, Jain T, Sandhu P, Galhotra V. Utility of magnetic resonance imaging in the differential diagnosis of tubercular and pyogenic spondylodiscitis. J Nat Sci Biol Med. 2015;6:388–93.
5. Ledbetter LN, Salzman KL, Shah LM. Imaging psoas sign in lumbar spinal infections: evaluation of diagnostic accuracy and comparison with established imaging characteristics. AJNR Am J Neuroradiol. 2016;37:736–41.
6. Kumar Y, Hayashi D. Role of magnetic resonance imaging in acute spinal trauma: a pictorial review. BMC Musculoskelet Disord. 2016;17:310. doi:10.1186/s12891-016-1169-6.
7. Adams A, Roche O, Mazumder A, Davagnanam I, Mankad K. Imaging of degenerative lumbar intervertebral discs; linking anatomy, pathology and imaging. Postgrad Med J. 2014;90:511–9.
8. Stabler A, Bellan M, Weiss M, Gartner C, Brossmann J, Reiser MF. MR imaging of enhancing intraosseous disk herniation (Schmorl's nodes). AJR Am J Roentgenol. 1997;168:933–8.
9. Shih TT, Chen PQ, Li YW, Hsu CY. Spinal fractures and pseudoarthrosis complicating ankylosing spondylitis: MRI manifestation and clinical significance. J Comput Assist Tomogr. 2001;25:164–70.
10. Lacout A, Lebreton C, Mompoint D, Mokhtari S, Vallee CA, Carlier RY. CT and MRI of spinal neuroarthropathy. AJR Am J Roentgenol. 2009;193:W505–14.
11. Artenstein AW, Friderici J, Holers A, Lewis D, Fitzgerald J, Visintainer P. Spinal epidural abscess in adults: a 10-year clinical experience at a tertiary care academic medical center. Open Forum Infect Dis. 2016;3:ofw191.
12. Patel A, Alton T, Bransford R, et al. Spinal epidural abscesses: risk factors, medical versus surgical management, a retrospective review of 128 cases. Spine J. 2014;14:326–30.
13. Stratton A, Gustafson K, Thomas K, James MT. Incidence and risk factors for failed medical management of spinal epidural abscess: a systematic review and meta-analysis. J Neurosurg Spine. 2017;26:81–9.
14. Alonge TO, Ogunlade SO, Omololu AB, Obajimi M. Infective lumbar discitis in a sickler–an occult 'typhoid' spine? West Afr J Med. 2003;22:267–8.
15. Sehn JK, Gilula LA. Percutaneous needle biopsy in diagnosis and identification of causative organisms in cases of suspected vertebral osteomyelitis. Eur J Radiol. 2012;81:940–6.
16. Sotgiu GG, Sulis G, Matteelli A. Tuberculosis-a World Health Organization Perspective. Microbiol Spectr. 2017;5. doi: 10.1128/microbiolspec.TNMI7-0036-2016.
17. Sharma A, Chhabra HS, Mahajan R, Chabra T, Batra S. Magnetic resonance imaging and GeneXpert: a rapid and accurate diagnostic tool for the management of tuberculosis of the spine. Asian Spine J. 2016;10:850–6.
18. De la Garza RR, Goodwin CR, Abu-Bonsrah N, Bydon A, Witham TF, Wolinsky JP, et al. The epidemiology of spinal tuberculosis in the United States: an analysis of 2002-2011 data. J Neurosurg Spine. 2017;26:507–12.
19. Principi N, Esposito S. Infectious discitis and spondylodiscitis in children. Int J Mol Sci. 2016;17:539.
20. Ratcliffe JF. The arterial anatomy of the adult human lumbar vertebral body: a microarteriographic study. J Anat. 1980;131(Pt1):57–79.
21. Moritani T, Kim J, Capizzano AA, Kirby P, Kademian J, Sato Y. Pyogenic and non-pyogenic spinal infections: emphasis on diffusion-weighted imaging for the detection of abscesses and pus collections. Br J Radiol. 2014;87:20140011.
22. Sundaram VK, Doshi A. Infections of the spine: a review of clinical and imaging findings. Appl Radiol. 2016;45:10–20.
23. Ansari S, Amanullah MF, Ahmad K, Rauniyar RK. Pott's spine: diagnostic imaging modalities and technology advancements. N Am J Med Sci. 2013;5:404–11.
24. Wu JS, Gorbachova T, Morrison WB, Haims AH. Imaging-guided bone biopsy for osteomyeltitis: are there factors associated with positive and negative cultures? Am J Roentgenol. 2007;188:1529–34.
25. Mahnken AH, Wildberger JE, Adam G, Stanzel S, Schmitz-Rode T, Gunther RW, et al. Is there a need for contrast-enhanced T1-weighted MRI of the spine after inconspicuous short tau inversion recovery imaging? Eur Radiol. 2005;15:1387–92.
26. Kumar Y, Wadhwa V, Phillips L, Pezeshk P, Chhabra A. MR imaging of skeletal muscle signal alterations: systematic approach to evaluation. Eur J Radiol. 2016;85:922–35.
27. Castillo M. Diffusion-weighted imaging of the spine: is it reliable? AJNR Am J Neuroradiol. 2003;24:1251–3.
28. Raya JG, Dietrich O, Birkenmaier C, Sommer J, Reiser MF, Baur-Melnyk A. Feasibility of a RARE-based sequence for quantitative diffusion-weighted MRI of the spine. Eur Radiol. 2007;17:2872–9.
29. Kumar Y, Khaleel M, Boothe E, Awdeh H, Wadhwa V, Chhabra A. Role of diffusion weighted imaging in musculoskeletal infections: current perspectives. Eur Radiol. 2017;27:414–23.
30. Glaziou P, Falzon D, Floyd K, Raviglione M. Global epidemiology of tuberculosis. Semin Respir Crit Care Med. 2013;34:3–16.
31. Alvi AA, Raees A, Khan Rehmani MA, Aslam HM, Saleem S, Ashraf J. Magnetic resonance image findings of spinal tuberculosis at first presentation. Int Arch Med. 2014;7:12.
32. Lee KY. Comparison of pyogenic spondylitis and tuberculous spondylitis. Asian Spine J. 2014;8:216–23.
33. Theodorou DJ, Theodorou SJ, Resnick D. Imaging in dialysis spondyloarthropathy. Semin Dial. 2002;15:290–6.

17

Two cases in which 3D MRI was used to differentiate between a disc mass that mimics a tumor and neurinoma

Jingyu Jia[1], Qiangqiang Wei[1], Tianlong Wu[2], Dingwen He[2] and Xigao Cheng[1*]

Abstract

Background: Since disc sequestration that mimics a tumor is rare and sometimes presents with an atypical appearance upon magnetic resonance imaging (MRI), it is often confused with other more common epidural and intradural neoplasms, particularly neurinoma. Open surgery is necessary due to the difficult of achieving a definitive diagnosis using computed tomography, MRI, and gadolinium- enhanced MRI prior to operation. Herein, we describe the use of coronal MR images of 3D fast-field echo with water selective excitation in the diagnosis of disc sequestration mimicking a tumor.

Case presentation: Two patients were admitted to our hospital with back pain, radiating pain, and hypoesthesia in the right lower limb. MRI revealed tumor-like masses in the lateral recess of L3 and posterior to the body of L4. The initial diagnosis indicated disc sequestration mimicking a tumor and neurinoma. The coronal MR images of 3D fast-field echo with water selective excitation showed a clear boundary between the tumor-like mass and the nerve root. Moreover, the mass was also completely separated from the dura. Therefore, neurinoma was excluded as a possible diagnosis prior to operation. Surgical excision to perform removal of the gross mass was performed in one patient. The histopathological diagnosis was consistent with the 3D fast-field echo with water-selective excitation MRI. Another patient was successfully treated by minimally invasive endoscopic surgery.

Conclusions: Disc sequestration that mimics a tumor is difficult to diagnose preoperatively. As a non–invasive strategy, coronal MR images of 3D fast-field echo with water selective excitation is a helpful imaging tool for differentiating between diagnosis of disc sequestration that mimics a tumor and neurinoma prior to operation. If the disc fragment of mimicking tumor can be identified prior to operation, open surgery may not be necessary for all patients. Minimally invasive endoscopic surgery also is an alternative strategy.

Keywords: Lumbar disc herniation, 3D fast-field echo with water selective excitation, Disc sequestration, Mimicking tumor

Background

Disc sequestration is defined as the migration of a herniated disc fragment into the epidural space such that it is completely separated from the parent disc [1]. Magnetic resonance imaging (MRI) is the first diagnostic tool and gold standard for evaluating spinal pathologies [2]. However, in rare cases, the appearance of disc sequestration upon MRI is similar to that of a common epidural tumor, such as neurinoma or meningioma [3–5]. In 1993, Emamian et al. [6] detailed one case of lumbar herniated disk mimicking a neurinoma. Since then, mimicking tumor discs have been reported in several case reports [1–5, 7–22]. Open surgery was performed in all cases [1–22] since the surgeons were unable to make a definitive diagnosis using computed tomography (CT), MRI, and gadolinium-enhanced (Gd) MRI before operation. Herein, the authors successfully identified the disc fragment that mimicked a neurinoma using the coronal MRI of 3D fast-field echo with water selective excitation prior to surgery (3D MRI).

* Correspondence: 228206846@qq.com
[1]Department of Orthopaedics, The Second Affiliated Hospital of Nanchang University, Nanchang City 330006, Jiangxi Province, China
Full list of author information is available at the end of the article

Case presentation

Case 1

A 57-year-old man with a 10-year history of intermittent pain of the lower back and a 7-month history of intermittent pain of the right lower limb was admitted to our clinic. He complained of increased pain and hypoesthesia of the right lower limb that had started 1 month prior. Physical examination revealed that the pain was located in the distribution of L4 and weakness of the left extensor digitorum longus. Using a 10-cm visual analog scale (VAS), the patient reported the intensity of his leg pain to be 7/10, with an Oswestry disability index (ODI) score of 70. Negative Lasegue's sign was shown bilaterally on the lower limbs. T1-weighted images (T1WI) of MRI revealed a tumor-like mass with signal intensity posterior to the body of L4 (Fig. 1b). But, the periphery of the mass demonstrated a hyperintense ring on T1WI (Fig. 1b). Similarly, the mass was hyperintense on T2-weighted images (Fig. 1a). We suspected neurinoma since the mass presented as a similar appearance as neurinoma on MRI (Fig. 1a–c). To further diagnose the mass, the coronal MRI of 3D fast-field echo with water selective excitation (3D MRI) was performed, which revealed a clear boundary between the mass and nerve root (Fig. 2). Meanwhile, the mass was also separated with dura (Fig. 2). Therefore, we excluded neurinoma as a possible diagnosis prior to operation. Surgical excision with gross removal of the mass was performed in our hospital (Fig. 3a). The histopathological diagnosis was consistent with a degenerated intervertebral disc (Fig. 3b). The patient's symptoms improved immediately after surgery. He identified the strength of the lower extremities improving and recovered fully after 5 months.

Case 2

A 63-year-old male was admitted to our hospital with back pain and radiating pain in the right lower limb that persisted for 3 months. Upon admission, his neurological examination revealed hypoesthesia of L3 and L4 in the right lower limb. Meanwhile, the patient presented a score of 6 on the VAS and a score of 64 on ODI. A negative Lasegue's sign was observed on the bilateral limbs. T2-weighted images (T2WI) in the axial planes revealed a dumbbell mass in the lateral recess (Fig. 4b). Gd MRI demonstrated a heterogeneous ring-like enhancement at the periphery of the mass (Fig. 4c). We suspected neurinoma and performed 3D MRI to confirm the diagnosis (Fig. 5). As in case 1, a clear boundary was detected between the mass and nerve root using 3D MRI (Fig. 5). Moreover, the mass was also separated with dura (Fig. 5). Minimally invasive endoscopic surgery was executed in the case (Fig. 6). The histopathological diagnosis confirmed that the mass was a degenerated intervertebral disc (Fig. 7). VAS and ODI score was 1 and 12 at 1 week postoperative follow-up, and 0 and 4 at 1 year postoperative follow-up. The VAS and ODI scores improved from preoperative levels, and there was no occurrence of postoperative complications. The patient remains symptom free at 1-year post-surgery.

MRI scan

Sequence development was conducted on a 3.0 T whole-body scanner (GE Medical Systems, UK) with a spine coil. Conventional axial T2 fast spin echo (4180/102) (repetition time ms/echo time ms), sagittal T2 fast spin echo (2200/120), and sagittal T1 fast spin echo (460/20) were used to acquire the original images. Then, 3D coronal CUBE-MRN sequence was acquired using the following acquisition parameters for a 1 mm-thick section

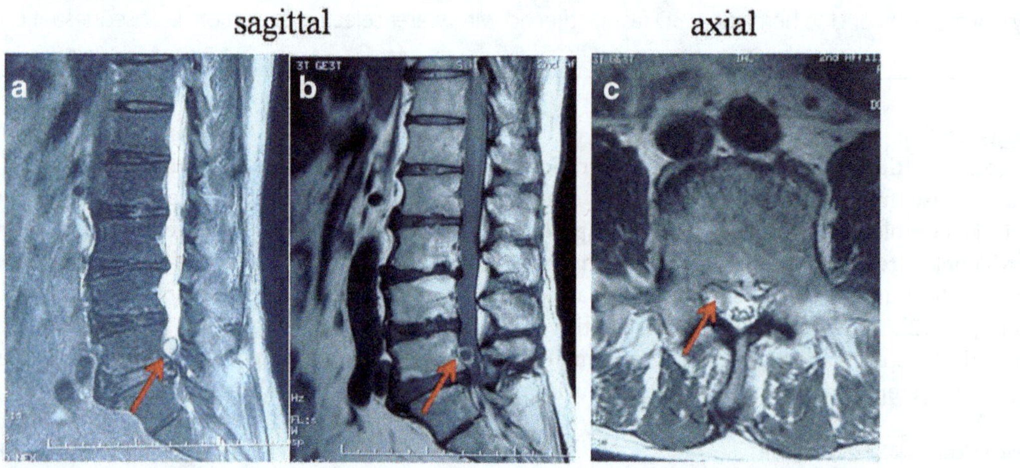

Fig. 1 Preoperative MRI of the lumbar spine without intravenous contrast. T2-weighted MRI in the sagittal and axial planes showed a mass that mimicked a neurinoma posterior to the body of L4 (**a** and **c**). T1-weighted MRI in the sagittal planes showed a tumor-like mass with signal intensity (**b**). Meanwhile, the periphery of the mass was hyperintense and ring-like on T1WI (**b**)

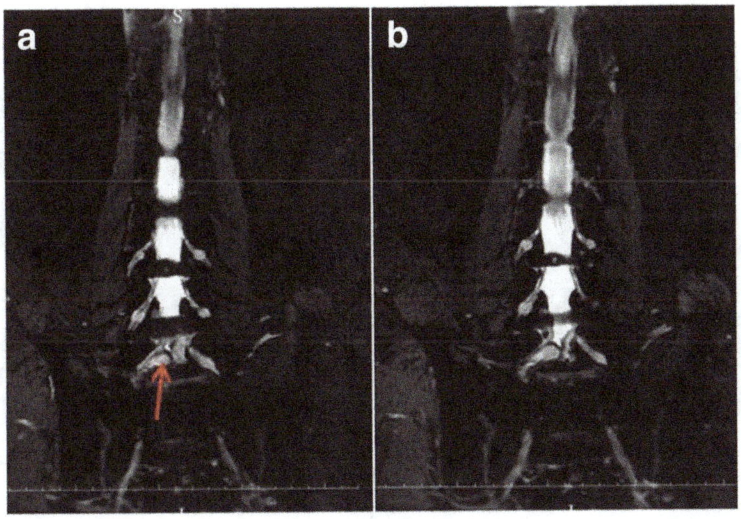

Fig. 2 Coronal MR images of 3D fast-field echo with water selective excitation. Clear boundary was observed between the mass and nerve root by coronal MR images (**a**). Meanwhile, it was found that the mass was also separated with dura (**b**)

without an overlapping section gap: a repetition time of 2000 ms, echo time of 32 ms, 352 × 256 matrix, 32 cm file of view, 20°flip angle, and 2 signal-intensity acquisitions. Original coronal fast spin echo images were acquired. We set the imaging plane to be parallel to the longitudinal axis of the lumbar spinal cord and centered on the level of the L3 vertebral body. The coronal image was reconstructed using maximum intensity projection and volume rendering technique on ADW version 4.6 software.

Discussion

Disc sequestration is defined as the migration of a herniated disc fragment into the epidural space such that it is completely separated from the parent disc [1]. Far migration of disc fragments and the variability in radiological appearance often result in diagnostic confusion prior to operation. A series of reports indicated that some sequestered disc fragments still can be misdiagnosed as other more common epidural and intradural neoplasms, even if CT, MRI, and Gd MRI have been performed before operation [1–19]. For example, Emamian et al. [6] reported one case in which a lumbar herniated disk mimicked a neurinoma in 1993. Subsequently, Sharma et al. [4], Ashkenazi et al. [8], and Levene et al. [5] also demonstrated three cases of disc sequestration that mimicked a nerve sheath tumor. Generally, disc fragments that mimic tumors appear hypointense on T1-weighted images and hyperintense on T2-weighted images. Following contrast medium administration, the patients in these cases presented with ring-like peripheral Gd enhancement. Although the ring-like peripheral enhancement is helpful for differentiating between disc fragments that mimic a tumor and metastatic tumors, hematomas, and meningioma, it is not specific. For example, ring-like peripheral enhancement can also be observed in neurinoma [4–8].

Like the previous reports, we were also unable to make a definitive diagnosis for the present cases depending on CT, MRI, and gadolinium-enhanced MRI before operation because of uncharacteristic radiological appearance.

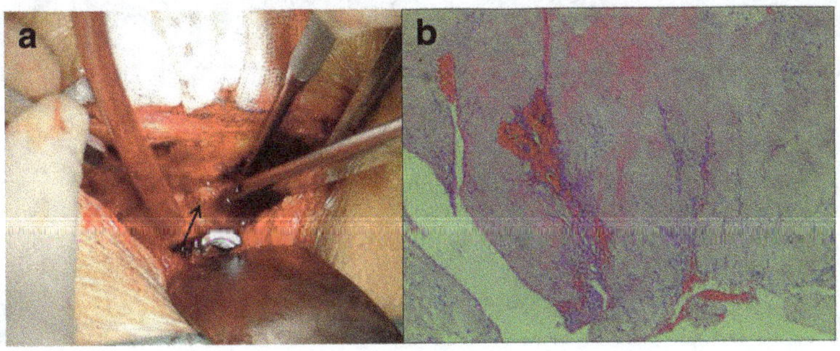

Fig. 3 Intraoperative view found the mass of mimicking tumor (black arrow) was disc fragment (**a**). The histopathological diagnosis confirmed the intraoperative observation that the mass was a disc fragment (**b**). (hematoxylin and eosin × 40)

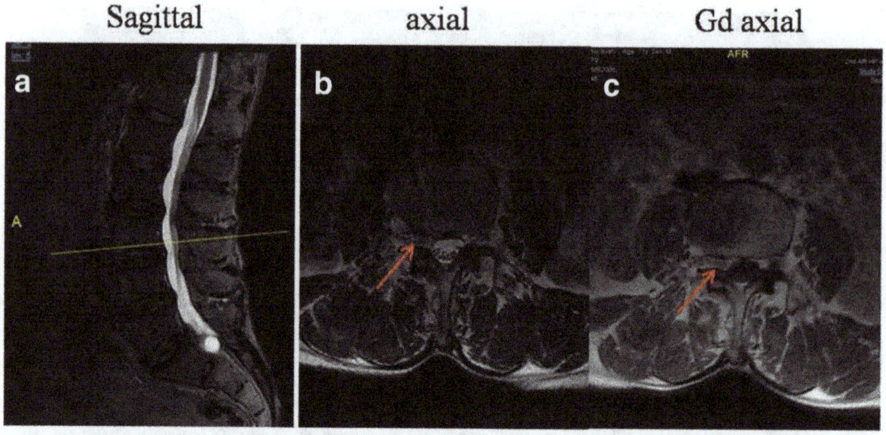

Fig. 4 Preoperative MRI of the lumbar spine without intravenous contrast and with gadolinium- enhanced MRI. T2-weighted MRI in the sagittal plane was used to aid in localization (**a**). T2-weighted images in the axial planes revealed a dumbbell mass in the lateral recess (**b**). Gadolinium-enhanced MRI demonstrated a heterogeneous ring-like enhancement at the periphery of the mass (**c**)

However, within this study we have demonstrated that the use of the coronal MR images of 3D fast-field echo with water selective excitation (3D MRI) was capable to differentiating a sequestered disc fragment from other neoplasms prior to operation.

A series of literatures [1–22] with respect to mimicking tumor disc have been published from 1993 to 2016. Open surgery was performed in all cases [1–22] since the surgeons were unable to make a definitive diagnosis depending on computed tomography (CT), MRI, and gadolinium-enhanced MRI before operation. If the disc fragment of mimicking tumor can be identified prior to operation, open surgery may not be necessary for all patients. We were demonstrated that minimally invasive endoscopic surgery is an alternative, less invasive option to open surgery.

In 2017, Takano et al. [22] successfully identified one patient with disc of mimicking tumor through discography and disco-CT. In this previous study, MRI showed a mass located posterolaterally to the left aspect of the dural sac at the L3 level in a 78-year-old man. The initial diagnosis indicated posterior epidural migration of lumbar disc fragments, malignancy, spontaneous hematoma, or epidural abscess. L3/4 discography clearly showed leakage of the contrast medium into the posterior dural space. Based on these findings, they diagnosed the patients with a neurological deficit due to posterior epidural migration of the lumbar disc fragments. The lesion was identified intraoperatively as a herniated-disc fragment. However, as an invasive technique, complications associated with discography are relatively common and include nerve root injury.

Unlike discography, 3D MRI is a non–invasive imaging examination modality. Compared to conventional MRI, 3D MRI can display the whole view of the nerve root, including the extraforaminal region [23]. Meanwhile, the 3D space location between the herniated disc and nerve

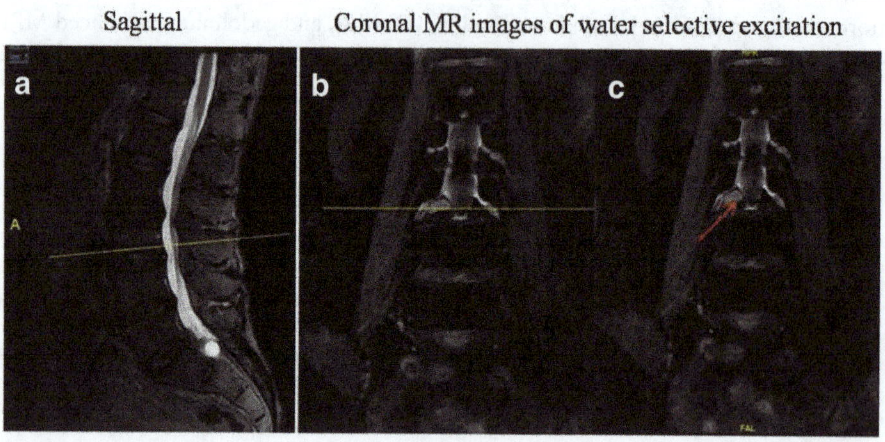

Fig. 5 Coronal MR images of 3D fast-field echo with water selective excitation. T2-weighted MRI in the sagittal and axial plane was used to aid in localization (**a** and **b**). A clear boundary was observed between the mass and nerve root by coronal MRI (**c**)

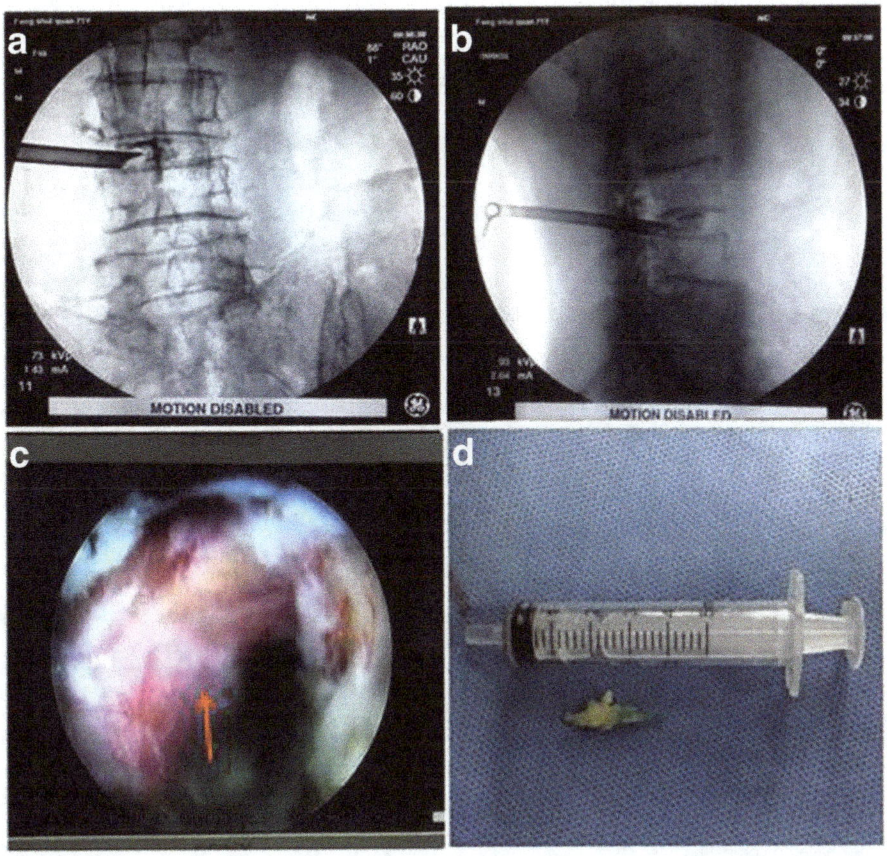

Fig. 6 Intraoperative C-arm image showed the placement of the cannula on anteroposterior and lateral views (**a** and **b**). The exiting nerve root (red arrow) was exposed (**c**) and the mass (**d**) was removed under invasive endoscopic surgery

root can also be clearly visualized. Although 3D MRI [24, 25] has been used to diagnose symptomatic extraforaminal disc herniation, spinal cord and nerve root compression in recent years, this is the first investigation to indicate that 3D MRI is a helpful imaging tool for differentiating between diagnosis of disc sequestration that mimics a tumor and neurinoma prior to operation.

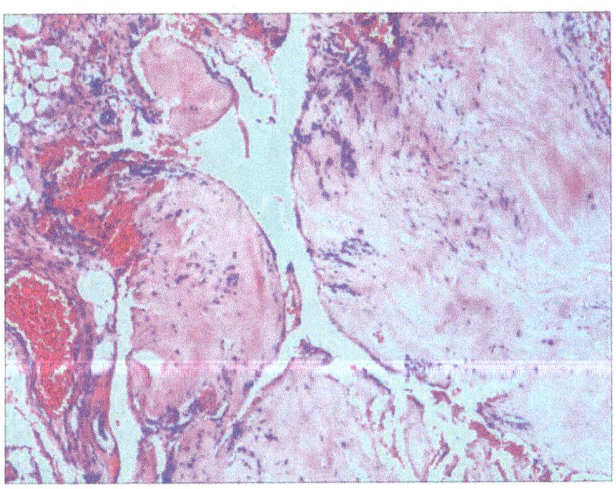

Fig. 7 The histopathological diagnosis confirmed that the mass was a degenerated intervertebral disc

Since the disc fragment appeared similar to a neurinoma on T1WI and T2WI of MRI in the present cases, neurinoma was speculated prior to operation by us. However, 3D MRI showed a clear boundary between the mass and nerve root. Moreover, the authors found that the mass was also completely separated from the dura in the 3D MRI view. As a result, we excluded neurinoma as a possible diagnosis prior to operation, and minimally invasive endoscopic surgery was performed in the patient. Postoperatively, histopathology confirmed that the mass was consistent with a degenerated intervertebral disc.

Conclusion

This case report indicates that 3D MRI as a non–invasive imaging examination is a helpful tool for differentiating between an epidural disc fragment that mimicked a tumor and neurinoma prior to operation. If the disc fragment of mimicking tumor can be identified prior to operation, open surgery may not be necessary for all patients. Further verification for the usefulness and deficiency of 3D MRI on differentiating the disc of mimicking tumor ought to be considered using larger sample size in future study.

Abbreviations

3D MRI: The coronal MRI of 3D fast-field echo with water selective excitation; CT: Computed tomography; MRI: Magnetic resonance imaging; ODI: Oswestry disability index; T1WI: T1-weighted images; T2WI: T2-weighted images; VAS: Visual analog scale

Acknowledgements

We thank Drs. Xi Xiong, Jian Cao and Shen Hu in the case management, including the systemic examination, follow-up visits, and advice regarding the clinical approach.

Funding

This work was supported by National Nature Science Foundation of China (81360268).

Authors' contributions

XC and JJ contributed substantially to the conception and design, data acquisition, analysis, and interpretation. They performed the surgery and were involved in drafting and revising the manuscript. QW, TW, WC and DH provided critical revision of the manuscript. All authors read and approved the final manuscript.

Consent for publication

The two patients provided informed, written consent to publish his clinical details and images.

Competing interests

The authors declare that they have no competing interests.

Author details

Department of Orthopaedics, The Second Affiliated Hospital of Nanchang University, Nanchang City 330006, Jiangxi Province, China. [2]Department of Orthopaedics, The Second Affiliated Hospital of Nanchang University, Nanchang City, Jiangxi Province, China.

References

1. Hoch B, Hermann G. Migrated herniated disc mimicking a neoplasm. Skelet Radiol. 2010;39(12):1245–9.
2. Li K, Li Z, Geng W, Wang C, Ma J. Postdural disc herniation at L5/S1 level mimicking an extradural spinal tumor. Eur Spine J. 2016;25(Suppl 1):80–3.
3. Ajayi O, Shoakazemi A, Tubbs RS, Moisi M, Rostad S, Newell DW. Atypical presentation of a sequestered posterolateral disc fragment. Cureus. 2016; 8(2):e502.
4. Sharma MS, Morris JM, Pichelmann MA, Spinner RJ. L5-S1 extraforaminal intraneural disc herniation mimicking a malignant peripheral nerve sheath tumor. Spine J. 2012;12(12):e7–e12.
5. Levene HB, Nimmagadda A, Levi AD. An unusual case of footdrop: anterior disc herniation mimicking a nerve sheath tumor. Neurosurgery. 2010;66(2):E419–20.
6. Emamian SA, Skriver EB, Henriksen L, Cortsen ME. Lumbar herniated disk mimicking neurinoma. Case report. Acta Radiol. 1993;34(2):127–9.
7. Bakar B, Sumer MM, Cila A, Tekkok IH. An extreme lateral lumbar disc herniation mimicking L4 schwannoma. Acta Neurol Belg. 2009;109(2):155–8.
8. Ashkenazi E, Pomeranz S, Floman Y. Foraminal herniation of a lumbar disc mimicking neurinoma on CT and MR imaging. J Spinal Disord. 1997;10(5):448–50.
9. Kuo CH, Chang PY, Wu JC, Huang WC, Tu TH, Cheng H. Lumbar disc mimicking tumor. J Neurosurg Spine. 2014;20(6):767–8.
10. Song KJ, Kim KB, Lee KB. Sequestrated thoracic disc herniation mimicking a tumoral lesion in the spinal canal–a case report. Clin Imaging. 2012;36(4):416–9.
11. Pillai SS. Intra-radicuar disc herniation mimicking a nerve root tumor. J Orthop Case Rep. 2012;2(1):7–10.
12. Liu CC, Huang CT, Lin CM, Liu KN. Intradural disc herniation at L5 level mimicking an intradural spinal tumor. Eur Spine J. 2011;20(Suppl 2):S326–9.
13. Ekşi MS, Yener U, Akakin A, Akakin D, Konya D. Posterior epidural disc herniation at L3-L4 mimicking a spinal tumor: a case report. J Neurosurg Sci. 2010;54(2):71–6.
14. Demirci A, Er U. A lumbar disc herniation mimicking spinal tumor with intra- and extradural components. Spine J. 2011;11(1):90–1.
15. Solmaz I, Onal MB, Civelek E, Sirin S, Kahraman S. Intramedullary lumbar lesion mimicking spinal cord tumor: a case of non-neoplastic intramedullary spinal cord lesion. Eur Spine J. 2010;19(Suppl 2):S169–73.
16. Stavrinou LC, Stranjalis G, Maratheftis N, Bouras T, Sakas DE. Cervical disc, mimicking nerve sheath tumor, with rapid spontaneous recovery: a case report. Eur Spine J. 2009;18(Suppl 2):176–8.
17. Lee JS, Suh KT. Intradural disc herniation at L5-S1 mimicking an intradural extramedullary spinal tumor: a case report. J Korean Med Sci. 2006;21(4):778–80.
18. Aydin MV, Ozel S, Sen O, Erdogan B, Yildirim T. Intradural disc mimicking: a spinal tumor lesion. Spinal Cord. 2004;42(1):52–4.
19. Saruhashi Y, Omura K, Miyamoto K, Katsuura A, Hukuda S. A migrated lumbar disc herniation simulating a dumbbell tumor. J Spinal Disord. 1999; 12(4):307–9.
20. Dimogerontas G, Paidakakos NA, Konstantinidis E. Voluminous free disk fragment mimicking an extradural tumor. Neurol Med Chir (Tokyo). 2012; 52(9):656–8.
21. Bose B. Thoracic extruded disc mimicking spinal cord tumor. Spine J. 2003; 3(1):82–6.
22. Takano M, Hikata T, Nishimura S, Kamata M. Discography aids definitive diagnosis of posterior epidural migration of lumbar disc fragments: case report and literature review. BMC Musculoskelet Disord. 2017;18(1):151.
23. Shen J, Wang HY, Chen JY, Liang BL. Morphologic analysis of normal human lumbar dorsal root ganglion by 3D MR imaging. AJNR Am J Neuroradiol. 2006;27(10):2098–103.
24. Byun WM, Jang HW, Kim SW. Three-dimension al magnetic resonance rendering imaging of lumbosacral radiculography in the diagnosis of symptomatic extraforaminal disc herniation with or without foraminal extension. Spine (Phila Pa 1976). 2012;37(10):840–4.
25. Taira G, Endo K, Ito K, Ichimaru K, Imakiire A, Miura Y. Diagnosis of lumbar disc herniation by three-dimensional MRI. J Orthop Sci. 1998;3(1):18–26.

18

Difference in whole spinal alignment between supine and standing positions in patients with adult spinal deformity using a new comparison method with slot-scanning three-dimensional X-ray imager and computed tomography through digital reconstructed radiography

Kazuhiro Hasegawa[1*], Masashi Okamoto[1], Shun Hatsushikano[1], Gabriel Caseiro[2] and Kei Watanabe[3]

Abstract

Background: A precise comparison of supine and standing whole spine alignment in both the coronal and sagittal planes, including the pelvic parameters, has not been reported. Furthermore, previous studies investigated positional differences in the Cobb angle only in young patients with idiopathic scoliosis. The difference in alignment has never been investigated in a population of patients with adult spinal deformity (ASD). In most cases, ASD patients are aware of the symptoms when standing and tend to stoop with back pain, whereas the symptoms disappear when lying on a bed. Therefore, it is important to elucidate the positional differences in the deformity in older adults. The purposes of this study are to establish a method for comparing whole spine alignment between supine and standing, and to clarify the positional difference of the alignment in the patients with ASD.

Methods: Twenty-four patients with ASD (mean age: 60.1 years, range 20–80 years; 24 women) were evaluated. A slot-scanning three-dimensional X-ray imager (EOS) was used to assess the whole spine in the standing position. Computed tomography was used to assess the whole spine in the supine position. The computed tomography DICOM dataset of the whole spine in the supine position was transformed to two-dimensional (coronal and sagittal) digital reconstructed radiography images. The digital reconstructed radiography images were input for three-dimensional measurement by the EOS software and compared with the standing whole spine alignment measured by EOS.

Results: The mean intraclass correlation coefficients (supine, standing) of intra-rater / inter-rater reliabilities for the measured parameters were 0.981, 0.984 / 0.970, 0.986, respectively. The Cobb and rotation angles of the major curve, mostly the thoracolumbar area, were significantly greater in the standing position than in the supine position. Lumbar lordosis during standing was significantly kyphotic. With respect to the pelvic parameters, the sacral slope was significantly smaller in the standing position than in the supine position. Pelvic tilt and pelvic incidence were significantly greater in the standing position than in the supine position.

(Continued on next page)

* Correspondence: kazu3795jp@yahoo.co.jp
[1]Niigata Spine Surgery Center, 2-5-22 Nishi-machi, Niigata City 950-0165, Japan
Full list of author information is available at the end of the article

(Continued from previous page)

Conclusions: The lumbar to pelvic parameters and the major curve in standing position significantly deteriorate compared with the supine position in patients with ASD.

Keywords: Adult spinal deformity, Computed tomography, Digital reconstructed radiolography, Slot-scanning 3D X-ray imager (EOS), Supine and standing position, Whole spinal alignment

Background

Spinal deformity is a three-dimensional abnormality. Alignment is usually assessed in standing radiographs in both the sagittal and coronal planes using the Cobb angle [4]. When a patient presents with neurologic symptoms, details of the abnormality are usually assessed by referring to computed tomography (CT) images or magnetic resonance images (MRI) obtained with the patient in a supine position. Previous studies of adolescent idiopathic scoliosis (AIS) report major Cobb angles 7–10° smaller in the supine position than in the standing position due to changes in the gravitational loading direction [1, 21, 28, 30]. Therefore, to understand the pathology of the whole spine, it is important to determine the difference in the curve measurement between the supine and standing positions, including alignment. A drawback of previous reports is the potential error related to different measurement methods used for X-ray and other imaging modalities (CT or MRI) to compare the Cobb angle, which may lead to misinterpretation or controversy [1, 20, 21, 28, 30].

To our knowledge, a precise comparison of supine and standing measurements using the same modality and measurement method to overcome this drawback has not been reported. Whole spine alignment in both the coronal and sagittal planes, including the pelvic parameters, with regard to a positional difference has not been investigated. Furthermore, previous studies investigated positional differences in the Cobb angle only in young patients with AIS. The difference in alignment has never been investigated in a population of patients with adult spinal deformity (ASD). In contrast to AIS, the chief complaint of patients with ASD is usually mechanical back pain with or without radicular pain to the lower extremities. In most cases, the patients are aware of the symptoms when standing and tend to stoop with back pain, whereas the symptoms disappear when lying on a bed. Therefore, it is important to elucidate the positional differences in the deformity in older adults.

The purposes of this study were to: 1) Establish a method of comparing whole spine alignment between the supine and standing positions with minimal measurement error; and 2) Clarify the difference in the whole spine alignment between the supine position and the weight-bearing standing position in adult-to-elderly patients with spinal deformity.

Methods

Measurement of standing whole spine alignment with the EOS system

Comparison of whole spine alignment between the supine and standing positions necessitates high reproducibility of the imaging technology. Conventional X-ray measurement with a cone-beam X-ray provides significant magnification of the subject within the margin of the cassette. Therefore, we used the EOS system (EOS Imaging, Paris, France) as a principal device for measuring whole spine alignment [16]. The EOS system is a slot-scanning three-dimensional (3D) X-ray imager developed in collaboration by multidisciplinary partners, radiation physics engineers, biomechanical engineers, medical radiologists, and orthopedic pediatric surgeons to overcome the limitations of conventional X-ray measurement. From the simultaneous anteroposterior and lateral X-rays of the whole body to the 3D bone external envelope technique, 3D reconstruction is possible at every level of the osteoarticular system and especially the spine in the standing position. The EOS allows for more precise bone reconstruction in orthopedics, especially at the level of the spine, pelvis, and lower limbs, with limited X-ray exposure compared with conventional X-rays and CT scans [6, 7, 9, 19].

Radiographs with the EOS system [3, 9] were routinely obtained, as follows: 1) EOS radiographs were made from the head, including the center of the auditory canal, to the feet. 2) Each patient was asked to stand comfortably on a force plate while placing their hands on their cheeks. 3) A mirror placed at eye level in the inner wall of the EOS cabin helped the patient maintain a horizontal gaze [16].

The default scan speed of the EOS system was 7.6 cm/s. Acquisition time was linked to scan height: Time of acquisition (s) = height of acquisition (cm)/7.6. Scan speed can be increased if the patient is restless and having difficulty keeping still during the acquisition. Nevertheless, subtle artifacts in the images can occur due to body sway during scanning, but these are minimized because of the rapid X-ray detection time (0.8333 ms) with no blurring of the images. Some accessories are available to stabilize the patient in the EOS cabin. A recent study demonstrated that motion artifacts do not affect spinal measurements [26].

Measurement of supine whole spine alignment with CT-generated digital reconstructed radiographs

Following EOS scanning, the whole spine, including the head and pelvis of the patient, was also scanned in the supine position with CT (Activion16, TSX-031A, Toshiba Medical Systems Corp., Tochigi, Japan). Currently, the most accurate 3D bone information may be obtained with CT imaging. To eliminate software-related bias and to guarantee equivalent computational methods during spinopelvic parameter comparisons between the supine position in the CT and the standing position in the EOS, the same analysis software must be used. Therefore, we chose to transform the CT dataset into an EOS-like dataset using the digitally reconstructed radiograph (DRR) technique. The DRR technique consists of simulating X-rays passing through the reconstructed CT volume based on an absorption-only optical model, thus generating an X-ray-like image. These biplanar projections were reconstructed using the same calibration parameters and geometry as the EOS cabin (Fig. 1). These projected anteroposterior and lateral DRRs, as well as those performed with the EOS system, were used as inputs for stereoradiographic spine modeling. Thus, for each position, 3D spine modeling was obtained using sterEOS software (sterEOS 1.6, EOS Imaging, Paris, France) [15] with both the EOS data (standing position) and the CT-generated DRRs (supine position), and compared between the two positions (Fig. 2).

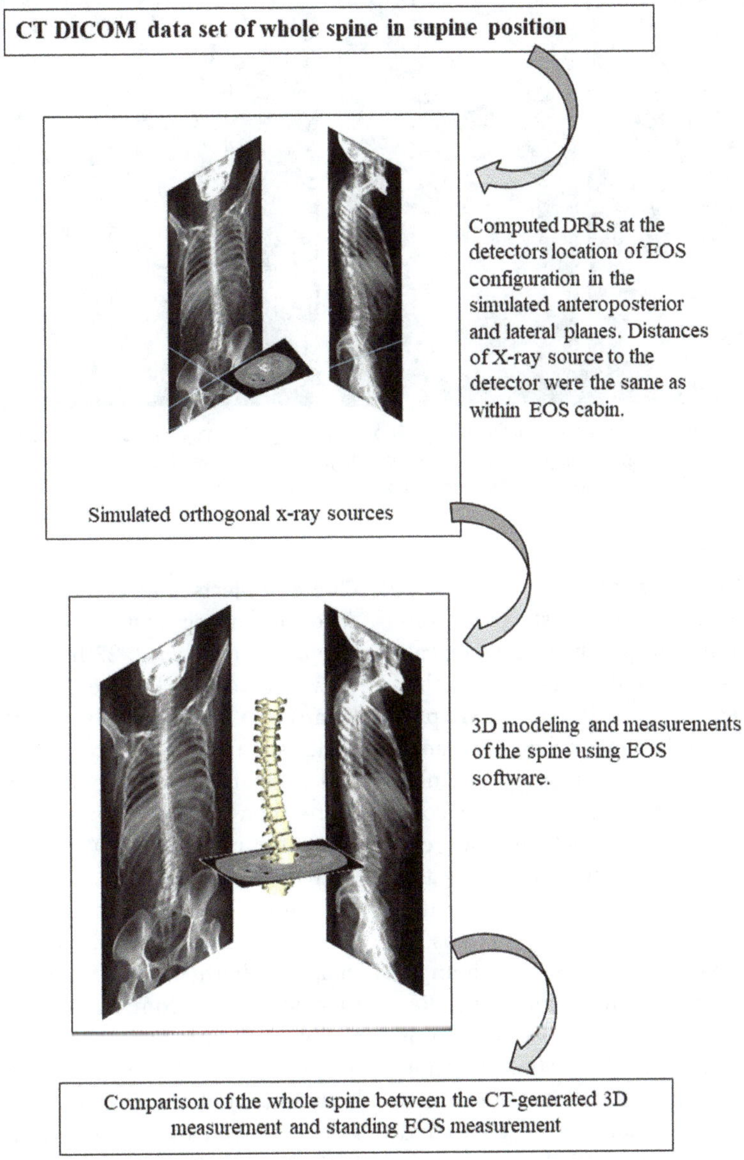

Fig. 1 Conversion of supine CT data into digital reconstructed radiography (DRR) for comparable EOS measurement

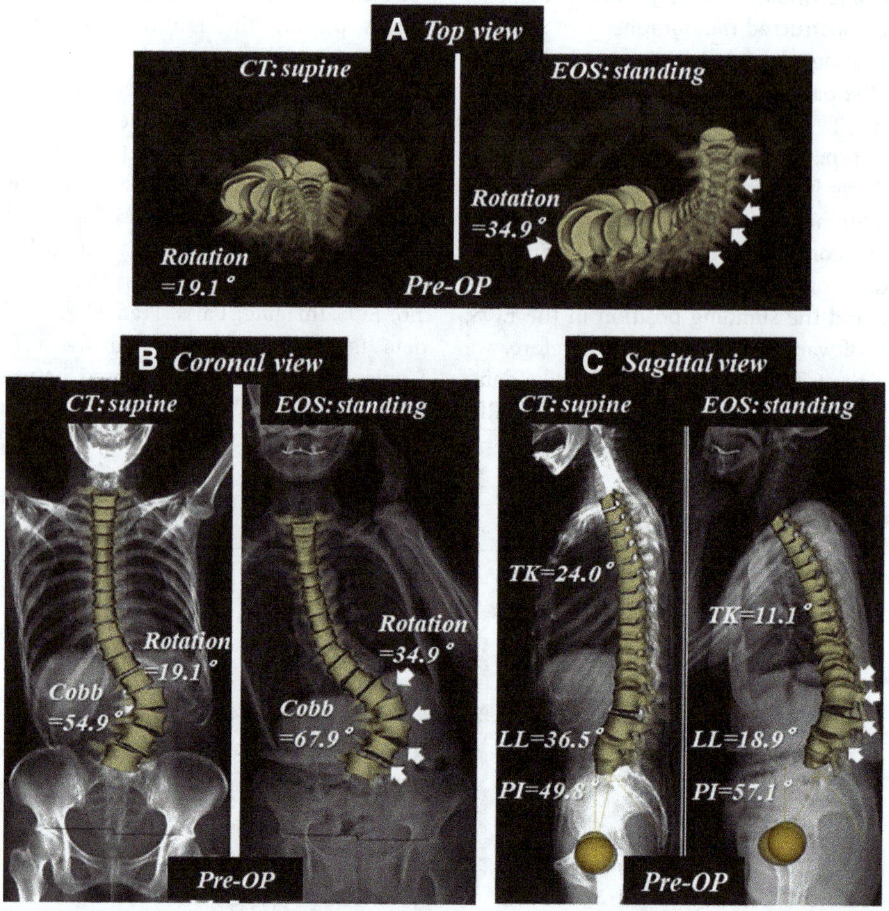

Fig. 2 Patient with degenerative kyphoscoliosis. Preoperative supine CT and standing EOS images. **a** Top view images. Arrows show deterioration of T1 off-set and thoraco-lumbar rotation in standing position. **b** Coronal images. Arrows show deterioration of thoraco-lumbar curve in standing position. **c** Sagittal images. Arrows show deterioration of thoraco-lumbar kyphosis in standing position

Spino-pelvic parameters for comparison

Using the full-spine workflow of the sterEOS software, the following spinopelvic parameters were calculated: kyphosis T1–T12 and T4–12, lumbar lordosis (LL) with respect to L1–L5 and L1–S1, pelvic tilt (PT), sacral slope (SS), and pelvic incidence (PI). PI is the angle between the line perpendicular to the sacral plate at its midpoint and the line connecting the midpoint of the sacral plate to the center of the axis connecting both acetabulae. PT is the angle defined between the line connecting the midpoint of the sacral plate to the center of the axis of both acetabulae and the vertical axis. SS is the angle between the sacral plate and the horizontal line. Regarding the deformity, the Cobb angle of the major curve (Cobb angle) and the axial vertebral rotation of the apex in the major curve (Rotation) were measured. All of the parameter results were compared between the supine (CT-generated DRR) and standing (EOS) positions.

Clinical subjects

After obtaining institutional review board approval (Approval number 2, 27th Dec., 2013, Institutional Review Board of Kameda Daiichi Hospital, Niigata, Japan), we prospectively enrolled patients with ASD under the following criteria: 1) diagnosis: degenerative and idiopathic spinal kyphoscoliosis with Cobb angle more than 30° or degenerative kyphosis with PI-LL mismatch more than 20°, 2) age: > 20 years old, 3) sex: woman, 4) candidate for surgical treatment, 5) a full-spine CT scan (acquired from auditory canals to the proximal third of the femur) and a full-spine EOS image in both preoperative and postoperative states, 6) study term: from April 2014 to March 2016. The following demographic characteristics were obtained for each patient: age, sex, weight, and height. The body mass index was calculated as the weight in kilograms divided by the square of the height in meters. Patients with transitional vertebrae were excluded for precise measurement and comparison between supine and standing positions. Regarding the gender difference, we found a significant difference between men and women in PT, pelvic thickness, SVA, and lower extremity alignment in the previous study [17]. If men are included, the result may be affected. Therefore, men are excluded in this study. Consequently, a total of 24 cases with a mean age of 60.1 years (range: 20–80 years; 24 women) were analyzed after obtaining of informed consent for participation in the study. We used the Japanese version of the Oswestry Disability Index (ODI) [12, 13] and Scoliosis Research Society-22 score (SRS-22) [2, 18] to assess the health-related quality of life. ODI and SRS-22 are the principal condition-specific outcome measures used in the management of low back disorders and spinal deformities, respectively. Normal values without symptoms are 0 (%) in the ODI and 5 in the SRS-22, with the worst values being 100 (%) in the ODI and 0 in the SRS-22.

Statistical analysis

JMP (version 9; SAS Institute, Cary, NC) and SPSS (IBM SPSS Statistics for Windows, Version 24.0, IBM Corp., Armonk, NY) were used for all statistical analyses. Mean, range, standard deviation (SD), standard error (SE), and the interquartile range, 25%/75%, were calculated for all the demographic and radiographic parameters. All variance-dependent variables were checked for normality and homogeneity of variance. Alpha was set at $p < 0.05$.

An intra-class correlation coefficient (ICC) was calculated to explore consistency within and between examiners for measurements with the original EOS images and the CT-generated DRRs. To evaluate intra-rater reliability, we compared the measurements obtained by two examiners who completed the EOS measurement training and had worked with these measurements for 3 years, and measured all the parameters of the 24 subjects twice with a 1-week interval. To evaluate inter-rater reliability, we compared the measurements obtained by the two examiners of all the parameters of the same 24 subjects in 1 week. An ICC value approaching 1.0 indicates less variability, better consistency, and a value over 0.8 is considered sufficiently reliable.

The values of all the alignment spinopelvic parameters were normally distributed, thus a paired-t-test was performed to compare between supine (CT-generated DRR) and standing (EOS) positions. Type I error (α), power ($1-\beta$), and post-hoc sample size for the statistical significance were calculated.

Results

Patient demographic data

Mean age and body mass index were 60.1 years (20–80) and 22.2 kg/m^2 (18.0–31), respectively. Mean value with SD, SE, and 25%/75% interquartile range of all the demographic and radiologic standard parameters are reported in Table 1. The mean ODI score was 31.4% (0–52%) and the mean SRS-22 (subtotal) score was 2.9 (1.8–4.4).

Table 1 Demographics of the subject and spinal alignment parameters in standing position measured by EOS (24 women)

	Mean	Range (min/max)	SD	SE	IQ 25%/75%*1
Age (years)	60.1	20 / 80	14.2	2.9	59.3 / 67
Body mass index*2	22.2	18.0 / 31.0	3.0	0.6	20.0 / 25.0
ODI*3 (%)	31.4	0 / 52	12.4	2.5	24.0 / 40.0
SRS-22*4	2.9	1.8 / 4.4	0.5	0.1	2.6 / 3.2
VAS*5	6.6	0 / 10	2.8	0.6	5.3 / 8.0
T1–12 kyphosis (°)	24.0	−6.8 / 56.2	15.5	3.2	11.1 / 37.6
T4–12 kyphosis (°)	17.8	−10.6 / 45.8	14.5	3.0	9.7 / 25.6
L1-S1 lumbar lordosis (°)	21.8	−32.6 / 63.3	25.5	5.2	5.8 / 44.6
L1-L5 lumbar lordosis (°)	8.5	−38.5 / 66.0	26.1	5.3	−9.6 / 33.5
Sacral slope (°)	27.0	0 / 60.4	14.1	2.9	18.1 / 32.9
Pelvic tilt (°)	30.7	3.8 / 48	10.6	2.2	25.3 / 37.8
Pelvic incidence (°)	57.7	33.6 / 80.8	10.9	2.2	53.0 / 65.0
Cobb's angle (°) *6	39.5	12.2 / 74.2	20.1	4.7	22.8 / 57.6
Rotation (°) *7	14.7	0.7 / 31.9	10.2	2.4	4.9 / 20.7

*1Interquartile range, 25%/75% values
*2The body mass index was calculated as the weight in kilograms divided by the square of the height in meters (kg/m^2)
*3The Oswestry Disability Index [12, 13]
*4Scoliosis Research Society – 22, subtotal [2, 18]
*5Visual analog scale, 0 is no pain and 10 is most severe pain
*6Cobb's angle of the major curve
*7Vertebral rotation of the apex in the major curve

Reliability of the measurements in the supine (CT-generated DRR) and standing (EOS) positions

The mean ICCs of intra-rater reliabilities for supine and standing positions were 0.98 (0.96–1.00) and 0.98 (0.96–1.00), respectively. The mean ICCs of inter-rater reliabilities for supine and standing positions were 0.97 (0.93–0.99) and 0.99 (0.97–1.00), respectively. Overall, the ICC data suggested excellent measurement consistency and reliability in both the standing and supine positions (Table 2).

Comparison of spinal and pelvic parameters between the supine and standing positions

Thoracic kyphosis in the standing position was not different from that in the supine position (Table 3, Fig. 3). On the other hand, LL at both in L1-L5 and L1-S1 levels was significantly smaller in the standing position than in the supine position. This means that the lumbar spine is more kyphotic in the standing position than in the supine position.

With regard to pelvic alignment, SS was significantly smaller in the standing position than in the supine position. In contrast to the SS value, PT was significantly greater in the standing position than in the supine position. PI was significantly greater in the standing position than in the supine position (Table 3, Fig. 3).

The Cobb and rotation angles of the major curve were significantly greater in the standing position than in the supine position. Statistical power was at least 0.8 in all parameters. Post hoc calculated sample size necessary for sufficient power was less than 24 for all parameters except for T1-T12 / T4-T12 kyphosis and Rotation.

Table 2 Comparison of Intra-Class Correlation Coefficient (ICC) and 95% confidential interval for all the parameters between supine (CT-based DRR) and standing (original EOS)

CT	ICC	95% CI	EOS	ICC	95% CI
Intra-rater reliability (two examiners, 24 subjects)					
T1-T12 TK	0.963	0.905 / 0.986	T1-T12 TK	0.980	0.955 / 0.991
T4-T12 TK	0.967	0.926 / 0.985	T4-T12 TK	0.989	0.976 / 0.995
L1-L5 LL	0.979	0.953 / 0.991	L1-L5 LL	0.986	0.968 / 0.994
L1-S1 LL	0.992	0.981 / 0.996	L1-S1 LL	0.991	0.980 / 0.996
PI	0.982	0.959 / 0.992	PI	0.981	0.956 / 0.992
SS	0.990	0.976 / 0.995	SS	0.984	0.964 / 0.993
PT	0.996	0.992 / 0.998	PT	0.998	0.996 / 0.999
Cobb angle	0.989	0.972 / 0.996	Cobb angle	0.991	0.976 / 0.996
Rotation	0.973	0.930 / 0.990	Rotation	0.955	0.887 / 0.983
Average	0.981	0.955 / 0.992	average	0.984	0.962 / 0.993
Inter-rater reliability (two examiners, 24 subjects)					
T1-T12 TK	0.932	0.850 / 0.970	T1-T12 TK	0.988	0.972 / 0.995
T4-T12 TK	0.971	0.935 / 0.987	T4-T12 TK	0.984	0.964 / 0.993
L1-L5 LL	0.964	0.919 / 0.984	L1-L5 LL	0.989	0.974 / 0.995
L1-S1 LL	0.986	0.963 / 0.994	L1-S1 LL	0.993	0.976 / 0.997
PI	0.969	0.821 / 0.990	PI	0.974	0.940 / 0.988
SS	0.964	0.466 / 0.991	SS	0.982	0.945 / 0.993
PT	0.992	0.846 / 0.998	PT	0.997	0.917 / 0.999
Cobb angle	0.992	0.928 / 0.998	Cobb angle	0.994	0.985 / 0.998
Rotation	0.963	0.905 / 0.986	Rotation	0.974	0.931 / 0.990
Average	0.970	0.848 / 0.989	average	0.986	0.956 / 0.994

Discussion

Adults with spinal deformities generally have a lower health-related quality of life. The present findings are consistent with findings of previous studies in that the patients in our population had poor low-back pain-related quality of life. Fairbank et al. [12] reported that the mean ODI score in a normal Caucasian population is 10.2. In addition, Tonosu et al. [27] reported that the mean ODI in a normal Japanese population is 8.73 (8.80 in men, 8.66 in women) when corrected for age, and a tendency for the ODI to gradually increase with advancing age. The mean ODI score in the present study (31.4%) was much greater than these values and mean SRS-22 score in our study (2.9) was lower than the normal value [5]. To clarify the pathology leading to the lower quality of life in patients with ASD, a precise comparison of supine and standing measurements using the same modality and measurement method is needed.

The difference in curve magnitude between standing and supine positions was studied previously in AIS patients. Keenan et al. [20] investigated the difference in the Cobb angle between the supine position (reconstructed CT) and standing position (conventional X-ray) in 52 patients with AIS having a mean age of 14.6 years. They reported a mean Cobb angle on standing radiographs of 51.9°, which was a significantly greater value than the mean Cobb angle on supine CT images of 40.5° [20]. The Cobb angle measurement, however, includes a fundamental error related to the selection of the vertebral endplates. In another study [24], spinal parameters were measured on 50 anteroposterior radiographs of scoliotic spines, on 6 separate occasions each by 4 orthopedic surgeons using the Cobb method; they reported that the 95% confidence limit for intraobserver variability was 4.9° and that for interobserver variability was 7.2°. Thus, due to the inherent inter- and intra-observer error in conventional X-ray measurements, it is difficult to conclude whether there are quantitative differences in the curve magnitude due to the positioning of the subjects.

In the present study, we transformed the CT dataset (supine position images) into an EOS-like dataset with the DRR technique, which generates two-dimensional X-ray-like images using the same calibration parameters and geometry as the EOS cabin. The projected anteroposterior and lateral DRRs were used as inputs for routine-like EOS stereoradiographic spine modeling with

Table 3 Comparison of the values of standard parameters between supine (CT-generated DRR) and standing (original EOS) positions by paired t-test

Parameters (°)	position	Image modality	Mean	Range (min/max)	SD	SE	95% CI[*1]	Type I error (α)
T1-T12 kyphosis	supine	CT	24.4	−2.2 / 44.7	10.9	2.2	19.8 / 29.0	*0.8581*
	standing	EOS	24.0	−6.8 / 56.2	15.5	3.2	17.5 / 30.5	
T4-T12 kyphosis	supine	CT	15.3	−10.3 / 35.7	11.1	2.3	10.7 / 20.0	*0.1641*
	standing	EOS	17.8	−10.6 / 45.8	14.5	3.0	11.7 / 24.0	
L1-S1 LL[*2]	supine	CT	**33.1**	−11 / 55.9	17.5	3.8	25.7 / 40.5	***0.0002***
	standing	EOS	**21.8**	−32.6 / 63.3	25.5	5.2	11.0 / 32.6	
L1-L5 LL	supine	CT	**18.9**	−20.3 / 45.1	16.9	3.5	11.7 / 26.0	***0.0010***
	standing	EOS	**8.5**	−38.5 / 66.0	26.1	5.3	−2.5 / 19.5	
SS[*3]	supine	CT	**34.1**	11.1 / 48.5	10.5	2.2	29.7 / 38.6	***0.0003***
	standing	EOS	**27.0**	0 / 60.4	14.1	2.9	21.1 / 33.0	
PT[*4]	supine	CT	**19.2**	5.2 / 37	7.5	1.5	16.1 / 22.4	***< 0.0001***
	standing	EOS	**30.7**	3.8 / 48	10.6	2.2	26.2 / 35.2	
PI[*5]	supine	CT	**53.4**	32.2 / 68.1	9.2	1.9	49.5 / 57.3	***0.0013***
	standing	EOS	**57.7**	33.6 / 80.8	10.9	2.2	53.1 / 62.3	
Cobb angle[*6]	supine	CT	**31.0**	6.8 / 57	15.3	3.6	23.4 / 38.7	***0.0001***
	standing	EOS	**39.5**	12.2 / 74.2	20.1	4.7	29.5 / 49.4	
Rotation[*7]	supine	CT	**11.7**	0.1 / 25.0	7.6	1.8	8.0 / 15.5	***0.0318***
	standing	EOS	**14.7**	0.7 / 34.9	10.2	2.4	9.7 / 19.8	

[*1]95% confidence interval
[*2]Lumbar lordosis
[*3]Sacral slope
[*4]Pelvic tilt
[*5]Pelvic incidence
[*6]Cobb's angle of major curve (°)
[*7]Vertebral rotation of the apex in the major curve (°)
Mean values with bold letters indicate statistically significance ($p < 0.05$) between supine (CT) and standing (EOS)

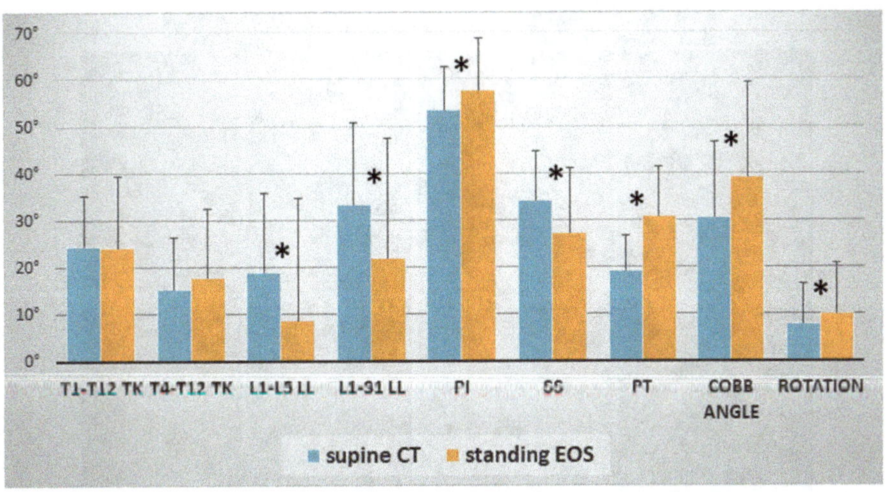

Fig. 3 Mean (+ standard deviation) values of spinopelvic parameters measured in supine (blue bars) and standing (orange bars) positions Asterisks denote statistically significant differences ($p < 0.05$) based on paired t-test

sterEOS software. The EOS data (standing position) and the CT-generated DRRs (supine position) were then compared. In the present study, we confirmed the reliability of this comparison method using repeatability tests with ICC in the 24 subjects, and found that the ICCs were excellent in all the values, both in CT-generated DRRs and EOS measurements. Thus, the inherent error due to measurement and different imaging modalities was overcome by the comparison with the EOS 3D measurement system.

In adult-to-elderly patients with spinal deformity, sagittal malalignment is more important than coronal alignment [14]. In contrast to AIS, adult-to-elderly patients with spinal deformity complain that they tend to stoop with back pain or radicular pain of the lower extremities, and the symptoms disappear when they lie down. Therefore, the positional change of the 3D whole spine alignment should be clarified, especially in aging adults. In the present study with patients having a mean age of 60.1 years, the Cobb angle and Rotation angle of the major curve, mostly the thoracolumbar area, were significantly greater in the standing position than in the supine position. Lumbar lordosis in the standing position was significantly more kyphotic and the pelvis was significantly more retroverted, with a smaller SS and greater PT, compared with that in the supine position. The axial skeleton of human beings is aligned as a chain of balance in the standing position with the "cone of economy" in healthy subjects [8]. The standing full-body sagittal alignment and balance in reference to the gravity line were recently described in a healthy adult population using EOS radiographs [17]. The results of the present study suggest that the "cone of economy" principle deteriorates in patients with spinal deformity, making it difficult to maintain the standing position due to back pain with or without radicular pain.

PI is a fundamental parameter for spinopelvic standing alignment [10, 11, 22], and is believed to be a constant value in each individual. The value was, however, significantly greater in the standing position than in the supine position. Mangion et al. [23] measured PI on radiographs of 30 fetuses, 30 children, and 30 adults, and found that PI considerably increases during the first few months of life, continues to increase during the early years, and stabilizes at around the age of 10 years. In our previous study [16], PI was positively correlated with age, even in healthy adult subjects. PI increased around 10° on average from 20 to 70 years of age, probably due to sacroiliac osteoarthritis [16]. This finding is compatible with a previous review article on sagittal pelvic alignment parameters, which described that PI tends to increase with age in both normal and scoliotic subjects [29]. In the present study, we demonstrated a significant difference in PI between the supine and standing positions. The reconstructed coronal CT image of a case with degenerative kyphoscoliosis (Fig. 4a) shows osteoarthritis of the sacroiliac joint with a vacuum

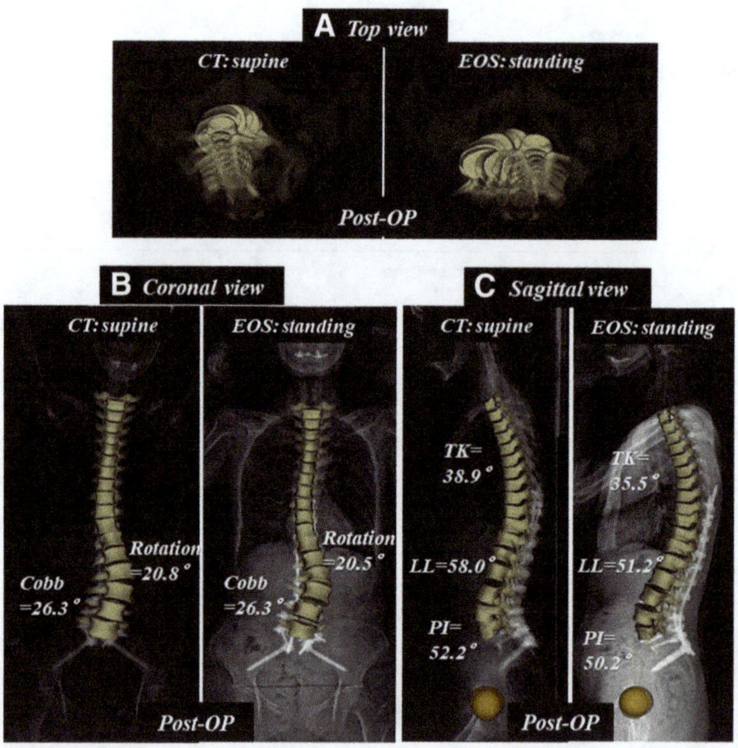

Fig. 4 Patient with degenerative kyphoscoliosis (Fig. 2) treated by posterior correction and fusion from T9 to pelvis. Postoperative supine CT and standing EOS images. **a** Top view images. **b** Coronal images. **c** Sagittal images

phenomenon, subchondral osteosclerosis, and cyst formation (Fig. 5a). The preoperative PI was 57.1° in standing EOS (49.8° in supine CT) and the PI decreased to 50.2° in standing EOS (52.2° in supine CT) following spinopelvic correction surgery with bilateral S2 alar-iliac fixations (Fig. 4b) [25]. Furthermore, the vacuum in the sacroiliac joint disappeared and the cyst became smaller after surgery as a result of fixation by the screws stabilizing the sacroiliac joints (Fig. 5b). Sacroiliac joints are the only sites that can move between the base of the sacrum and the

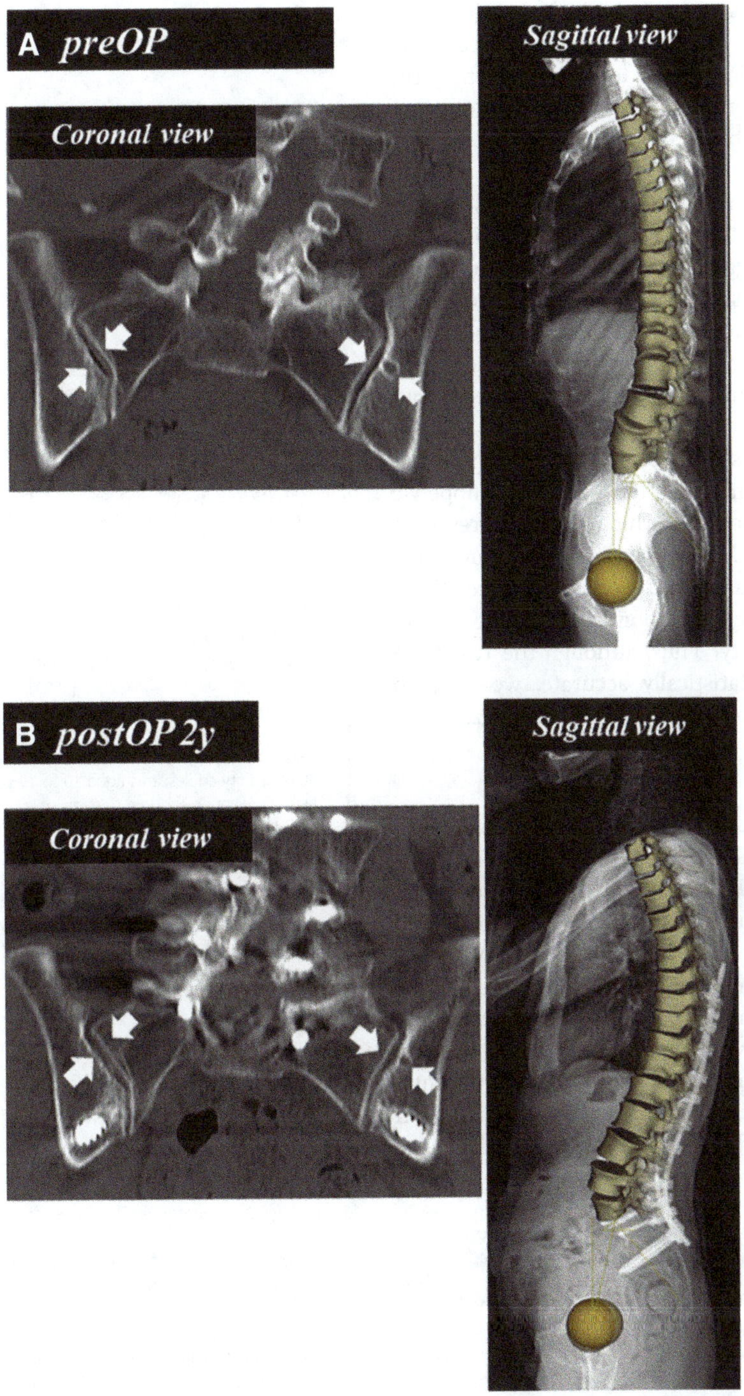

Fig. 5 Reconstructive coronal reconstructed CT images of bilateral sacro-iliac joints and corresponding EOS images of the patient (Figs. 2 and 4). **a** Preoperative images. Arrows indicate vacuum in the bilateral sacro-iliac joints and subchondral cyst. **b** Images postoperative 2 years. Arrows indicate vanished vacuum in the joints and diminished subchondral cyst

acetabulum, thereby affecting the PI value. Therefore, our data suggest that the sacroiliac joint moves abnormally due to osteoarthritic changes in ASD cases, leading to changes in the PI between the supine and standing positions. The high ICC for both the supine and standing position values suggests that the difference is a true difference, and not due to measurement variability. PI is considered a set characteristic of the individual spinopelvic shape, but it can change due to degenerative processes of the spine. Thus, it is important to remember that the aging and degenerative processes affect the whole spinopelvic alignment and balance in reference to patient positioning.

The findings in the present study offer a basic pathology of ASD with positional change in thoraco-lumbar to pelvic alignment, suggesting that a main focus of the correction and fusion surgery is the lumbar to pelvic area and further extension of the fusion to upper thoracic area is not necessary. Furthermore, we believe that the results contribute not only for spine surgeons but also for the professionals involved in the conservative management of patients with back pain and spine deformities by keeping in mind the sagittal spinopelvic profile in the supine position which could represent a starting point. Potential limitations of this study are, however, the wide age range of the patients but relatively small sample size. Aging and spondylotic change affect the spino-pelvic flexibility. Thus, although the results in the present study is statistically accurate, we need to continue the investigation with further sample size.

Conclusion

We established a method for comparing spinopelvic alignment between the supine and standing positions by converting CT DICOM data into an EOS-like dataset, a DRR technique. Comparison revealed that the Cobb angle and axial apical rotation of the major curve, mostly in the thoracolumbar area, were significantly greater in the standing position than in the supine position. Lumbar lordosis in the standing – weight-bearing – position was significantly less lordotic and the pelvis was significantly more retroverted, with a smaller SS, greater PT, and even greater PI, compared with that in the supine position.

Abbreviations

AIS: Adolescent idiopathic scoliosis; ASD: Adult spinal deformity; Cobb angle: The Cobb angle of the major curve; CT: Computed tomography; DRR: Digitally reconstructed radiograph; ICC: Intra-class correlation coefficient; LL: Lumbar lordosis; MRI: Magnetic resonance image; ODI: Oswestry disability index; PI: Pelvic incidence; PT: Pelvic tilt; Rotation: The apical vertebral rotation in the major curve; SD: Standard deviation; SE: Standard error; SRS-22: Scoliosis Research Society-22 score; SS: Sacral slope

Acknowledgments

The authors are deeply grateful to the great mentor, Prof. Jean Dubousset (Académie Nationale de Médecine, Paris, France), for his thoughtful advice.

Funding

None of the authors has received any grant or financial support for the present study.

Authors' contributions

KH: Protocol/project development, Data analysis, Manuscript writing/editing. MO: Data collection and management, Data analysis. SH: Data collection and management, Data analysis. GC: Data analysis, Manuscript editing. KW: Protocol/project development, Manuscript editing. All authors read and approved the final manuscript.

Consent for publication

Not applicable.

Competing interests

The authors declares that they have no competing interests.

Author details

[1]Niigata Spine Surgery Center, 2-5-22 Nishi-machi, Niigata City 950-0165, Japan. [2]EOS imaging, Paris, France. [3]Department of Orthopaedic Surgery, Niigata University Medical and Dental Hospital, Niigata, Japan.

References

1. Adam C, Izatt M, Askin G. Design and evaluation of an MRI compatible axial compression device for 3D assessment of spinal deformity and flexibility in AIS. Stud Health Technol Inform. 2010;158:38–43.
2. Asher M, Lai SM, Burton D, et al. The reliability and concurrent validity of the Scoliosis Research Society-22 patient questionnaire for idiopathic scoliosis. Spine. 2003;28:63–9.
3. Carreau JH, Bastrom T, Petcharaporn M, et al. Computer-generated, three-dimensional spine model from biplanar radiographs: a validity study in idiopathic scoliosis curves greater than 50 degrees. Spine Deformity. 2014;2:81–8.
4. Cobb J. Outline for the study of scoliosis. Instr Course Lect. 1948;5:261–75.
5. Daubs MD, Hung M, Neese A, et al. Scoliosis Research Society-22 results in 3052 healthy adolescents aged 10 to 19 years. Spine. 2014;39:826–32.
6. Delin C, Silvera S, Bassinet C, et al. Ionizing radiation doses during lower limb torsion and anteversion measurements by EOS stereoradiography and computed tomography. Eur J Radiol. 2014;83:371–7.
7. Deschenes S, Charron G, Beaudoin G, et al. Diagnostic imaging of spinal deformities: reducing patients radiation dose with a new slot-scanning X-ray imager. Spine. 2010;35:989–94.
8. Dubousset J. Three-dimensional analysis of the scoliotic deformity. In: Weinstein SL, editor. Pediatric spine: principles and practice. New York: Raven Press; 1994. p. 479–83.
9. Dubousset J, Charpak G, Dorion I, et al. Le système EOS: Nouvelle imagerie ostéo-articulaire basse dose en osition debout. E-mèmoire de l'Académie Nationale de. Chirurgie. 2005;4:22–7.
10. Duval-Beaupère G, Schmidt C, Cosson PH. A Barycentremetric study of the sagittal shape of spine and pelvis: the conditions required for an economic standing position. Ann Biomed Eng. 1992;20:451–62.
11. Duval-Beaupère G, Legaye J. Composante sagittale de la statique rachidienne. Rev Rhumatisme. 2004;71:105–19.
12. Fairbank JCT, Pynsent PB. The Oswestry disability index. Spine. 2000;25: 2940–53.
13. Fujiwara A, Kobayashi N, Saiki K, et al. Association of the Japanese Orthopaedic Association Score with the Oswestry disability index, Roland-Morris disability questionnaire, and short-form 36. Spine. 2003;28:1601–7.
14. Glassman SD, Bridwell K, Dimar J, et al. The impact of positive sagittal balance in adult spinal deformity. Spine. 2005;30:2024–9.
15. Glaser DA, Doan J, Newton PO. Comparison of 3-dimensional spinal reconstruction accuracy. Spine. 2012;37:1391–7.
16. Hasegawa K, Okamoto M, Hatsushikano S, et al. Normative values of spino-pelvic sagittal alignment, balance, and health-related quality of life in relation to age in a cohort of healthy adult subjects. Eur Spine J. 2016;25:3675–86.

17. Hasegawa K, Okamoto M, Hatsushikano S, et al. Standing sagittal alignment of the whole axial skeleton in reference to the gravity line in humans. J Anat. 2017;230:619–30. https://doi.org/10.1111/joa.12586.
18. Hashimoto H, Sase T, Arai Y, et al. Validation of a Japanese version of the Scoliosis Research Society-22 patient questionnaire among idiopathic scoliosis patients in Japan. Spine. 2007;32:E141–6.
19. Hui SC, Pialasse JP, Wong JY, et al. Radiation dose of digital radiography (DR) versus micro-dose x-ray (EOS) on patients with adolescent idiopathic scoliosis: 2016 SOSORT- IRSSD "John Sevastic award" winner in imaging research. Scoliosis Spinal Disord. 2016;11:46.
20. Keenan BE, Izatt MT, Askin GN, et al. Supine to standing cobb angle change in idiopathic scoliosis: the effect of endplate pre-selection. Scoliosis. 2014;9:16.
21. Lee MC, Solomito M, Patel A. Supine magnetic resonance imaging cobb measurements for idiopathic scoliosis are linearly related to measurements from standing plain radiographs. Spine. 2013;38:E656–61.
22. Legaye J, Duval-Beaupere G, Hecquet J, et al. Pelvic incidence: a fundamental pelvic parameter for three-dimensional regulation of spinal sagittal curves. Eur Spine J. 1998;7:99–103.
23. Mangione P, Gomez D, Senegas J. Study of the course of incidence angle during growth. Eur Spine J. 1997;6:163–7.
24. Morrissy RT, Goldsmith GS, Hall EC, et al. Measurement of the cobb angle on radiographs of patients who have scoliosis. Evaluation of intrinsic error. J Bone Joint Surg Am. 1990;72:320–7.
25. O'Brien JR, Yu WD, Bhatnagar R, et al. An anatomic study of the S2 iliac technique for lumbopelvic screw placement. Spine. 2009;34:E439–42.
26. Simon AL, Ferrero E, Noelle Larson A, et al. Stereoradiography imaging motion artifact: does it affect radiographic measures after spinal instrumentation? Eur Spine J. 2016. https://doi.org/10.1007/s00586-016-4462-z.
27. Tonosu J, Takeshita K, Hara N, et al. The normative score and the cut-off value of the Oswestry disability index (ODI). Eur Spine J. 2012;21:1596–602.
28. Torell G, Nachemson A, Haderspeck-Grib K, et al. Standing and supine cobb measures in girls with idiopathic scoliosis. Spine. 1985;10:425–7.
29. Vrtovec T, Janssen MMA, Likar B, et al. A review of methods for evaluating the quantitative parameters of sagittal pelvic alignment. Spine J. 2012;12: 433–46.
30. Wessberg P, Danielson BI, Willen J. Comparison of cobb angles in idiopathic scoliosis on standing radiographs and supine axially loaded MRI. Spine. 2006;31:3039–44.

19

Measuring the morphological characteristics of thoracolumbar fascia in ultrasound images

Kyra De Coninck*, Karen Hambly, John W. Dickinson and Louis Passfield

Abstract

Background: Chronic lower back pain is still regarded as a poorly understood multifactorial condition. Recently, the thoracolumbar fascia complex has been found to be a contributing factor. Ultrasound imaging has shown that people with chronic lower back pain demonstrate both a significant decrease in shear strain, and a 25% increase in thickness of the thoracolumbar fascia. There is sparse data on whether medical practitioners agree on the level of disorganisation in ultrasound images of thoracolumbar fascia. The purpose of this study was to establish inter-rater reliability of the ranking of architectural disorganisation of thoracolumbar fascia on a scale from 'very disorganised' to 'very organised'.

Methods: An exploratory analysis was performed using a fully crossed design of inter-rater reliability. Thirty observers were recruited, consisting of 21 medical doctors, 7 physiotherapists and 2 radiologists, with an average of 13.03 ± 9.6 years of clinical experience. All 30 observers independently rated the architectural disorganisation of the thoracolumbar fascia in 30 ultrasound scans, on a Likert-type scale with rankings from 1 = very disorganised to 10 = very organised. Internal consistency was assessed using Cronbach's alpha. Krippendorff's alpha was used to calculate the overall inter-rater reliability.

Results: The Krippendorf's alpha was .61, indicating a modest degree of agreement between observers on the different morphologies of thoracolumbar fascia.The Cronbach's alpha (0.98), indicated that there was a high degree of consistency between observers. Experience in ultrasound image analysis did not affect constancy between observers (Cronbach's range between experienced and inexperienced raters: 0.95 and 0.96 respectively).

Conclusions: Medical practitioners agree on morphological features such as levels of organisation and disorganisation in ultrasound images of thoracolumbar fascia, regardless of experience. Further analysis by an expert panel is required to develop specific classification criteria for thoracolumbar fascia.

Keywords: Inter-observer reliability, Thoracolumbar fascia, Ultrasound imaging

* Correspondence: K.De-Coninck@kent.ac.uk
School of Sport and Exercise Sciences, University of Kent, Medway Building, Chatham Maritime, Chatham, Kent ME4 4AG, UK

Background

A growing body of evidence supports the notion that the thoracolumbar fascia, an anatomical structure consisting of layers of dense connective tissue in the lumbar area of the trunk, is clinically important in people with chronic lower back pain [1–8]. The thoracolumbar fascia has been shown to play an important role in force transmission between lower limbs and trunk in both ex-vivo cadaver studies [9, 10] and in-vivo research during walking [11, 12]. Subcutaneous fascial bands have been found to mechanically link the skin, subcutaneous layers and deeper muscles. The differences in morphological characteristics of subcutaneous fascial planes may reflect how mechanical forces are distributed across various tissues [13]. However, what is not clear, is whether medical practitioners are able to agree on these different morphological features in ultrasound images of thoracolumbar fascia.

The architecture of the thoracolumbar fascia is complex, it consists of layers of dense collagenous connective tissue, interspersed with loose connective tissue which allows the dense layers to slide and hence play a role in trunk mobility. The thoracolumbar fascia is continuous with the aponeuroses of major trunk muscles which are instrumental in movement and vertebral control [8, 9]. It has been hypothesised that fibrosis, densification and thickening in the thoracolumbar fascia may be the result of an inflammatory response or soft tissue injury [1, 14–17]. For instance, a recent animal study demonstrated that an induced soft tissue injury in the lumbar region, when combined with movement restriction, lead to fibrosis, and significant thickening of thoracolumbar fascia [18]. An earlier pioneering ultrasound based human study concluded that the thoracolumbar fascia in people with chronic lower back pain demonstrated 25% greater thickness compared to a matched control group [4]. A follow-up investigation found that thoracolumbar fascia shear strain during passive trunk flexion, was reduced in people with chronic lower back pain by 56% [19]. In both aforementioned studies, Langevin's research team found significant differences not only in fascial thickness and echogenicity, but also in disorganisation of the architecture of the connective tissues of people with chronic lower back pain. Even though the clinical relevance of fascial tissues has been established [20], to date no classification of thoracolumbar fascia has been developed. In order to develop a classification system, a level of inter-observer reliability of the different types of architecture of thoracolumbar fascia needs to be established.

The aim of this study was to determine the inter-rater reliability for the rating of morphological characteristics of thoracolumbar fascia in ultrasound images, on Likert-type scale, by a range of clinicians.

Methods

Participants

The study was approved by the University of Kent's Ethics Committee and conducted in compliance with the Helsinki Declaration. Informed consent was obtained from all participants.

The inclusion criteria for participants were: medical professionals in the orthopaedic, sports medicine or sport rehabilitation field, with or without ultrasound experience or training. Twenty raters were recruited at a European Sports Medicine symposium to rate the scans independently, in a group setting. Subsequently, a further 10 participants were recruited through opportunistic sampling (see Table 1 for characteristics). This group viewed the scans individually on a standard size desktop PC computer (screen size 50 × 28 cm). These participants received the same presentation on thoracolumbar fascia. All scans were anonymised and displayed in randomised order. All participants viewed all 30 scans. Participants were asked about clinical training, years of clinical experience, musculoskeletal ultrasound training, and frequency of ultrasound image usage for diagnostic purposes in clinical practice.

Ultrasound image data acquisition

Images were taken at the intervertebral level 2–3, as fascial planes are the most parallel to the skin at this level [4]. The interspinous ligament between lumbar vertebrae 2 and 3, and the superficial border of posterior paraspinal muscles were identified using a validated protocol [21]. One focal region was set as close as possible to the thoracolumbar complex. Bi-lateral parasagittal (longitudinal) images were taken 2 cm lateral of the intervertebral disc space between lumbar vertebrae 2 and 3. The image acquisition was based on a validated protocol [4]. All images presented to raters were

Table 1 Characteristics of raters

Clinical training	$N = 30$
MD	21 (70%)
Physiotherapists	7 (23%)
Radiologists	2 (6%)
Years of clinical experience	13.03 (± SD 9.6)
USI training & experience	$N = 30$
Trained & experienced	12 (40%)
Untrained & unexperienced	17 (57%)
not known	1 (3%)
Frequency of USI usage	$n = 12$ (40%)
daily	4 (33%)
weekly	4 (33%)
monthly	4 (33%)

USI = ultrasound imaging

obtained using uniform settings, a frequency of 18 MHz was used, with a depth of 3 cm, which allow optimum image quality for subcutaneous structures [22]. See Fig.1 for example of ultrasound image and anatomical orientation.

Each ultrasound image was obtained using B-Mode imaging, with a MyLabGold25 semi-portable ultrasound scanner (Easote, Rimini, Italy). A 4 cm, 18 MHz linear array transducer (Easote LA435) was used for all images.

Selection of ultrasound images for reliability study

Initially, a single investigator selected 40 scans from a data-base of 308 bi-lateral scans of 154 male and female subjects with and without lower back pain from a larger prior study. A focus group then viewed the 40 images and selected 30 scans. Both the individual investigator and the focus group were instructed to select scans which, in their opinion, represented both 'organised' perimuscular fascia and 'disorganised' perimuscular fascia, with a range in between. 'Organised' was defined as 'being able to draw a rectangular box' around the hyperechoic zone, 'disorganised' was described as 'not being able to draw a rectangular box' around the hyperechoic zone. All raters were blind to any pathology or background information related to the scans. These 30 scans were deemed to represent the range of morphologies from very disorganised to very organised and a range of scans in between (Fig. 2).

Inter-observer reliability rating protocol

In inter-observer reliability studies, it is vital that raters apply coding to data they understand [23]. For this reason, a 20 mins presentation about the thoracolumbar fascia was delivered, this facilitated anatomical orientation and exposed the participants to a representative

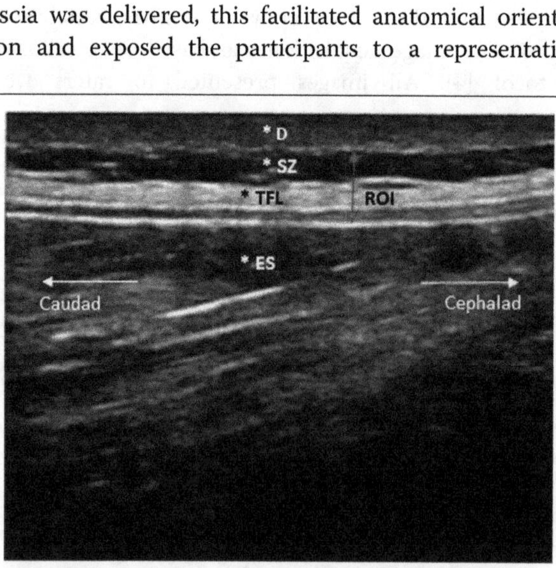

Fig. 1 Anatomical orientation and delineation of the zones rated. *D = dermins. *SZ = subcuteanouz zone. *TFL = thoracolumbar fascia. *ES = erector spinae. ROI = region of interest, zones rated

range of ultrasound images prior to rating. Participants were not given examples of actual ratings, only of the range of images they would be rating, to avoid bias. (See Fig. 1 for anatomical orientation and region of interest). Scans were projected on a standard sized screen (133 × 100 cm).

Table 1 shows that 57% had no training or experience in ultrasound imaging, 40% had experience ranging from monthly to daily evaluations of ultrasound imaging, 1 participant did not respond to this question, no observers had experience in evaluating ultrasound images of thoracolumbar fascia.

Participants were instructed to rank the region of interest (ROI in Fig. 1) which included the thoracolumbar fascia (* thoracolumbar fascia in Fig. 1) and the subcutaneous zone (*SZ in Fig. 1) on a Likert-type scale. A Likert scale with rating points from 1 to 10 was used, point 1 was labelled as 'very disorganised' and point 10 as 'very organised', the intermediate points were numbered but remained unlabelled. Participants were familiarised to the definition of thoracolumbar fascia organisation and disorganisation. For instance, 'very organised' was defined as 'to be able to draw a rectangular shaped box around the hyperechoic area of thoracolumbar fascia' (see Fig. 1).

Participants viewed scans sequentially in a time frame of 30 s to 1 min. They were able to modify responses, request to re-assess a scan, and make written comments about their decisions. Participants could not discuss ratings with each other, in order to avoid bias. All responses were anonymised prior to analysis.

Statistical analysis

Inter-rater reliability was assessed from the total raw scores of all 899 decisions, and the raw scores divided into 4 sub-groups using Cronbach's alpha, to assess internal consistency among observers [24, 25]. The Cronbach's alpha coefficient was calculated using SPSS (version 21) statistical software. Standard error of measurement (SEM) was calculated as the square root of error variance in accordance with de Vet's guidelines [26]. The Krippendorff's alpha for ordinal measures was used to assess inter-observer agreement [23, 27] and was calculated using a custom-designed online calculator [28]. As Likert scales are an ordinal measurement, the median and interquartile range for the total of scans was calculated, as well as for each scan individually [29, 30].

Participant ratings of scans were categorised into four groups [30–32]. Group 1 (very disorganised) consisted of all scans with a median rating of 1 to 3. Group 2 (somewhat disorganised) consisted of all median ratings from 4 to 5. Group 3 (somewhat organised) consisted of all median ratings from 6 to 7. Group 4 (very organised) consisted of all median ratings from 8 to 10 (Fig. 2). The Cronbach's alpha and

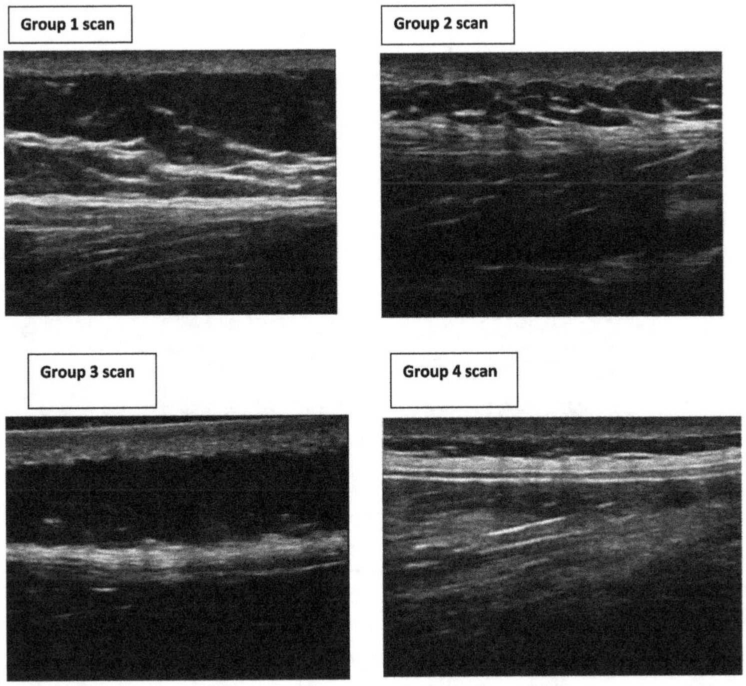

Fig. 2 A range of different thoracolumbar fascia morphologies. Sub-groups of different TLF morphologies. Group 1 = example of 'very disorganised', Group 2 = 'somewhat disorganised' Group 3 = 'somewhat organised', Group 4 = 'very organised' . The sub-grouping was based on the median scores for each scan

Krippendorf's alpha were calculated using the original raw scores from individual raters for each scan.

Results

Results of descriptive analysis

The median (m = 5) and interquartile range (IQR = 4) of the total ratings were calculated (range = 1–10), as well as for each group (Table 2 and Fig. 3).

Results of inter-rater reliability analysis

All participants assessed all scans, except one participant who did not complete one rating. The Cronbach's alpha was 0.98, which is considered excellent according to the Landis and Koch criteria [33]. Observers without ultrasound imaging experience scored a Cronbach's alpha = 0.96, observers with ultrasound imaging experience scored a Cronbach's alpha = 0.95, both in the excellent range. Scores between 4 sub-groups are reported in Table 2. The Krippendorff's alpha for ordinal measures was .61, with an error variance of 0.63, indicating a modest degree of agreement.

Discussion

In this study we found that medical practitioners agree on different morphological features in ultrasound images of thoracolumbar fascia such as levels of organisation and disorganisation. This agreement is independent of experience in ultrasound image rating. We found that the knowledge gap between musculoskeletal (MSK)-trained radiologists, MSK-trained medical doctors and physiotherapists on the one hand, and clinicians untrained and inexperienced in MSK ultrasound, did not affect the inter-observer agreement.

It is important to establish internal consistency before images can be used for research or clinical evaluation to ensure validity [24]. The measurement error was smaller

Table 2 Inter-rater reliability scores for all data and sub-groups

Group	Decisions (%)	Median (IQR)	Cronbach's alpha	Landis and Koch criteria [33]	SEM
All data	899	5 (4)	.98	excellent	0.10
Group 1	300 (32.8%)	2 (3)	.70	excellent	0.40
Group 2	209 (22.6%)	5 (3)	.68	good	0.17
Group 3	150 (20.3%)	7 (3)	.47	moderate	0.56
Group 4	240 (24.2%)	8 (2)	.56	moderate	0.50

SEM standard error of measurement, *Group 1* very disorganised, *Group 2* somewhat disorganised, *Group 3* somewhat organised, *Group 4* very organised

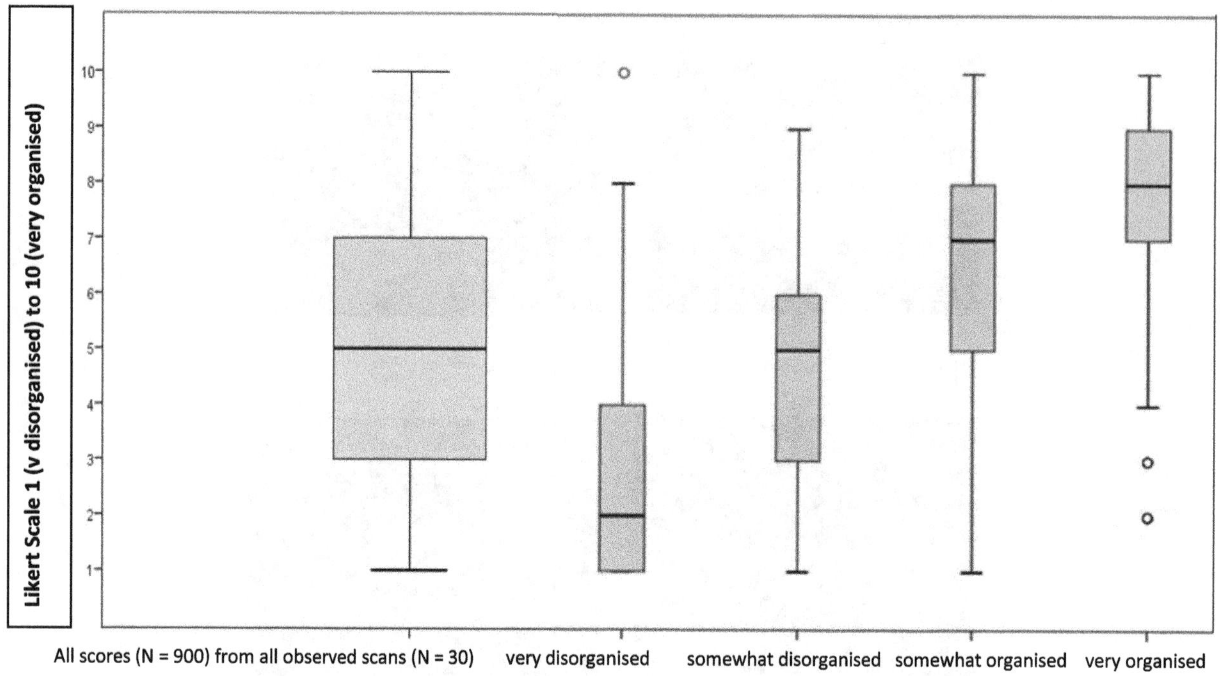

Fig. 3 Box-plots of all ratings, and ratings for each sub-group. Boxplots for total scores of the ratings (899 decisions) and ratings for each sub-group. Central tendency is the median, distribution is the interquartile range

in both groups of disorganised scans, and higher in the more organised groups. This could be an indication that it may be easier to interpret disorganisation or irregular shapes rather than organisation or regular shapes. The modest Krippendorf's alpha for the ratings suggests that a minimal amount of measurement error was introduced by the independent observers, and therefore statistical power for subsequent analyses is not substantially reduced.

In this cohort, the differences in ultrasound experience do not appear to impact on consistency. We did not observe any raters who systematically under- or over-rated the images. Novice raters have demonstrated good to excellent reliability in measuring abdominal and lumbar muscle thickness obtained by ultrasound scans [34, 35]. However, a straightforward comparison between quantitative measures of lumbar and abdominal muscle tissue, commonly found in the literature on rehabilitation of lower back pain, and this study's qualitative ratings of subcutaneous connective tissue requires caution. Substantial observer variability can occur, even at the expert level of image interpretation [36]. Interestingly, in this study, experienced radiologists agreed with the interpretation of clinicians relatively inexperienced in the reading of ultrasound images. The American College of Radiology Imaging Network (ACRIN) has highlighted that in order to improve the research in interpretation of medical images, observers in reliability studies should ideally reflect a broad range of experience to provide a sufficient level of generalisability [37].

In multi-reader medical image interpretation, the phenomenon of 'groupthink', has been identified, where the opinion of novice raters might be influenced by senior or experienced raters [36]. In order to avoid a situation of potential pseudo-consensus, all raters viewed the scans independently without discussing decisions with each other.

This study has a number of limitations. First, it involved a small cohort size of both observers and scans. The results are encouraging and should be validated in a larger cohort [37]. Secondly, the study relied on static ultrasound images. Future studies may consider functional and dynamic measurements. Finally, we did not determine the frequency in which raters interpret the same image differently. This needs to be taken into account for future studies.

Conclusion

Medical practitioners agree on morphological features such as levels of organisation and disorganisation in ultrasound images of thoracolumbar fascia, regardless of experience. These findings will be useful for the establishment of a clinical diagnostic scale and the further development of using ultrasound as a decision-making tool for researchers and clinicians.

Acknowledgements
The authors thank Karthik Muthumayandi for assistance with development of electronic data collection, and Dr. Samantha L Winter for helpful discussions during manuscript preparation.

Authors' contributions
KDC conceived the study, participated in study design, collected the data, analysed the data and drafted the manuscript. KH participated in study concept and design, reviewed the manuscript. JWD participated in study design, analysis, interpretation and manuscript preparation. LP participated in study design and manuscript preparation. All authors read and approved the final manuscript.

Consent for publication
Consent for publication was sought from all participants whose images are contained in this manuscript.

Competing interests
The authors declare they have no competing interests.

References
1. Langevin HM, Sherman KJ. Pathophysiological model for chronic low back pain integrating connective tissue and nervous system mechanisms. Med Hypotheses. 2007;68:74–80.
2. Yahia LH, Rhalmi S, Newman N, Isle M. Sensory innervation of human thoracolumbar fascia. Acta Orthop Scand. 1992;63:195–7.
3. Taguchi T, Tesarz J, Mense S. The Thoracolumbar Fascia as a Source of Low Back Pain. In: Huijing PA, Hollander P, Findley TW, Shleip R, editors. Fascia Research II - Basic Science and Implications for Conventional and Complementary Healthcare. Munich: Elsevier GmbH; 2009. p. 251.
4. Langevin HM, Stevens-Tuttle D, Fox JR, Badger GJ, Bouffard NA, Krag MH, Wu J, Henry SM. Ultrasound evidence of altered lumbar connective tissue structure in human subjects with chronic low back pain. BMC Musculoskelet Disord. 2009;10:151.
5. Tesarz J, Hoheisel U, Wiedenhöfer B, Mense S. Sensory innervation of the thoracolumbar fascia in rats and humans. Neuroscience. 2011;194:302–8.
6. Hoheisel U, Taguchi T, Treede RD, Mense S. Nociceptive input from the rat thoracolumbar fascia to lumbar dorsal horn neurones. Eur J Pain. 2011;15: 810–5.
7. Wilke J, Schleip R, Klingler W, Stecco C. The lumbodorsal fascia as a potential source of low back pain: a narrative review. Biomed Res Int. 2017; 2017. https://doi.org/10.1155/2017/534 9620.
8. Willard FH, Vleeming A, Schuenke MD, Danneels L, Schleip R. The thoracolumbar fascia: anatomy, function and clinical considerations. J Anat. 2012;221:507–36.
9. Barker PJ, Hapuarachchi KS, Ross JA, Sambaiew E, Ranger TA, Briggs CA. Anatomy and biomechanics of gluteus maximus and the thoracolumbar fascia at the sacroiliac joint. Clin Anat. 2014;27:234–40.
10. Macintosh JE, Bogduk N, Gracovetsky S. The biomechanics of the thoracolumbar fascia. Clin Biomech. 1987;2:78–83.
11. Vleeming A, Pool-Goudzwaard AL, Stoeckart R, van Wingerden JP, Snijders CJ. The posterior layer of the thoracolumbar fascia. Its function in load transfer from spine to legs. Spine (Phila Pa 1976). 1995;20:753–8.
12. Carvalhais VO, Do C, Ocarino J de M, Araujo VL, Souza TR, PLP S, Fonseca ST. Myofascial force transmission between the latissimus dorsi and gluteus maximus muscles: an in vivo experiment. J Biomech. 2013;46:1003–7.
13. Li W, Ahn AC, Weitz D, Mahadevan L, Barnett R, Zhang M. Subcutaneous fascial bands—a qualitative and morphometric analysis. PLoS One. 2011;6: e23987.
14. Pavan PG, Stecco A, Stern R, Stecco C. Painful connections: densification versus fibrosis of fascia. Curr Pain Headache Rep. 2014;18:441.
15. Diviti S, Gupta N, Hooda K, Sharma K, Lo L. Morel-lavallee lesions-review of pathophysiology, clinical findings, imaging findings and management. J Clin Diagnostic Res. 2017;11:TE01–4.
16. Corey SM, Vizzard MA, Bouffard NA, Badger GJ, Langevin HM. Stretching of the back improves gait, mechanical sensitivity and connective tissue inflammation in a rodent model. PLoS One. 2012;7:e29831.
17. Schilder A, Hoheisel U, Magerl W, Benrath J, Klein T, Treede R-D. Sensory findings after stimulation of the thoracolumbar fascia with hypertonic saline suggest its contribution to low back pain. Pain. 2014;155:222–31.
18. Bishop JH, Fox JR, Maple R, Loretan C, Badger GJ, Henry SM, Vizzard MA, Langevin HM. Ultrasound evaluation of the combined effects of thoracolumbar fascia injury and movement restriction in a porcine model. PLoS One. 2016;11: e0147393.
19. Langevin HM, Fox JR, Koptiuch C, Badger GJ, Greenan-Naumann AC, Bouffard NA, Konofagou EE, Lee W-N, Triano JJ, Henry SM. Reduced thoracolumbar fascia shear strain in human chronic low back pain. BMC Musculoskelet Disord. 2011;12:203.
20. Klingler W, Velders M, Hoppe K, SR PM. Clinical Relevance of Fascial Tissue and dysfunctions. Curr Pain Headache Rep. 2014;18:439.
21. Stokes M, Hides MJ, Elliott J, Kiesel MSK, Hodges CP, Hons B. Rehabilitative ultrasound imaging of the posterior Paraspinal muscles. J Orthop Sport Phys Ther. 2007;37:581–95.
22. Kremkau F. Diagnostic ultrasound: principles and instruments. 7th ed. St. Louis, Mo: Saunders; 2006.
23. Krippendorff K. Reliability in content analysis: some common misconceptions and recommendations. Hum Commun Res. 2004;30:411–33.
24. Tavakol Mohsen DR. Making sense of Cronbach's alpha. Int J Med Educ. 2011;2:53–5.
25. Cronbach LJ, Shavelson RJ. My current thoughts on coefficient alpha and successor procedures. Educ Psychol Meas. 2004;64:391–418.
26. de Vet HCW, Terwee CB, Knol DL, Bouter LM. When to use agreement versus reliability measures. J Clin Epidemiol. 2006;59:1033–9.
27. Hayes AFKK. Answering the call for a standard reliability measure for coding data. Commun Methods Meas. 2007;1:77–89.
28. Freelon D. ReCal OIR: ordinal, interval, and ratio intercoder reliability as a web service. Int J Internet Sci. 2013;8:10–6.
29. Jamieson S. Likert scales: how to (ab)use them. Med Educ. 2004;38:1217–8.
30. Norman G. Likert scales, levels of measurement and the "laws" of statistics. Adv Heal Sci Educ. 2010;15:625–32.
31. LaValley MP, Felson DT. Statistical presentation and analysis of ordered categorical outcome data in rheumatology journals. Arthritis Rheum. 2002; 47:255–9.
32. Hallgren KA. Computing inter-rater reliability for observational data: an overview and tutorial. Tutor Quant Methods Psychol. 2012;8:23–34.
33. Landis JR, Koch GG. The measurement of observer agreement for categorical data. Biometrics. 1977;33:159–74.
34. Teyhen DS, George SZ, Dugan JL, Williamson J, Neilson BD, Childs JD. Inter-rater reliability of ultrasound imaging of the trunk musculature among novice raters. J Ultrasound Med. 2011;30:347–56.
35. Wilson A, Hides JA, Blizzard L, Callisaya M, Cooper A, Srikanth VK. Measuring ultrasound images of abdominal and lumbar multifidus muscles in older adults: a reliability study. Man Ther. 2016;23:114–9.
36. Bankier AA, Levine D, Halpern EF, Kressel HY. Consensus interpretation in imaging research: is there a better way? Radiology. 2010;257:14–7.
37. Obuchowski NA. How many observers are needed in clinical studies Peter Hogg. Am J Roentgenol. 2004;182(April):867–9.

20

Prevalence of diffuse idiopathic skeletal hyperostosis (DISH) assessed with whole-spine computed tomography in 1479 subjects

Akihiko Hiyama*, Hiroyuki Katoh, Daisuke Sakai, Masato Sato, Masahiro Tanaka and Masahiko Watanabe

Abstract

Background: Computed tomography (CT) analyses have reported that the prevalence of diffuse idiopathic skeletal hyperostosis (DISH) in Japan is 8.7–27.1%. However, these data were obtained using chest-abdominal CT, and no evaluations of sagittal, coronal, and axial images using whole-spine CT have been reported. The aim of this study was to investigate the prevalence and characteristic of DISH by whole spinal CT.

Methods: Participants were patients who had experienced trauma who had undergone whole-spine CT scanning based on the initial clinical practice guidelines for trauma in our institute from April 2015 to February 2018. The subjects were > 20 years old and 1479 were included in the analysis. The presence and distribution of DISH and clinical parameters such as age and sex were reviewed retrospectively according to the location of DISH.

Results: The overall prevalence of DISH was 19.5% ($n = 289$). Subjects with DISH were older than those without. DISH was located in the thoracic spine in 65.1% and thoracolumbar spine in 24.2% of patients. More than 80% of ligamentous ossifications associated with DISH occurred at T8 ($n = 255$, 88%), T9 ($n = 262$, 91%), and T10 ($n = 247$, 85%). Most of the ossification occurred to the right anterior of the vertebral body, and there were few ossifications in the areas in contact with the artery and vein.

Conclusions: The prevalence of DISH based on whole-spine CT was 19.5%. Ossification was noted more often at T8, T9, and T10, and to the right anterior of the vertebral body. It is for the first time report that we have studied the location of ossification in detail using the axial images of whole spine CT. We hope this study will enhance the understanding of the characteristics of DISH.

Keywords: Diffuse idiopathic skeletal hyperostosis (DISH), Computed tomography (CT), Prevalence, Thoracic spine

Background

Recently, much attention has focused on vertebral fractures accompanying diffuse idiopathic skeletal hyperostosis (DISH). That is, an ankylosed spine tends to fracture as result of minor injuries such as falling because of stress concentration. Such fractures can cause reverse chance fractures that can lead to spinal paralyses, and are often resistant to conservative treatment [1–3]. Like other conditions with ligament ossification, DISH is thought to result from a multifactorial process whose etiology is not easily identified. In Japan, which is experiencing an aging society, the prevalence of minor paralysis caused by trauma is on the rise.

Proposed by Resnick et al. in 1975, DISH is a degenerative disease in which the spinal longitudinal ligaments and entheses gradually become ossified [4]. The pathogenetic mechanisms responsible for DISH are poorly understood, but genetic, metabolic, endocrine, anatomic, environmental, and toxic factors may contribute to its' development [5, 6]. Moreover, DISH is a condition of the elderly and is rarely seen before middle age. It is more common in males than in females with male/female ratios ranging between 2:1 and 7:1 [7, 8]. The

* Correspondence: a.hiyama@tokai-u.jp
Department of Orthopaedic Surgery, Tokai University School of Medicine, 143 Shimokasuya, Isehara, Kanagawa 259-1193, Japan

criteria most often used to diagnose DISH was first reported by Resnick and Niwayama in 1976 [9], before computed tomography (CT) was available as a diagnostic tool. However, when examining the prevalence of DISH, the problem is that the criteria also differs according to the article [9, 10].

The prevalence of DISH reported both in Japan and internationally varies widely between 3.8–25% [8, 9, 11–15]. It is considered to occur more frequently in Caucasians than in people of Asian and Black ethnicity. However, some groups have suggested that this considerable variation could be attributed to the incomplete diagnosis of DISH based on X-ray alone. CT provides far more detailed imaging of the intervertebral disc spaces and bridging ossifications, but there are only a few reports on CT-based diagnosis of DISH. Analyses using CT have reported that the prevalence of DISH in Japan averages 8.7% (13% for males, 2.5% for females) and may be as high as 27.1% (38.7% for males, 13.9% for females) [12, 16]. However, these data were obtained using chest-abdominal CT, and evaluations using sagittal, coronal, and axial whole-spine CT have not been reported. Most of the patients surveyed so far have been older than 40 years and, therefore, the true prevalence is unknown. The purpose of this study was to use whole-spine CT to investigate the prevalence and characteristics of DISH in trauma patients examined in an emergency critical care setting. In addition, we hope this study will enhance the understanding of the characteristics of DISH.

Methods

Our institution is a tertiary emergency medical facility that treats over 800 patients with severe trauma a year. The patients included in this study were those who had undergone whole-spine CT scanning during the period between April 2015 to February 2018 based on the clinical practice guidelines for trauma patients at our institute. The patients were aged over 20 years and their mean age was 54.7 years.

A total of 1479 subjects were included in the analysis: 1023 males and 456 females. The presence and distribution of DISH, and their clinical parameters such as age and sex were reviewed retrospectively and classified according to the location of DISH. The numbers of subjects in the age groups 20–39, 40–49, 50–59, 60–69, 70–79, 80–89, and ≥90 years were described in Table 1.

Table 1 Distribution of study population according to sex

Age group, yrs	Male	Female	ALL
20–39	286	93	379
40–49	167	60	227
50–59	160	46	206
60–69	167	70	237
70–79	162	98	260
80–89	70	77	147
90-	11	12	23
	1023	456	1479

Computed tomography (CT) examination

All CT scans were performed on a multidetector CT (120 kV, 380 mA, 0.6 mm slice; SOMATOM Definition AS; Siemens Healthcare, Forchheim, Germany) equipped with a 128-slice multidetector array. The diagnosis of DISH was based on whole-spine CT according to the criteria proposed by Resnick and Niwayama [9]: flowing ligamentous ossification in ≥4 contiguous vertebrae of the spine, with preserved intervertebral disc space, and the absence of inflammatory changes in the apophyseal joints or the sacroiliac region. The reconstructed CT sagittal, coronal, and axial images (Fig. 1) were used rather than X-ray to evaluate the continuous ligament ossification. All CT data were evaluated by authors. For testing the reliability of diagnoses, the testers read the same images of 20 patients to check inter-observer agreement. We also used intra-observer error at different time points, and the interval was found to be longer than one month by the first author. Differences were settled by consensus to minimize intra- and inter-observer bias and errors. Finally all images were reviewed by the first author.

Statistical analysis

Statistical analysis was performed using SPSS software for Windows (v. 20.0; IBM Corp., Armonk, NY, USA). All values are expressed as mean ± standard deviation. We studied statistical differences between the group with and without DISH. Analysis of DISH prevalence in males and females was performed using the chi-squared test. Analysis of variance with a post hoc test (Mann–Whitney *U* test) was used for comparisons. *P*-values < 0.05 were considered significant.

Results

The Kappa coefficient of inter- and intra-observer agreements were 0.79 and 0.89, respectively.

The demographics of the subjects included in this study are shown in Table 2. The prevalence of DISH was 19.5% (289/1479). The subjects with DISH were significantly older than those without: 71.7 and 50.6 years, respectively ($P < 0.001$). The prevalence of DISH increased with age. The prevalence of DISH in subjects aged ≥70 years was 40.9% (176/430), indicating that one in two people ≥70 years had DISH. In addition, the prevalence of DISH increased with age in both males and females (Fig. 2a). The results showed that the prevalence rates classified by age groups 20–39, 40–49, 50–59, 60–69,

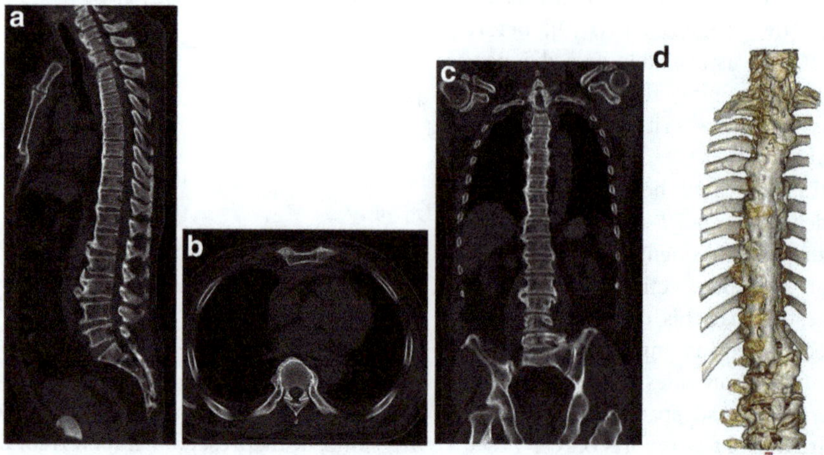

Fig. 1 CT images of a patient with DISH. Reconstructed CT of sagittal (**a**), axial (**b**), coronal (**c**) and 3D (**d**) views in a patient with DISH

70–79, 80–89, and ≥90 years were 0.3, 4.8, 18.1, 32.3, 50.0, 51.4, and 63.6% in male and 0, 3.3, 10.9, 20.0, 19.4, 36.4, and 41.7% in female, respectively. There were a significantly greater number of subjects with DISH in their 70s using the chi-squared test.

Among the 289 subjects with DISH, 216 (prevalence 216/1023 = 21.1%) were male and 73 (73/456 = 16.0%) were female (Fig. 2b). This tendency for a higher frequency in male was a significant ($P < 0.05$). In addition, when analyzed with subjects ≥40 years as in previous reports, the prevalence of DISH in 737 males and 363 females was 29.2% (215/737) and 20.1% (73/363), respectively, also showing a significant sex difference ($P < 0.01$) (data not shown).

Table 2 Distribution of study population according to DISH(+) or (−)

	DISH (+)	DISH (−)	ALL
Sex	N	N	N (%)
Male	216	807	1023 (69.2)
Female	73	383	456 (30.8)
Male to Female	3.0: 1	2.1: 1	2.3: 1
Age, Mean	71.7	50.6	54.7
Age group, yrs	N (%)	N (%)	N
20–39	1 (0.3)	378 (99.7)	379
40–49	10 (4.4)	217 (95.6)	227
50–59	34 (16.5)	172 (83.5)	206
60–69	68 (28.7)	169 (71.3)	237
70–79	100 (38.5)	160 (61.5)	260
80–89	64 (43.5)	83 (56.5)	147
90-	12 (52.2)	11 (47.8)	23
Total (%)	289 (19.5)	1190 (80.5)	1479

DISH diffuse idiopathic skeletal hyperostosis, *N* number

We classified DISH into six types according to location in which ossification along the aspect of ≥4 contiguous vertebral bodies was observed: (1) cervical—ossification only in the cervical region (C1–C7); (2) cervicothoracic—ossification only in the cervicothoracic region (C1–T12); (3) thoracic—ossification only in the thoracic region (T1–T12); (4) thoracolumbar—ossification only in the thoracolumbar region (T1–L5); (5) lumbar—ossification only in the lumbar region (L1–L5); and (6) whole spine—ossification in the entire spine (C1–L5). Figure 3 shows the prevalence of DISH classified by location in the spine: 65.1% were thoracic, and 24.2% were thoracolumbar. The prevalence of cervical and lumbar spine involvement was low.

Evaluation of the fused segments from the cervical to lumbar spine for all subjects revealed that the eighth thoracic (T8) to the 10th thoracic (T10) levels were the levels most involved, with more than 80% of the ligamentous ossifications associated with DISH located at T8 (n = 255segments/289subjects, 88%), T9 (n = 262segments/289subjects, 91%), or T10 (n = 247segments/289subjects, 85%) (Fig. 3). Of the 233 cases with consecutive ossification at T8–T10, the apex of thoracic kyphosis was located at T8–T10 in 142 subjects (60.9%) (Table 3).

Axial images of the ossification lesions at T9 (Fig. 4a) were studied further focusing on the location of the ossification, revealing that the ossification at T9 was observed in almost all cases in area 1, which is the right anterior region of the vertebra (98.3%) (Fig. 4b). As age increased, ossification in the left anterior region also appeared (Table 4). In a few subjects, the ossification was observed in the area in contact with the aorta and the azygous vein (Fig. 4c). The average number of vertebral bodies continuously bridged by ossification of the anterior longitudinal ligament was 7.9, and involvement of

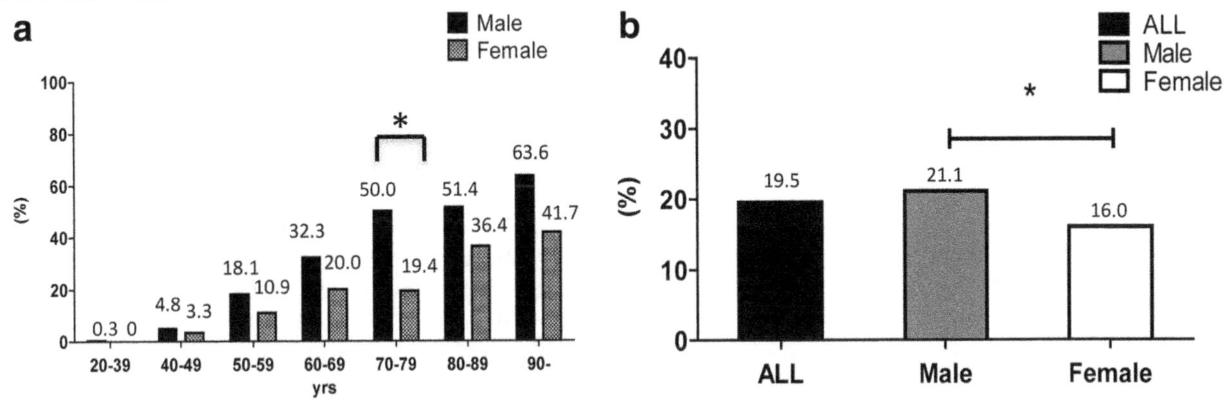

Fig. 2 Prevalence of DISH detected by CT. **a** Age distribution of the prevalence of DISH detected by CT. The prevalence of DISH increased with age in both males and females. **b** Comparison of the prevalence of DISH between male and female

≥12 vertebrae was seen in 47 of the 289 patients (16.3%). The average numbers of ossified vertebrae according to the age groups 20–49 ($n = 11$), 50–59 ($n = 34$), 60–69 ($n = 68$), 70–79 ($n = 100$), 80–89 ($n = 64$), and ≥90 ($n = 12$) years were 6.8 ± 2.0, 6.8 ± 2.6, 7.4 ± 3.2, 8.3 ± 3.5, 8.3 ± 4.2, and 9.4 ± 3.6, respectively, showing that the number of vertebrae with ligamentous ossification increased with age.

Discussion

DISH is a common condition in the elderly, but DISH is still insufficiently investigated and understood. In this study, CT images of the whole spine were used to determine the prevalence of DISH in 1479 patients aged > 20 years. While the prevalence of DISH has been reported to vary widely from 3.8 to 25%, it was 19.5% in these subjects. Factors that may affect the prevalence of DISH include differences in ethnic and genetic background, diagnostic imaging methods, patient age, and lifestyle habits. The prevalence of DISH in Japan, which would exclude the effects of race and genetic factors, has been reported to range from 8.7 to 27.1% [12, 13, 16]. Based on chest X-rays of 1363 patients, Weinfeld et al. showed that the prevalence differed between ethnic groups [14]. They reported DISH to be less common in the black, Native-American and Asian populations.

The prevalence of DISH may differ between past and present reports because of advances in diagnostic imaging (Additional file 1). In past reports, DISH was identified by X-ray alone, which resulted in lower prevalence than that identified by recent reports of DISH identified through examination of chest CT. Hirasawa et al. compared the prevalence of DISH evaluated by reconstructed CT of the chest to pelvis against plain radiography of the chest and abdomen [12], and found that the prevalence of DISH based on CT was 27.1% and that based on X-ray was 17.6%. Mori et al. reported that the prevalence of DISH was 8.7% using chest CT performed for investigation of pulmonary disease [16], which was smaller than that reported by Hirasawa et al. [12]. The

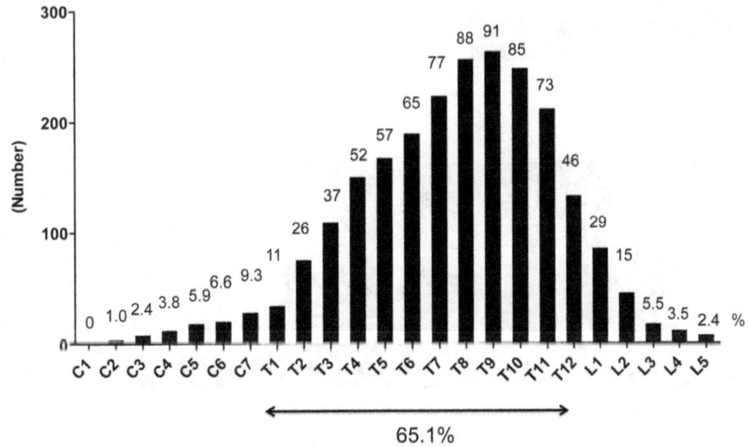

Fig. 3 Prevalence of DISH classified by location in the spine. The levels of fused segments are shown from the cervical to lumbar spine, and involved mainly T8–10

Table 3 Among 233 subjects who had consecutive ossification in T8 - T10, 142 subjects were found at the apex of the thoracic kyphosis at T8 - T10

Apex of kyphosis	N	%	
T5	1	0.4	
T6	11	4.7	
T7	37	15.9	
T8	68	29.2	
T9	47	20.2	142 (60.9%)
T10	27	11.6	
T11	25	10.7	
T12	11	4.7	
L1	5	2.1	
L3	1	0.4	
	233		

N number

differences in prevalence between these studies may relate to the sample size: that Mori et al. evaluated a large number of subjects (3013 cases), but was a patient-based and not a population-based study [16]. They acknowledged that the relationship between pulmonary disease and ossification of the spinal ligaments, including DISH, could have affected the prevalence data. Moreover, the study by Mori et al. included only chest CT and was not based on CT of the chest to pelvis, which may account for the differences from the study by Hirasawa et al. [12]. Our findings and those of previous reports indicate that most cases of DISH occur in the middle and lower thoracic spine. This means that when making the diagnosis, evaluation using whole-spine CT will be more effective than X-ray [12, 16]. On the accuracy of DISH diagnosis by CT, intra- and inter-observer error by review of CT was also less than that of X-ray [12]. From these data, we think that CT may be a most suitable modality for the evaluation of DISH. Thus, analysis of the prevalence of DISH and its characteristics from the analysis using CT is considered to be useful for analyzing the treatment and pathology.

Another possible reason for the difference in prevalence of DISH is age of the study population. Most previous reports only included people older than 40 years with an average of 65 years [8, 13, 17], whereas in this study, we included younger patients (> 20 years) for an average age of 54.7 years old.

One limitation of our study is that the patients' past history was not analyzed; in particular, the presence of metabolic disease, because the distribution of these patients may affect the prevalence of DISH. Although the pathogenesis of DISH has not been fully elucidated, DISH may be related to modern lifestyle-related diseases such as obesity and metabolic syndrome, and the prevalence rate of DISH may be higher in those with metabolic disease. Some have suggested that its prevalence

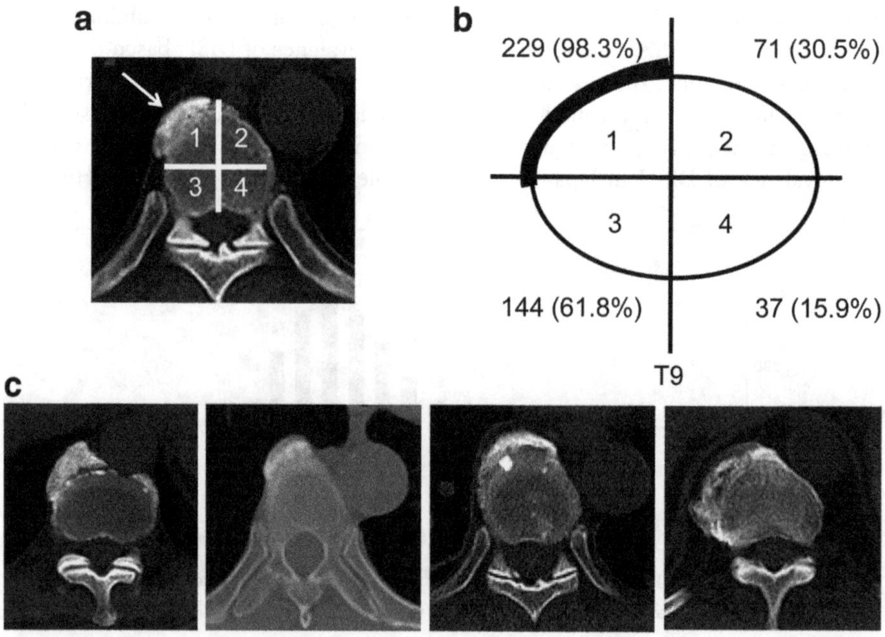

Fig. 4 Axial (AX) image of the areas showing ossification at T9. **a** A 58-year-old man presented with DISH between T7–11. The vertebral body was divided into 4 areas from the AX image of T9. In this case ossification was observed in area 1 (arrow). **b** Location of ossification on vertebral body: Area 1, right anterior; Area 2, left anterior; Area 3, right posterior; Area 4, left posterior. **c** Ossification was rarely found in vertebral bodies contacting with the aorta and the azygous vein

Table 4 Axial image of the lesion of ossification at the T9 level among 233 subjects who had consecutive ossification in T8 - T10

		T9 Lesion				T9 Lesion			
		1	2	3	4	1	2	3	4
Age, yrs		N				%			
20–39	1	1	0	0	0	100	0	0	0
40–49	7	6	1	3	1	85.7	14.3	42.9	14.3
50–59	24	24	3	18	1	100.0	12.5	75.0	4.2
60–69	54	52	6	24	3	96.3	11.1	44.4	5.6
70–79	86	85	25	56	10	98.8	29.1	65.1	11.6
80–89	51	51	29	35	18	100.0	56.9	68.6	35.3
90-	10	10	7	8	4	100.0	70.0	80.0	40.0
	233	229	71	144	37	98.3	30.5	61.8	15.9

N number

may increase in the coming decades because of the relationship between DISH and such modern lifestyle-related diseases [5, 6, 18, 19]. We could not investigate any possible associations between such factors and DISH because no clinical background information except for age and sex were available in our retrospective study.

Other studies have reported a higher prevalence of DISH in males than in females. The Research on Osteoarthritis/Osteoporosis Against Disability (ROAD) study of Kagotani et al. investigated the prevalence of DISH in 1647 people who underwent whole-spine X-ray [13]. Their logistic regression analysis revealed that the prevalence of DISH was associated with male sex (odds ratio (OR): 5.55) and presence of severe lumbar spondylosis (OR: 5.50). It appears that male tend to be more likely to develop DISH than female regardless of ethnicity or genetic factors. In our study, there was a tendency for the prevalence of DISH to be higher in males than in females, but the difference was small than in previous studies. It is possible that this result may have been affected by the inclusion of younger patients than in previous studies.

The most common site of DISH is the thoracic spine. We found that most of the ossification occurred in the middle and lower thoracic spine: T8 (88%), T9 (91%), and T10 (85%). It is interesting that DISH occurs at these sites. Hirasawa et al. and Kagotani et al. also found that DISH frequently occurred at T7–10 [12, 13]. Hirasawa et al. reported that more than 80% of DISH occurred at T8/9 or T9/10, which may reflect an anatomical effect; these vertebrae are susceptible to compressive mechanical stress because T8 is located almost at the peak of the physiological spinal kyphosis. Accordingly, DISH seems to arise mainly from the thoracic spine and may extend to the cervical and/or lumbar spine because of mechanical stress. Similar results were obtained in this study when the peak of spinal kyphosis was evaluated by supine CT. Interestingly, most of the ossification occurred to the right anterior of the vertebral body, and there were few ossifications in the area in contact with the arteries and veins. Previous study also demonstrated that the location of ossification was termed as anteolateral or right-sided hyperostosis [10]. Arterial blood flow and blood pressure may be affecting the ossification progress of DISH. Unfortunately we do not know about this mechanism from this study. However, it is for the first time report that we have studied the location of ossification in detail using the axial images of whole spine CT.

To date, the current knowledge on the pathogenesis of DISH is very limited. Some groups have reported that the pathogenesis of DISH is based on the excess of growth factors that might induce transformation of mesenchymal cells into fibroblasts and osteoblasts [20–22]. We think that it is need further analysis of these molecular mechanisms, which is important to clarify the etiology of DISH in the future. Okada et al. reported that the thoracolumbar junction (T11–L2) was the most frequently fractured level (54.8%) in patients with DISH [1]. The fact that vertebral body fractures associated with DISH are more frequent in the thoracolumbar junction may be related to the fact that most of DISH occurs from T8 to T10. However, in this cross-sectional study, it was impossible to evaluate whether DISH occurred first in the thoracic spine and then secondarily in the cervical or lumbar spine.

This study has some limitations. First, we did not have access to clinical data such as the presence of diabetes, which is a risk factor associated with DISH. This was a retrospective study and it was not possible to investigate all subjects. Second, there may have been selection bias in the inclusion of subjects due to the fact that they were all trauma patients, but we did not have access to data about each patient before their trauma. DISH patients are usually asymptomatic, and health checks of the general population will be an excellent way to evaluate the prevalence of DISH. Finally, the radiation exposure experienced in whole-spine CT imaging in normal subjects is a health risk that must be considered. Some researchers agree that, when used correctly, such scans can save lives. However, according to some estimates, the radiation exposure a patient receives from a full-body CT scan is often 500 times that of an X-ray. Despite these limitations, our data suggest that the prevalence of DISH in Japan is larger than in past reports. We believe that prospective multicenter studies are needed to determine the prevalence and pathogenesis of DISH.

Conclusions

The prevalence of DISH based on whole-spine CT was 19.5%, which is similar to that reported by other studies. Most ossification occurred at levels T8–10 and in the right anterior region of the vertebral body.

Abbreviations

CT: Computed tomography; DISH: Diffuse idiopathic skeletal hyperostosis; ROAD: Research on Osteoarthritis/Osteoporosis Against Disability

Funding

Non financial associations that may be relevant or seen as relevant to the submitted manuscript.

Authors' contributions

All authors have read and approved the manuscript. AH conceived and designed the study and interpreted the results; HK analyzed the data and interpreted the results; DS acquired the data and interpreted the results; MS acquired the data and interpreted the results; MT analyzed and acquired the data; MW conceived and designed the study and interpreted the results.

Competing interests

The authors AH, HK, DS, MS, MT and MW declare that they have no competing interests.

References

1. Okada E, Tsuji T, Shimizu K, Kato M, Fukuda K, Kaneko S, Ogawa J, Watanabe K, Ishii K, Nakamura M, et al. CT-based morphological analysis of spinal fractures in patients with diffuse idiopathic skeletal hyperostosis. J Orthop Sci. 2017;22(1):3–9.
2. Balling H, Weckbach A. Hyperextension injuries of the thoracolumbar spine in diffuse idiopathic skeletal hyperostosis. Spine. 2015;40(2):E61–7.
3. Rustagi T, Drazin D, Oner C, York J, Schroeder GD, Vaccaro AR, Oskouian RJ, Chapman JR. Fractures in spinal ankylosing disorders: a narrative review of disease and injury types, treatment techniques, and outcomes. J Orthop Trauma. 2017;31(Suppl 4):S57–74.
4. Resnick D, Shaul SR, Robins JM. Diffuse idiopathic skeletal hyperostosis (DISH): Forestier's disease with extraspinal manifestations. Radiology. 1975; 115(3):513–24.
5. Littlejohn GO. Insulin and new bone formation in diffuse idiopathic skeletal hyperostosis. Clin Rheumatol. 1985;4(3):294–300.
6. Vezyroglou G, Mitropoulos A, Antoniadis C. A metabolic syndrome in diffuse idiopathic skeletal hyperostosis. A controlled study. J Rheumatol. 1996;23(4): 672–6.
7. Julkunen H, Heinonen OP, Knekt P, Maatela J. The epidemiology of hyperostosis of the spine together with its symptoms and related mortality in a general population. Scand J Rheumatol. 1975;4(1):23–7.
8. Kim SK, Choi BR, Kim CG, Chung SH, Choe JY, Joo KB, Bae SC, Yoo DH, Jun JB. The prevalence of diffuse idiopathic skeletal hyperostosis in Korea. J Rheumatol. 2004;31(10):2032–5.
9. Resnick D, Niwayama G. Radiographic and pathologic features of spinal involvement in diffuse idiopathic skeletal hyperostosis (DISH). Radiology. 1976;119(3):559–68.
10. Mata S, Chhem RK, Fortin PR, Joseph L, Esdaile JM. Comprehensive radiographic evaluation of diffuse idiopathic skeletal hyperostosis: development and interrater reliability of a scoring system. Semin Arthritis Rheum. 1998;28(2):88–96.
11. Cassim B, Mody GM, Rubin DL. The prevalence of diffuse idiopathic skeletal hyperostosis in African blacks. Br J Rheumatol. 1990;29(2):131–2.
12. Hirasawa A, Wakao N, Kamiya M, Takeuchi M, Kawanami K, Murotani K, Matsuo T, Deie M. The prevalence of diffuse idiopathic skeletal hyperostosis in Japan - the first report of measurement by CT and review of the literature. J Orthop Sci. 2016;21(3):287–90.
13. Kagotani R, Yoshida M, Muraki S, Oka H, Hashizume H, Yamada H, Enyo Y, Nagata K, Ishimoto Y, Teraguchi M, et al. Prevalence of diffuse idiopathic skeletal hyperostosis (DISH) of the whole spine and its association with lumbar spondylosis and knee osteoarthritis: the ROAD study. J Bone Miner Metab. 2015;33(2):221–9.
14. Weinfeld RM, Olson PN, Maki DD, Griffiths HJ. The prevalence of diffuse idiopathic skeletal hyperostosis (DISH) in two large American Midwest metropolitan hospital populations. Skelet Radiol. 1997;26(4):222–5.
15. Westerveld LA, van Ufford HM, Verlaan JJ, Oner FC. The prevalence of diffuse idiopathic skeletal hyperostosis in an outpatient population in the Netherlands. J Rheumatol. 2008;35(8):1635–8.
16. Mori K, Kasahara T, Mimura T, Nishizawa K, Nakamura A, Imai S. Prevalence of thoracic diffuse idiopathic skeletal hyperostosis (DISH) in Japanese: results of chest CT-based cross-sectional study. J Orthop Sci. 2017;22(1):38–42.
17. Oudkerk SF, de Jong PA, Attrach M, Luijkx T, Buckens CF, Mali WP, Oner FC, Resnick DL, Vliegenthart R, Verlaan JJ. Diagnosis of diffuse idiopathic skeletal hyperostosis with chest computed tomography: inter-observer agreement. Eur Radiol. 2017;27(1):188–94.
18. Laroche M, Moulinier L, Arlet J, Arrue P, Rousseau H, Cantagrel A, Mazieres B. Lumbar and cervical stenosis. Frequency of the association, role of the ankylosing hyperostosis. Clin Rheumatol. 1992;11(4):533–5.
19. Sarzi-Puttini P, Atzeni F. New developments in our understanding of DISH (diffuse idiopathic skeletal hyperostosis). Curr Opin Rheumatol. 2004;16(3): 287–92.
20. Iwasawa T, Iwasaki K, Sawada T, Okada A, Ueyama K, Motomura S, Harata S, Inoue I, Toh S, Furukawa KI. Pathophysiological role of endothelin in ectopic ossification of human spinal ligaments induced by mechanical stress. Calcif Tissue Int. 2006;79(6):422–30.
21. Denko CW, Malemud CJ. Body mass index and blood glucose: correlations with serum insulin, growth hormone, and insulin-like growth factor-1 levels in patients with diffuse idiopathic skeletal hyperostosis (DISH). Rheumatol Int. 2006;26(4):292–7.
22. Eckertova M, Krskova K, Penesova A, Radikova Z, Zlnay D, Rovensky J, Zorad S. Impaired insulin secretion and uptake in patients with diffuse idiopathic skeletal hyperostosis. Endocr Regul. 2009;43(4):149–55.

21

Evaluation of the theoretical optimal angle of the tibial tunnel in transtibial anatomic posterior cruciate ligament reconstruction by computed tomography

Xiaohui Zhang[1,2†], Yuanjun Teng[1,2†], Xinxin Yang[1,2], Rui Li[1,2], Chongwen Ma[1,2], Hong Wang[1,2], Hua Han[1,2*], Bin Geng[1,2] and Yayi Xia[1,2*]

Abstract

Background: "Killer turn" effect is a critical explanation for the recurrent posterior laxity following transtibial posterior cruciate ligament (PCL) reconstruction, which affected by the angle of the tibial tunnel. Meanwhile, excessive tunnel angle would have an adverse impact on the healing of tendon to bone. The purpose was to evaluate the theoretical optimal angle of the tibial tunnel in transtibial anatomic PCL reconstruction.

Methods: The measurements were performed on CT sagittal plane, including the thickness of cancellous bone (L1), the theoretical optimal angle of the tibial tunnel (TOA, which was measured between tibial plateau and the extension cord connecting the center of PCL insertion site with a point 5 mm superior from marrow cavity vertex), L2 - the distance from anterior tunnel aperture to anterior end of tibial plateau, L3 - the distance from anterior tunnel aperture to tibial tuberosity (lowest edge of patellar ligament attachment).

Results: The value of TOA and L3 were 35.4 ± 7.9 ° and 26.8 ± 11.4 mm, respectively. L1 and L2 were higher in males than females (L1, $P = 0.002$; L2, $P = 0.046$). Regarding age, L1, TOA, L2 and L3 were higher in the 46–60 years group than 31–45 years group ($P = 0.02$, $P = 0.001$, $P = 0.038$, $P = 0.032$, respectively). With regard to height, L1 was lower in group I - < 1.66 m than group II - 1.66 to 1.75 m and group III - > 1.75 m (I v II, $P = 0.015$, I v III, $P = 0.026$). L2 was also lower in group I than group II and group III (I v II, $P = 0.026$, I v III, $P = 0.006$). TOA and L3 showed no significant differences among sex and height groups ($P > 0.05$).

Conclusions: TOA (35.4 ° ± 7.9 °) and L3 (26.8 ± 11.4 mm) could be used as a reference for ideal tibial tunnel placement in transtibial anatomic PCL reconstruction, so as to prevent recurrent PCL laxity and ensure good graft healing. However, further clinical validation is needed.

Keywords: Posterior cruciate ligament, Reconstruction, Tunnel angle, Computed tomography

Background

The transtibial tunnel technique has been commonly used for posterior cruciate ligament (PCL) reconstruction, in which the graft is pulled through and fixed in the tibial tunnel. Although the subjective knee scores were improved [1], clinical outcomes were not as predictable as that in anterior cruciate ligament (ACL) reconstruction [2–4]. Previous studies have demonstrated that the recurrent posterior laxity is one of the most common residual problems in PCL-reconstructed knees, which is related to thinning and elongation of the graft [1, 5, 6]. Inevitably, the graft will produce an acute bend around the proximal posterior tibia in transtibial tunnel technique [6, 7]. The acute bend is termed as "killer turn". The more acute the "killer turn" for the graft emerging into the joint from a tibial tunnel, the higher risk of abrasion against the anterior 'lip' of the internal tibial tunnel aperture, thus leading

* Correspondence: 13993166655@126.com; xiayayilzu@sina.com
†Xiaohui Zhang and Yuanjun Teng contributed equally to this work.
[1]Department of Orthopaedics, Lanzhou University Second Hospital, Lanzhou University, No. 82 Cuiyingmen, Chengguan District, Lanzhou City, Gansu Province 730030, People's Republic of China
Full list of author information is available at the end of the article

to the enlargement of the tunnel inlet and attenuation of the graft [8].

Furthermore, previous studies had shown that the fixation strength of interference screw was significantly related to local thickness of cortical bone [9, 10]. And they recommended that fixation site should be placed away from the joint line. Accordingly, numerous surgeons tend to increase the tibial tunnel angle to achieve a smaller "killer turn" effect and stronger graft fixation. Whereas, several investigators had found in animal studies that the graft healing in cancellous-filled femoral tunnel was superior to that in marrow-dominated tibial tunnel [11–13]. They concluded that the healing of tendon-to-bone was highly correlated with peri-graft bone mass and connectivity, especially the cancellous bone architecture at the graft site. Because of the tibial marrow cavity, the peripheral cancellous bone mass of PCL graft would decrease with the increases in tibial tunnel angle. Thus leading to an adverse impact on graft healing. Therefore, there should be a compromise between reducing the "killer turn" angulation, increasing fixation strength and decreasing quality of bony tunnel. We speculated that the optimal position of the graft within the tibial tunnel was the proximal vertex of the tibial marrow cavity, which not only improve the "killer turn" angulation and fixation strength but also produce the satisfactory healing of tendon-to-bone. The theoretical optimal angle (TOA) is formed between the tibial tunnel through the proximal vertex of the tibial marrow cavity and tibial plateau.

The purpose of this study was to evaluate TOA of the tibial tunnel in transtibial anatomic PCL reconstruction through computed tomography (CT) measurements on the tibial anatomic characteristics.

Methods

Samples selection

After approved by the regional ethics committee of our institution, we retrospectively reviewed 963 CT images of the knee between January 2015 and August 2017 in our institution. Indications for CT were different from the aim of this study. Inclusion criteria: (1). patients accepted ultrahigh resolution CT examination of the knee; (2). the age range of patients is 18 years to 60 years; (3). scanning direction of CT was paralleled to anterior tibial crest, the selected sagittal section contained PCL tibial attachment and highest vertex of the tibial marrow cavity. Exclusion criteria: patients with displaced fractures involving knee, congenital skeletal dysplasia, previous knee surgery, inflammation or tuberculosis of bone and joint, tumor around the knee joint, and any knee abnormalities caused by disease.

Computed tomography imaging

All included patients accepted standard clinical knee CT performed on a 64-multi-detector-row CT (SOMATOM Sensation, Siemens AG, Wittelsbacherplatz 2, Muenchen, Germany). Scanning parameters included a gantry rotation speed of 1.00 s/rotation, 0.3 mm collimation width × 12 detectors, a CT pitch factor of 0.90 and a field of view of 25–30 cm. CT dose index (CTDI) volume was 20.9 mGy. Each patient was fixed in a supine position with the knee extended naturally.

Measurements of the tibial anatomic characteristics

The measurements of the tibial anatomic characteristics were performed with the ST-PACS CDMedical software Vision 3.1 (Crealife, Beijing, China) by two independent, blinded observers. All CT images were evaluated by observer 1, and observer 2 measured 100 cases randomly selected from all specimens and blinded to results from observer 1. After 1 month, observer 1 measured 50 cases again which were randomly selected from all images. In this way, the intra- and inter-observer reliability were determined.

The measurements were taken on sagittal section that provided the most inclusive and wide PCL tibial attachment, including the thickness of cancellous bone (L1), the theoretical optimal angle of the tibial tunnel relative to plateau (TOA, producing the minimal "killer turn" effect on the premise of the satisfactory tunnel bone quality), L2 - the distance from anterior tunnel aperture to anterior end of tibial plateau, L3 - the distance from anterior tunnel aperture to tibial tuberosity (lowest edge of patellar ligament attachment). Surgeons could easily locate the tibial tunnel position during transtibial PCL reconstruction by measuring L2 and L3.

L1 was measured from the proximal vertex of the tibial marrow cavity to tibial plateau along the anatomic axis of marrow cavity, the proximal vertex was observed on sagittal section (Fig. 1). Subsequently, TOA was measured between tibial plateau and the extension cord that connecting the center of PCL insertion site with a point 5 mm superior from the marrow cavity vertex (Fig. 1).As described by Lee et al. [14], we chose the point 5 mm superior from the marrow cavity vertex because a 10-mm-diameter tibial tunnel was usually used in PCL reconstruction. L2 was measured from anterior end of tibial plateau to anterior tunnel aperture (Fig. 1). L3 was measured from the lowest edge of patellar ligament attachment site on tibia to anterior tunnel aperture (Fig. 2).

Statistical analysis

All statistical analysis were performed using SPSS software (version 22.0, Inc., Chicago, IL, USA). The measurement

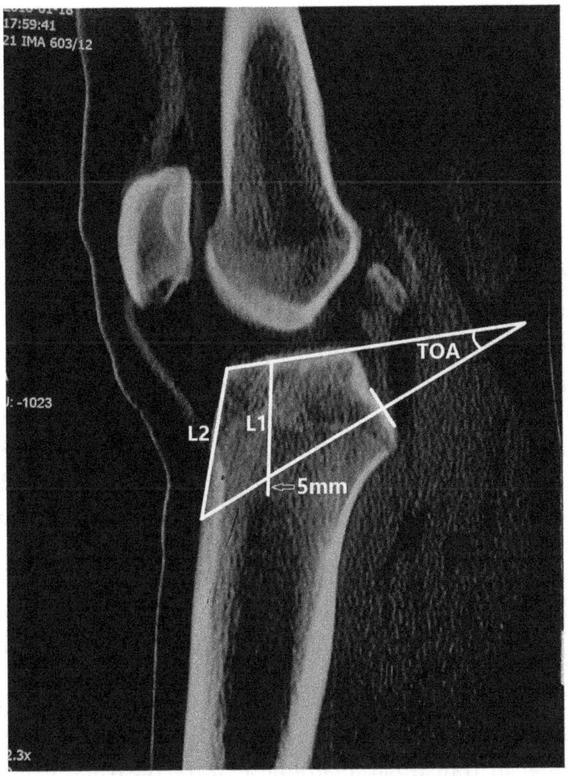

Fig. 1 CT sagittal section: L1 was measured from the proximal vertex of the tibial marrow cavity to the tibial plateau along the anatomic axis of the marrow cavity; TOA was measured between the tibial plateau and the extension cord that connecting the center of PCL insertion site with a point 5 mm superior from the marrow cavity vertex (hollow white arrows); L2 was measured from from anterior tunnel aperture to anterior end of tibial plateau

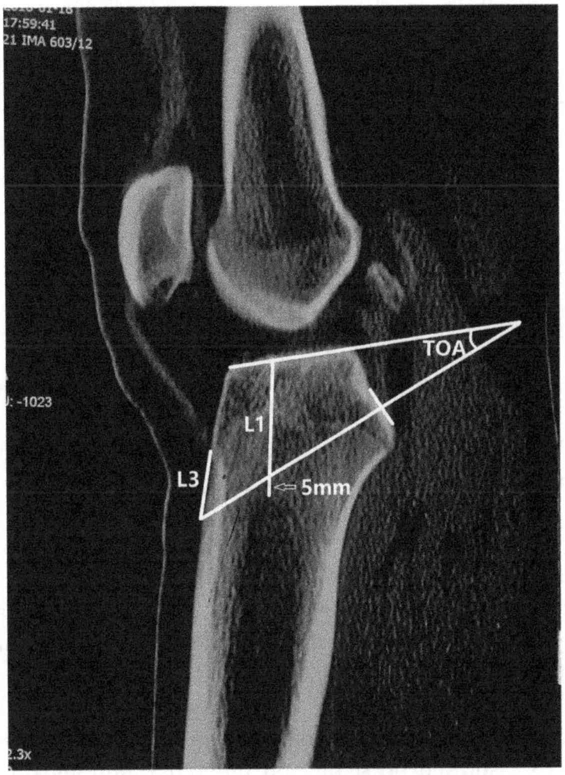

Fig. 2 CT sagittal section: L3 was measured from anterior tunnel aperture to tibial tuberosity (lowest edge of patellar ligament attachment)

results were shown as arithmetic mean ± standard deviation, to check up the data of all groups with normal test. All data were analyzed for the cohort as a whole, including age, height, and sex cohorts. One-way analysis of variance (ANOVA) was used to assess parameters among age cohorts and height cohorts, while independent t test between males and females. $P < 0.05$ was considered statistically significant. The intraclass correlation coefficients (ICCs) were used to analyze the calculation of intra- and inter-observer reliability. The ICCs ranges from 0.00 (no agreement) to 1.00 (perfect agreement).

Results

In total, 408 knees were included in the present study (based on inclusion and exclusion criteria). There were 230 left knees and 178 right knees. The number was slightly higher in male patients (225) than that in female patients (183). The average age of patients was 38.3 ± 14.1 years (18–60 years in males, 18–60 years in females).

Based on sex, Table 1 showed the tibial anatomic parameters. The average value of TOA and L3 were 35.4 ± 7.9 ° and 26.8 ± 11.4 mm, respectively. There were no significant differences between sex groups ($P > 0.05$). The value of L1 and L2 were significant higher in males than that in females (L1, $P = 0.002$; L2, $P = 0.046$).

Regarding age, the relative results were shown in Table 2. We stratified the cases into three groups: the young (18–30 years old, $n = 153$), the middle-aged (31–45 years old, $n = 104$), the elderly (46–60 years old, $n = 151$). In total, the value of L1, TOA, L2 and L3 were significant higher in the middle-aged than the young ($P = 0.02$, $P = 0.001$, $P = 0.038$, $P = 0.032$, respectively). No significant differences were found in

Table 1 Descriptive statistics of the proximal tibial parameters between males and females

Parameter	Mean Standard ± Deviation			P
	Total (n = 408)	Male (n = 225)	Female (n = 183)	
L1 (mm)	40.1 ± 7.6	41.1 ± 7.0	38.8 ± 8.0	.002
TOA (°)	35.4 ± 7.9	35.1 ± 7.2	35.8 ± 8.6	.352
L2 (mm)	47.0 ± 11.1	48.0 ± 10.8	45.8 ± 11.3	.046
L3 (mm)	26.8 ± 11.4	27.2 ± 10.9	27.3 ± 12.0	.463

L1 the thickness of cancellous bone, *TOA* the theoretical optimal angle, *L2* the distance from anterior tunnel aperture to anterior end of tibial plateau, *L3* the distance from anterior tunnel aperture to the tibial tuberosity (lowest edge of patellar ligament attachment)

Table 2 Anatomic parameters of the proximal tibia among three age groups

Age group (years)		Mean Standard ± Deviation			
		L1 (mm)	TOA (°)	L2 (mm)	L3 (mm)
Total	The Young 18–30 (n = 153)	39.2 ± 6.5	34.0 ± 6.7	45.6 ± 9.6	25.4 ± 10.6
	The Middle-aged 31–45 (*n* = 104)	41.6 ± 7.2*	37.3 ± 7.3*	48.9 ± 10.6*	28.7 ± 9.9*
	The Elderly 46–60 (*n* = 151)	39.9 ± 8.6	35.5 ± 9.1	47.2 ± 12.6	26.9 ± 12.9

Compared to the young, *$P < 0.05$. *L1* the thickness of cancellous bone, *TOA* the theoretical optimal angle, *L2* the distance from anterior tunnel aperture to anterior end of tibial plateau, *L3* the distance from anterior tunnel aperture to the tibial tuberosity (lowest edge of patellar ligament attachment)

the value of measurements between the elderly and other age groups ($P > 0.05$).

With regard to height, we stratified the cases into three groups: I- < 1.66 m (n = 161), II - 1.66 to 1.75 m (n = 207) and III - > 1.75 m (n = 40), as shown in Table 3. The mean value of L1 was significant lower in group I than that in group II and group III (I *v* II, P = 0.015, I *v* III, P = 0.026). Similarly, the average value of L2 was also significant lower in group I than that in group II and group III (I *v* II, P = 0.026, I *v* III, P = 0.006). But there were no differences between group II and group III ($P > 0.05$). Interestingly, the average value of TOA and L3 showed no significant differences among three height groups ($P > 0.05$).

Inter- and intra-observer reliability of measurements were analyzed by ICCs. Table 4 shows the values were range from 0.641 to 0.909, indicating good reliability.

Discussion

Present study evaluated the theoretical optimal angle (TOA) of the tibial tunnel on CT sagittal plane in transtibial anatomic PCL reconstruction. And the corresponding distance of TOA from anterior tunnel aperture to anterior end of tibial plateau (L2) and tibial tuberosity (L3) were also measured.

Previous studies have shown that clinical outcomes of PCL reconstruction were not so desirable compared with ACL reconstruction [2–4]. Many researchers believed that the "killer turn" for the graft emerging into the joint from a tibial tunnel could result in graft abrasion and tunnel inlet enlargement, which were critical causes to recurrent laxity after transtibial PCL reconstruction [6–8]. Meanwhile, animal studies suggested that the graft fixation strength with interference screw within the tibial tunnel was closely related to local thickness of cortical bone [9, 10, 15]. Therefore, surgeons tend to increase the tunnel angle to relieve the "killer turn" effect and increase the fixation strength. However, studies on rabbit models had shown that the peri-graft cancellous bone mass significantly influenced the healing of tendon-to-bone [11, 12]. For human tibias, the farther away from the knee joint line, the less the cancellous bone mass in proximal half. To our knowledge, this study firstly proposed the theoretical optimal angle of the tibial tunnel in transtibial anatomic PCL reconstruction that taking the "killer turn" effect, the graft fixation strength with interference screw and the healing of tendon-to-bone into account.

This study demonstrated that the average value of TOA, L2 and L3 were 35.4 ± 7.9 °, 47.0 ± 11.1 mm and 26.8 ± 11.4 mm, respectively. In other words, the graft will be located in marrow-dominated tunnel rather than cancellous-filled tunnel if a value of tunnel is higher than the corresponding limit. Thus, we speculated that there would be an adverse impact on the healing of tendon to bone according to the previous rabbit studies though they did not research tunnel angle [11, 12]. There is value in defining the optimal distances from anterior end of tibial plateau (L2) and tibial tuberosity (L3) to anterior tunnel aperture, but L2 is hard to clinically use due to difficulty in accuracy of palpation of tibial plateau. Actually, L3 could be positioned effortlessly on most people. Interestingly, L2 was influenced by sex, age and height of a different degree in the present study, while TOA and

Table 3 Descriptive statistics of the proximal tibial parameters among three height groups

Height group (m)		Mean Standard ± Deviation			
		L1 (mm)	TOA (°)	L2 (mm)	L3 (mm)
Total	I- < 1.66 m (*n* = 161)	38.6 ± 8.2	35.5 ± 8.9	45.2 ± 11.6	25.7 ± 12.2
	II - 1.66 to 1.75 m (n = 207)	40.8 ± 6.7*	35.3 ± 7.1	47.8 ± 10.4*	27.0 ± 10.2
	III - > 1.75 m (*n* = 40)	42.4 ± 7.9*	35.4 ± 7.5	50.5 ± 11.5*	29.9 ± 13.2

Compared to I, *$P < 0.05$. *L1* the thickness of cancellous bone, *TOA* the theoretical optimal angle, *L2* the distance from anterior tunnel aperture to anterior end of tibial plateau, *L3* the distance from anterior tunnel aperture to the tibial tuberosity (lowest edge of patellar ligament attachment)

Table 4 Inter- and intraobserver reliability agreements of the proximal tibial parameters based on ICCs[a]

Parameter	Interobserver	Intraobserver
L1 (mm)	0.909	0.903
TOA (°)	0.721	0.641
L2 (mm)	0.793	0.859
L3 (mm)	0.817	0.891

[a] *ICCs* intraclass correlation coefficients, *L1* the thickness of cancellous bone, *TOA* the theoretical optimal angle, *L2* the distance from anterior tunnel aperture to anterior end of tibial plateau, *L3* the distance from anterior tunnel aperture to the tibial tuberosity (lowest edge of patellar ligament attachment)

L3 were only influenced by age. Thus, TOA and L3 were relative constant references. X-ray measurement would be more accurate than direct vision or palpation to determine the value of TOA and L3 during PCL reconstruction. As a result, theoretical TOA (calculated by choice of ideal tunnel placement on sagittal CT images on this study) for transtibial anatomic PCL reconstruction was 35.4 ± 7.9 °. There was no effect of sex and height on TOA but it might be influenced by age.

Limitations

A few limitations were present in our imageology study: (1) This study was conducted through CT images measurements, there were no definite CT data threshold to distinguish the cancellous bone and marrow cavity. Nevertheless, the deviation could be relieved by ultrahigh resolution CT of the knee in the study and our ICCs analysis also proved the good reliability of results. (2) The measurements were carried out in a single sagittal CT section without anatomic study, small deviation may exist. (3) We did not calculate a sample size. When we performed height subgroup analysis, the sample size of group III (> 1.75 m) was small. (4) The choice of an ideal tunnel placement is a theoretical study by imageology, there is no clinical validation presented. However, our results should be paid more attention by surgeons. In future, the authentic optimal position of the tibial tunnel should be comprehensively evaluated involving postoperative follow up, histological analysis, biomechanical study, etc.

Conclusions

In summary, through the computed tomography (CT) measurements on the tibial anatomic characteristics, we found that the theoretical optimal angle of the tibial tunnel relative to tibial plateau and the corresponding distance from anterior tunnel aperture to the tibial tuberosity respectively were 35.4 ± 7.9 ° and 26.8 ± 11.4 mm in transtibial anatomic PCL reconstruction. However, further clinical validation is needed.

Abbreviations

ACL: Anterior cruciate ligament; CT: Computed tomography; ICCs: Intraclass correlation coefficients; L1: The thickness of cancellous bone; L2: The distance from anterior tunnel aperture to anterior end of tibial plateau; L3: The distance from anterior tunnel aperture to tibial tuberosity (lowest edge of patellar ligament attachment); PCL: Posterior cruciate ligament; TOA: The theoretical optimal angle of the tibial tunnel relative to tibial plateau

Acknowledgements

We wish to thank the timely help given by Meng Wu and Xiangdong Yun in revising the manuscript.

Funding

This work was supported by the Natural Science Foundation of China [81874017], the Cuiying Science and Technology Innovation Project of Lanzhou University Second Hospital [CY2017-ZD02; CY2017-QN12], the Research Project of Gansu Province Chinese Medicine Administration [GZK-2017-51]. The funding body made no other contributions to any aspects of this study.

Authors' contributions

XHZ, YJT, HH and YYX designed the study; XHZ, YJT, XXY, CWM, BG, HW and RL collected the data; XHZ, YJT, XXY, CWM, HH, HW, BG and YYX analyzed and interpreted the data; XHZ, YJT, XXY, HW, CWM and RL wrote the initial draft; XHZ, YJT, HH, BG, RL and YYX ensured the accuracy of the data. All authors read and approved the final manuscript.

Consent for publication

Not applicable.

Competing interests

The authors declare that they have no competing interests.

Author details

[1]Department of Orthopaedics, Lanzhou University Second Hospital, Lanzhou University, No. 82 Cuiyingmen, Chengguan District, Lanzhou City, Gansu Province 730030, People's Republic of China. [2]Orthopedics Key Laboratory of Gansu Province, Lanzhou University Second Hospital, Lanzhou University, No. 82 Cuiyingmen, Chengguan District, Lanzhou City, Gansu Province 730030, People's Republic of China.

References

1. Hermans S, Corten K, Bellemans J. Long-term results of isolated anterolateral bundle reconstructions of the posterior cruciate ligament: a 6- to 12-year follow-up study. Am J Sports Med. 2009;37(8):1499–507.
2. Ochiai S, Hagino T, Senga S, Yamashita T, Haro H. Treatment outcome of reconstruction for isolated posterior cruciate injury: subjective and objective evaluations. J Knee Surg. 2018. https://doi.org/10.1055/s-0038-1653947.
3. Chahla J, Moatshe G, Cinque ME, Dornan GJ, Mitchell JJ, Ridley TJ, Single-Bundle LPRF. Double-bundle posterior cruciate ligament reconstructions: a systematic review and meta-analysis of 441 patients at a minimum 2 Years' follow-up. Arthroscopy. 2017;33(11):2066–80.
4. Margheritini F, Rihn JA, Mauro CS, Stabile KJ, Woo SL, Harner CD. Biomechanics of initial tibial fixation in posterior cruciate ligament reconstruction. Arthroscopy. 2005;21(10):1164–71.
5. Kitamura N, Yasuda K, Tohyama H, Yamanaka M, Tanabe Y. Primary stability of three posterior cruciate ligament reconstruction procedures: a biomechanical in vitro study. Arthroscopy. 2005;21(8):970–8.
6. Weimann A, Wolfert A, Zantop T, Eggers AK, Raschke M, Petersen W. Reducing the "killer turn" in posterior cruciate ligament reconstruction by fixation level and smoothing the tibial aperture. Arthroscopy. 2007;23(10):1104–11.
7. McAllister DR, Markolf KL, Oakes DA, Young CR, McWilliams J. A biomechanical comparison of tibial inlay and tibial tunnel posterior cruciate ligament reconstruction techniques: graft pretension and knee laxity. Am J Sports Med. 2002;30(3):312–7.

8. Li Y, Zhang J, Song G, Li X, Feng H. The mechanism of "killer turn" causing residual laxity after transtibial posterior cruciate ligament reconstruction. Asia Pac J Sports Med Arthrosc Rehabil Technol. 2016;3:13–8.
9. Harvey AR, Thomas NP, Amis AA. The effect of screw length and position on fixation of four-stranded hamstring grafts for anterior cruciate ligament reconstruction. Knee. 2003;10(1):97–102.
10. Amis AA. The strength of artificial ligament anchorages. A comparative experimental study. J Bone Joint Surg Br. 1988;70(3):397–403.
11. Wen CY, Qin L, Lee KM, Wong MW, Chan KM. Grafted tendon healing in tibial tunnel is inferior to healing in femoral tunnel after anterior cruciate ligament reconstruction: a histomorphometric study in rabbits. Arthroscopy. 2010;26(1):58–66.
12. Wen CY, Qin L, Lee KM, Chan KM. Peri-graft bone mass and connectivity as predictors for the strength of tendon-to-bone attachment after anterior cruciate ligament reconstruction. Bone. 2009;45(3):545–52.
13. Grassman SR, McDonald DB, Thornton GM, Shrive NG, Frank CB. Early healing processes of free tendon grafts within bone tunnels is bone-specific: a morphological study in a rabbit model. Knee. 2002;9(1):21–6.
14. Lee YS, Ra HJ, Ahn JH, Ha JK, Kim JG. Posterior cruciate ligament tibial insertion anatomy and implications for tibial tunnel placement. Arthroscopy. 2011;27(2):182–7.
15. Nagarkatti DG, McKeon BP, Donahue BS, Fulkerson JP. Mechanical evaluation of a soft tissue interference screw in free tendon anterior cruciate ligament graft fixation. Am J Sports Med. 2001;29(1):67–71.

22

Morphology of intervertebral disc ruptures evaluated by vacuum phenomenon using multi-detector computed tomography: association with lumbar disc degeneration and canal stenosis

Koichiro Murata[1†], Koji Akeda[1*†], Norihiko Takegami[1], Kevin Cheng[2], Koichi Masuda[2] and Akihiro Sudo[1]

Abstract

Background: The progression of intervertebral disc (IVD) degeneration leads to rupture within IVD tissues. The location and appearance of areas of gaseous radiolucency in the IVD, known as vacuum phenomena (VPs), are considered to indirectly indicate the position and extent of IVD rupture. The clinical significance of VPs in degenerated IVDs is not fully understood. The purpose of this study is to assess and classify the morphology of IVD ruptures by the presence of intradiscal VPs, and to examine the association between morphological VP-positive IVD ruptures and degenerative lumbar diseases.

Methods: IVD rupture was evaluated by the presence of VPs using computed tomography (CT) imaging. VP shape (spot, linear, island) was classified using sagittal imaging, and VP distribution (A-N: anterior AF-NP; N: NP only; N-P: NP-posterior AF; A-N-P: anterior and posterior AF-NP) was classified using axial imaging. The disc height index (DHI) was calculated from lateral radiographs. Disc degeneration and lumbar spinal stenosis were evaluated by MRI grade.

Results: In the VP shape analysis, the island type was the most common, followed by linear and spot types. In the VP distribution analysis, A-N was the most common group, followed by N, N-P and A-N-P. Intra- and inter-observer reliabilities were statistically sufficient to classify different rupture shapes and distributions. The DHI tended to be lower in discs that contained VPs, especially in the anterior AF area. The shape and distribution of intradiscal VPs were significantly associated with the degree of disc degeneration and lumbar spinal stenosis graded by MRI. Discs with VPs extending from the NP into the anterior and/or posterior AF had a significantly higher proportion of advanced disc degeneration (Pfirrmann's classification: grades IV and V).

Conclusions: This is the first study to analyze the morphology of IVD rupture evaluated by the presence of intradiscal VPs using CT imaging. This classification can comprehensively present the shape and axial distribution of VPs within IVDs. Intradiscal VPs are associated with the progression of disc degeneration and lumbar spinal stenosis.

Keywords: Intervertebral disc, Intervertebral disc degeneration, Intervertebral disc vacuum phenomenon, Computed tomography, Lumbar spinal stenosis

* Correspondence: k_akeda@clin.medic.mie-u.ac.jp
†Koichiro Murata and Koji Akeda contributed equally.
[1]Department of Orthopaedic Surgery, Mie University Graduate School of Medicine, 2-174 Edobashi, Tsu City, Mie 514-8507, Japan
Full list of author information is available at the end of the article

Background

The intervertebral disc (IVD) consists of an outer annulus fibrosus (AF), which is rich in collagens accounting for its tensile strength, and an inner nucleus pulposus (NP), which contains large proteoglycans that retain water to maintain the osmotic pressure required for resistance against loading by compression. IVD degeneration is biochemically characterized by decreases in proteoglycan and water content in the NP, as well as collagen degeneration in the AF. The progression of IVD degeneration is known to lead to ruptures (including tears and/or cleft formation) within IVD tissues [1, 2].

Several authors have reported the morphological features of IVD ruptures [1–3], and have suggested the possibility that disc ruptures may be related to low back pain and/or the pathogenesis of degenerative lumbar diseases. IVD vacuum phenomena (VPs) refer to the radiographic appearance of a lucency caused by the presence of gas, usually in the lumbar region; this is one of the characteristics of IVD degeneration [4]. The location and appearance of gas is considered to indirectly indicate the position and extent of rupture within the IVD. However, only a few studies have reported the clinical relevance of intradiscal VPs [5, 6]. There have been no reports evaluating the types and distribution of intradiscal VPs or the association of intradiscal VPs and disc degeneration and/or degenerative disc diseases. Although magnetic resonance imaging (MRI) plays an important role in evaluating IVD pathologies [7], including tissue degeneration, it is less accurate than computed tomography (CT) for detecting VPs [8].

The purposes of this study were (1) to evaluate and classify the morphology of IVD rupture by the presence of VPs using multi-detector computed tomography (MDCT) imaging, and (2) to examine the association between morphological IVD rupture and radiological lumbar disc degeneration and canal stenosis.

Methods

Subjects

This IRB-approved retrospective study was conducted on spinal computed tomography (CT) images of 99 consecutive patients (48 men and 51 women) who underwent spinal surgery. The overall average age of the patients was 67.5 years-old (range, 23–90). A total of 590 discs from T12/L1 to L5/S1 were analyzed. The clinical diagnoses of the patients were as follows: 74 lumbar spinal stenosis (LSS), 15 lumbar disc herniation (LDH), 7 cervical spinal diseases, and 3 others (Table 1). Multi-detector CT (MDCT) (slice increment: 1.0 mm, slice thickness: 1.0 mm; Asteion TSX-021B, Toshiba Medical Systems Co., Otawara, Tochigi, Japan) was performed for all patients. Lateral lumbar spine radiography was also performed in 75 patients and magnetic resonance imaging (MRI) in 74 patients. All radiological images were taken within three-months before surgery.

Table 1 Patient demography

Diagnosis	Subjects (male/female)	Average age
LSS	74 (34/40)	71.5 (23–90)
LDH	15 (9/6)	53.6 (36–77)
Cervical diseases	7 (6/1)	62 (44–88)
Others	3 (2/1)	61.3 (50–67)
Total	99 (51/48)	67.5 (23–90)

Computed tomography (CT) images of 99 patients (51 men and 48 women) with spinal diseases were reviewed. The overall average age was 67.5 years-old (range: 23–90). The clinical diagnoses of the patients were 74 lumbar spinal stenosis (LSS), 15 lumbar disc herniation (LDH), 7 cervical spinal diseases, and 3 others

Morphological classification of VPs

Intradiscal VPs were evaluated by the presence of areas of gaseous radiolucency using MDCT imaging. The morphological classification of intradiscal VPs included two separate categories, VP shape and rupture distribution.

VP shape

VP shape was evaluated using mid-sagittal imaging (Fig. 1). VP shapes were categorized according to three classifications: spot, linear, and island. A spot-type VP was defined as a point-like VP less than 2 mm in diameter. A linear-type rupture was defined as a radiating VP whose width was less than 2 mm. An island-type rupture was defined as a VP forming a wide cleft (> 2 mm).

VP distribution

VP distribution was classified using mid-axial imaging of intervertebral space (Fig. 2). The IVD was divided into three areas: nucleus pulposus (N), anterior annulus fibrosus (A), and posterior annulus fibrosus (P) on axial CT images of the disc. Using these divisions, the distribution of the intradiscal VPs was classified into four categories created by combinations of the three areas: 1) **A-N** indicates a VP in both the anterior annulus fibrosis and nucleus pulposus, 2) **N** indicates a VP in only the nucleus pulposus, 3) **N-P** indicates a VP in both the nucleus pulposus and the posterior annulus fibrosis, and 4) **A-N-P** indicates a VP in the anterior and posterior annulus fibrosus as well as the nucleus pulposus.

Disc height index (DHI)

Using lateral lumbar spine radiographs of each subject, anterior disc height (Ha), posterior disc height (Hp), superior disc depth (Ds) and inferior disc depth (Di) were measured. Disc height was expressed as the DHI, which was calculated as: $[(Ha + Hp) / (Ds + Di)] \times 100$ [9].

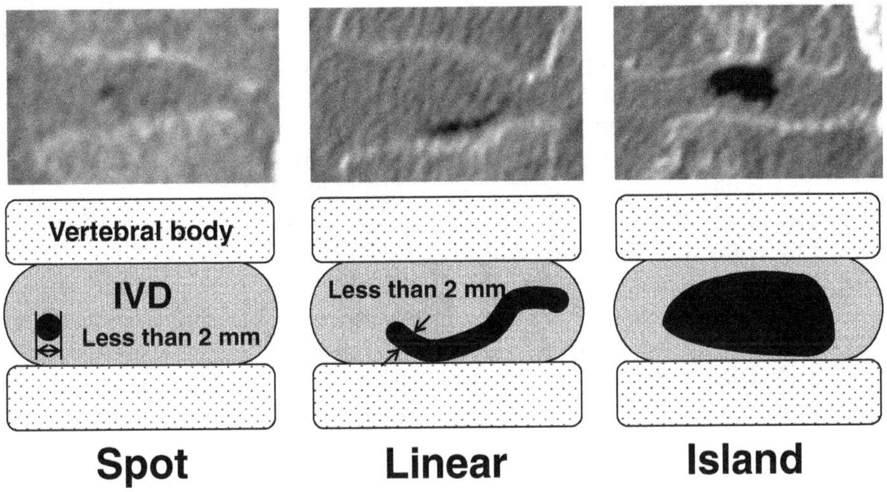

Fig. 1 Shape type of vacuum phenomena. The presence of vacuum phenomena (VPs) was classified into three types (spot, linear, and island) using sagittal imaging by multi-detector computed tomography (MDCT)

Classification of disc degeneration

The degree of disc degeneration was evaluated by sagittal T2-weighted lumbar MRI, and was graded according to Pfirrmann's classification from Grades I to V [10]. Grades IV and V were defined as advanced stages of IVD degeneration.

Classification of lumbar spinal stenosis (LSS)

The extent of lumbar spinal stenosis was graded from A to D using the method based on the morphologic appearance of the dural sac (cerebrospinal fluid / rootlet ratio) on T2-weighted axial imaging [11]. Grades C and D were defined as severe stenosis.

Data analysis

Two observers (orthopaedic surgeons) assessed the CT classifications of VP shape and distribution. The reliability of the CT classifications using CT images from 55 randomly selected VP-positive discs (52 patients) was evaluated using agreement percentage and kappa statistics for both intra- and inter-observers [12]. The agreement was regarded as "substantial" when the kappa values were more than 0.61 [13].

Statistical analysis

Differences in the proportion of CT-classifications between males and females, and among age groups were statistically analyzed using the chi-square test or Fisher's

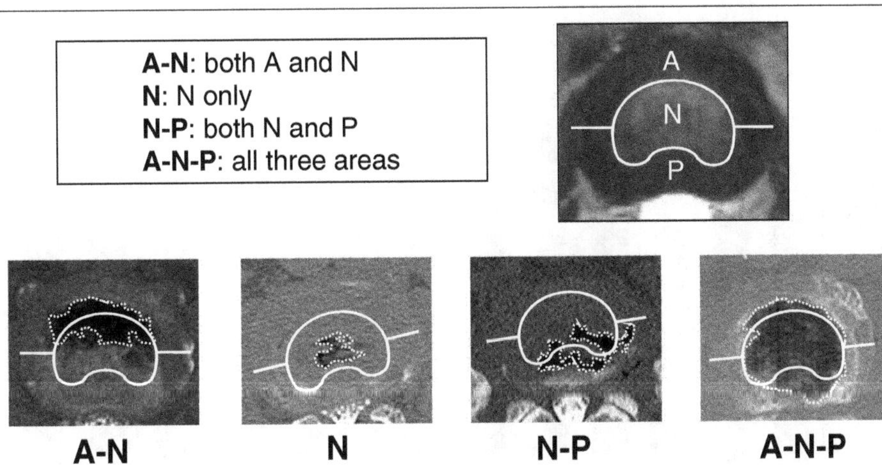

Fig. 2 Distribution of vacuum phenomena. The distribution of vacuum phenomena (VPs) was classified using axial imaging by multi-detector computed tomography (MDCT). The intervertebral disc (IVD) was divided into three areas (nucleus pulposus: N; anterior annulus fibrosus: A; and posterior annulus fibrosus: P). Then, the distribution of intradiscal VPs was classified into four groups using combinations of these areas

exact test. Statistically significant differences between the presence of VPs and DHI were assessed using one-way ANOVA followed by post hoc multiple comparisons using the Bonferroni method. The association between the morphology of ruptures (shape and distribution) and the MRI grading of disc degeneration or lumbar spinal stenosis was statistically assessed by the Fisher's exact test followed by a post hoc test. The post hoc test was performed to assess the probability values for each combination of independent category levels by using a Bonferroni correction to control for type I error inflation [14, 15]. All the statistical analyses were performed using IBM SPSS Statistics (IBM Japan, Tokyo or IBM Corp., Armonk, NY, USA).

Results

A VP was found in 226 discs (38.3%) of the 590 discs analyzed. The number of VP-positive discs was highest in the L4/5 level and lowest in the T12/L1 level (n [% of total VP-positive discs]: T12/L1: 19 [8.4%]; L1/2: 34 [15.0%]; L2/3: 40 [17.7%]; L3/4: 36 [16.0%]; L4/5: 54 [23.9%]; L5/S1: 43 [19.0%]) (Fig. 3a). The number of VPs was highest in the seventy (71–80 years-old) age group, followed by eighty, sixty, fifty and under fifty age groups (% of total VP-positive discs: 21–50 years-old: 3 [1.3%], 51–60: 13 [5.8%]; 61–70: 61 [27.0%]; 71–80: 93 [41.6%]; 81–90: 55 [24.3%]) (Fig. 3b). The percentage of VP-positive discs by age group was highest in the eighty age group, followed by seventy, sixty, fifty and under fifty age groups (% of VP-positive discs by age group: 21–50 years-old: 4.6%, 51–60: 21.7%; 61–70: 35.7%; 71–80: 46.1%; 81–90: 61.1%).

Intra- and inter-observer agreement of VP shape type

Intra- and inter-observer agreement of the VP shape type was "substantial" with kappa values 0.75–0.76 and 0.67, and with % agreements 87.3–89.1% and 83.6, respectively. In the VP distribution analysis, intra- and inter-observer agreement was also "substantial" with kappa values 0.64–0.65 and 0.70, and with % agreements 74.5–76.4 and 80.0%, respectively.

Prevalence of various VP types and distribution

VP shape type analysis revealed that among the total number of VP-positive discs, the island type was the most common (119 discs [53%]), followed by linear (61 discs [27%]) and spot (46 discs [20%]). There was no significant difference in the proportion of each VP shape between males (Spot: 18%; Linear: 26%; Island 56%) and females (Spot: 23%; Linear: 28%; Island 49%) ($P = 0.47$) (Fig. 4a). No significant differences in these proportions were identified among all age groups ($P = 0.5$), and the island type had the highest proportion in all age groups more than 51 years-old (Fig. 4b).

The analysis of VP distribution revealed that A-N was the most common area group (95 discs [42%]), followed by N (71 discs [32%]), N-P (37 discs [17%]) and A-N-P (23 discs [9%]) area groups. There were no significant differences in the proportion of each VP distribution between males (A-N: 39%; N: 32%; N-P: 16%; A-N-P: 13%) and females (A-N: 46%; N: 30%; N-P: 17%; A-N-P: 6%) ($P = 0.23$) (Fig. 5a). No significant differences in these proportions were found in all age groups ($P = 0.52$) (Fig. 5b).

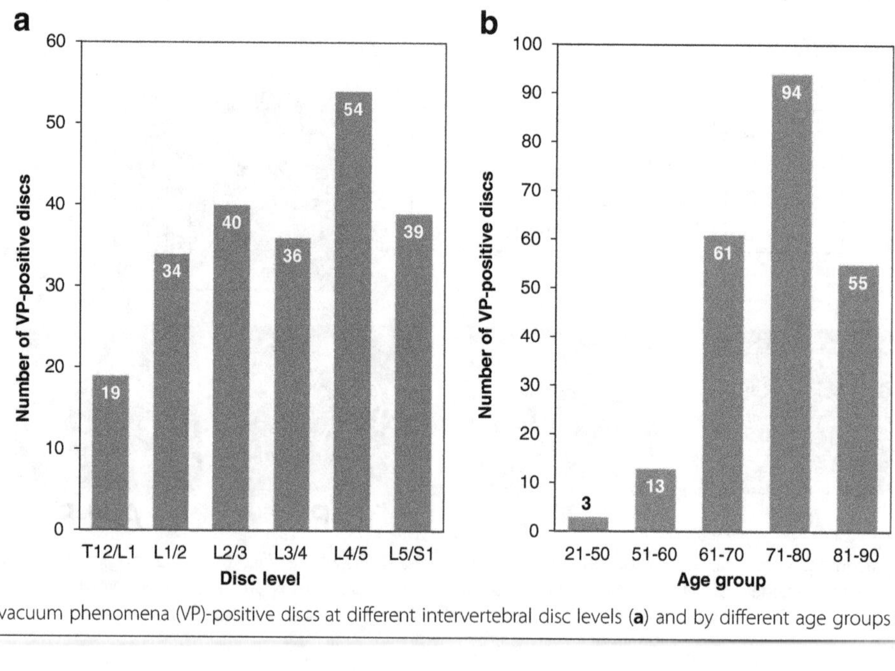

Fig. 3 Number of vacuum phenomena (VP)-positive discs at different intervertebral disc levels (**a**) and by different age groups (**b**)

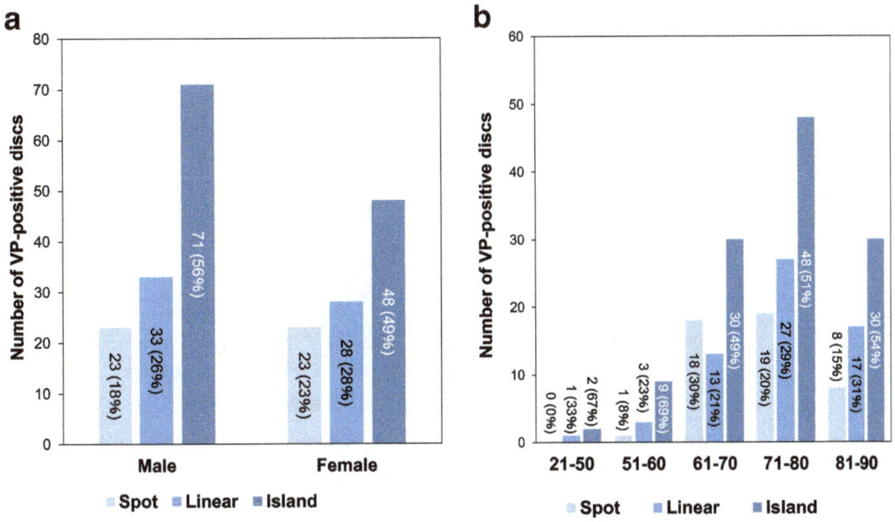

Fig. 4 Characteristics of intradiscal vacuum phenomena (VPs) in shape classification. **a** Number of vacuum phenomena (VPs) positive-discs by shape classification in males and females. **b** Number of VP-positive discs by age group by VP shape classification. The counts of VP-positive discs are written in the graph. Percentages in parentheses indicate the proportion of VP-positive discs of each rupture shape compared with the total number of VP-positive discs by gender (**a**) and by age group (**b**)

Association between the shape and distribution of VPs

A Pearson's chi-square test revealed a significant association between the shape and distribution of VPs ($P < 0.0001$).

Spot type VPs tended to be distributed in the A-N (% of total number of VP-positive discs: 9.7%) and N (8.4%) areas with high frequency; however no significant differences were identified in this distribution trend (Fig. 6). Linear type VPs were most highly distributed in the N (15.0%) area with statistical significance ($P < 0.0001$), followed by A-N (8.8%), then N-P (3.1%) areas (Fig. 6). No linear type VPs were found in the A-N-P area ($P < 0.0001$). Island type VPs were most highly distributed in the A-N (23.5%) area, however no statistical difference was identified ($P = 0.8$). There was a significantly lower frequency of the island type located in the N area (8.0%, $P < 0.0001$), and a significantly higher frequency in the A-N-P area (10.2%, $P < 0.004$).

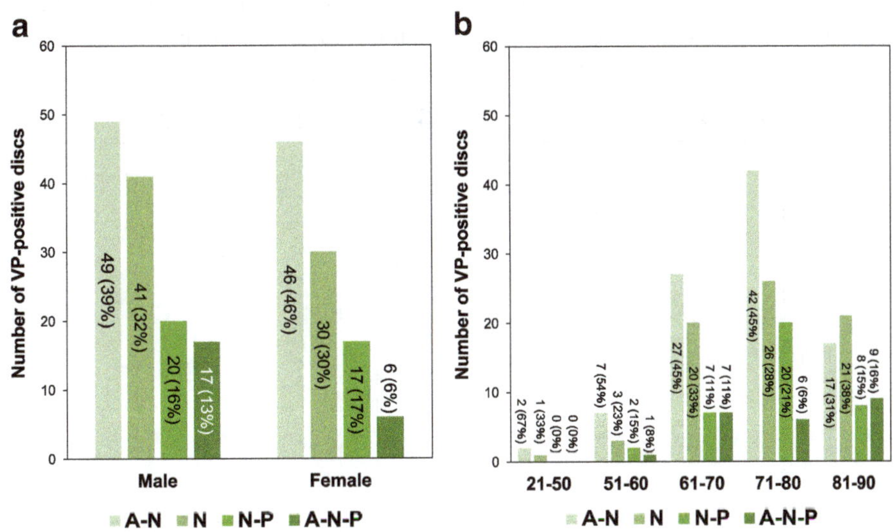

Fig. 5 Characteristics of intradiscal vacuum phenomena by distribution. **a** Number of vacuum phenomenon (VP)-positive discs in males and females. **b** Number of vacuum phenomena (VPs) by age group in VPs distribution. The counts of VP-positive discs are written in the graph. Percentages in parentheses indicate the proportion of VP-positive discs of each rupture shape compared with the total number of VP-positive discs by gender (**a**) and by age group (**b**). VP: vacuum phenomenon; VP-: non-ruptured group; Nucleus pulposus: N; anterior annulus fibrosus: A; and posterior annulus fibrosus: P

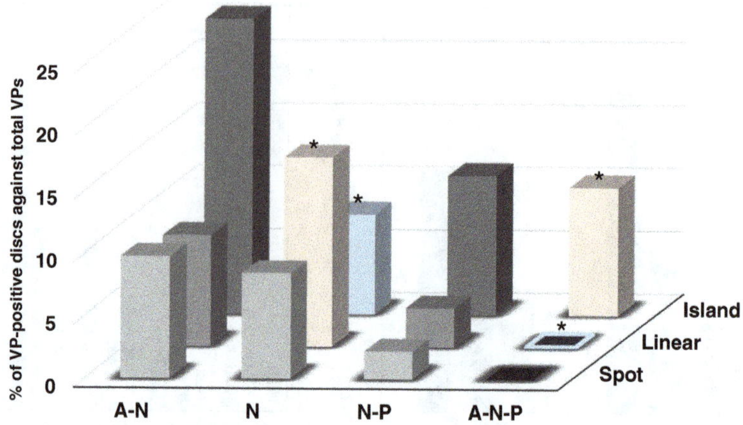

Fig. 6 Association between vacuum phenomenon shape type and distribution. The percentage of vacuum phenomenon (VP)-positive discs of the total number of VP-positive discs in each combination of shape and distribution classification is presented. Nucleus pulposus: N; anterior annulus fibrosus: A; and posterior annulus fibrosus: P. $*P < 0.004$ (by Bonferroni correction)

Association of VP type and distribution with disc height

In the VP shape type analysis (Fig. 7a), the DHI of the VP-negative (−) group was significantly higher than that of the island type group ($P < 0.01$); however no significant differences were found with linear and spot types. Among the VP-positive (+) discs, the DHI tended to be highest in spot type VPs, lower in linear VPs, and lowest in island VPs. The DHI in the island type groups was significantly lower than that of the other groups ($P < 0.01$) (Fig. 7a).

In the VP distribution study (Fig. 7b), the DHI in A-N and A-N-P area groups was significantly lower than that of the VP (−) group ($P < 0.01$, respectively; Fig. 7b). In addition, the DHI in A-N and A-N-P area groups was significantly lower than that of the N distribution ($P < 0.01$).

Association of VP shape type and distribution with disc degeneration

In the VP shape type analysis (Table 2A), the Fisher's exact test showed a significant association between VP shapes and MRI grades of disc degeneration ($P < 0.0001$). The results of the post-hoc test showed that VP (−) discs had a significantly higher proportion of discs with MRI grade 2 (percentages of the raw marginal total: 20.6%) and grade 3 (28.8%), but significantly lower with grade 5 (10.5%) (Table 2A, Fig. 8a). The proportion of spot type discs was highest in MRI grade 4 (53.6%); however those discs showed no significant association with MRI grading (Table 2A, Fig. 8a). In the linear type, the proportion of discs with MRI grade 5 (44.4%) was highest and significantly higher than other MRI grades ($P < 0.0001$).

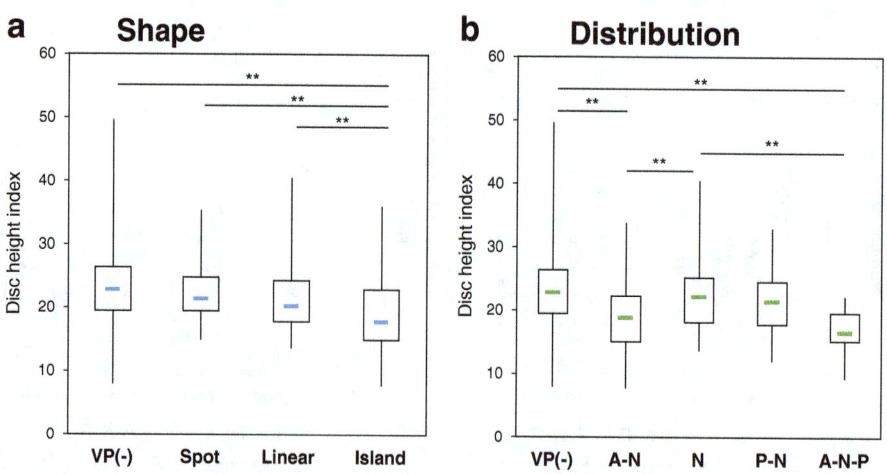

Fig. 7 Association of disc height with shape type of vacuum phenomenon. **a** Shape type analysis. The disc height index (DHI) in the island type group was significantly lower than that of the other groups. $**P < 0.01$. **b** Distribution analysis. The DHI tended to be lower in the areas including the anterior AF. $**P < 0.01$. VP: vacuum phenomenon; VP-: non-ruptured group; Nucleus pulposus: N; anterior annulus fibrosus: A; and posterior annulus fibrosus: P

Table 2 Association between intradiscal vacuum phenomena (VPs) and disc degeneration

A: Shape		MRI Pfirrmann's classification of disc degeneration					Total
		I	II	III	IV	V	
VP (−)	Count (% raw)	8 (3.0%)	**55 * (20.6%)**	**77 * (28.8%)**	99 (37.1%)	**28 * (10.5%)**	267
	Exp. Count	4.8	**34.5**	**59.3**	102.3	**66.0**	
	Corrected *P*-value	0.02	**< 0.0001**	**< 0.0001**	0.51	**< 0.0001**	
Spot	Count(% raw)	0 (0%)	1 (2.6%)	13 (34.2%)	20 (52.6%)	4 (10.5%)	38
	Exp. Count	0.7	4.9	8.4	14.6	9.4	
	Corrected *P*-value	0.38	0.05	0.06	0.06	0.03	
Linear	Count (% raw)	0 (0%)	1 (2.2%)	8 (17.8%)	16 (35.6%)	**20 * (44.4%)**	45
	Exp. Count	0.8	5.8	10.0	17.2	**11.1**	
	Count (% raw)	0.03	0.02	0.45	0.69	**0.0012**	
Island	Count (% raw)	0 (0%)	**0 * (0%)**	**0 * (0%)**	34 (37.4%)	**57 * (62.6%)**	91
	Exp. Count	1.7	**11.8**	**20.2**	34.9	**22.5**	
	Corrected *P*-value	0.15	**< 0.0001**	**< 0.0001**	0.83	**< 0.0001**	
B: Distribution		MRI Pfirrmann's classification of disc degeneration					Total
		I	II	III	IV	V	
VP (−)	Count (% raw)	8 (3.0%)	**55 # (20.6%)**	**77 # (28.8%)**	99 (37.1%)	**28 # (10.5%)**	267
	Exp. Count	4.8	**34.5**	**59.3**	102.3	**66.0**	
	Corrected *P*-value	0.02	**< 0.0001**	**< 0.0001**	0.51	**< 0.0001**	
A-N	Count (% raw)	0 (0%)	2 (2.7%)	10 (13.5%)	26 (35.1%)	**36 # (48.6%)**	74
	Exp. Count	1.3	9.6	16.4	28.4	**18.3**	
	Corrected *P*-value	0.20	0.004	0.45	0.53	**< 0.0001**	
N	Count (% raw)	0 (0%)	0 (0%)	9 (16.4%)	28 (50.9%)	18 (32.7%)	55
	Exp. Count	1.0	7.1	12.2	21.1	13.6	
	Corrected *P*-value	0.28	0.0023	0.26	0.04	0.14	
N-P	Count (% raw)	0 (0%)	0 (0%)	2 (7.1%)	11 (39.3%)	**15 # (53.6%)**	28
	Exp. Count	0.5	3.6	6.2	10.7	**6.9**	
	Corrected *P*-value	0.46	0.004	0.05	0.91	**0.00025**	
A-N-P	Count (% raw)	0 (0%)	0 (0%)	0 (0%)	5 (29.4%)	**12 # (70.6%)**	17
	Exp. Count	0.3	2.2	3.8	6.5	**4.2**	
	Corrected *P*-value	0.2	0.004	0.05	0.53	**< 0.0001**	

The results of a contingency-table test are presented. **A:** VP shape analysis. **B:** VP distribution analysis. Percentages of the raw marginal total (% raw) are in parentheses. Exp. Count: expected count; VP (−): non-ruptured group; Nucleus pulposus: N; anterior annulus fibrosus: A; and posterior annulus fibrosus: P. $^{*}P < 0.0025$, $^{\#}P < 0.002$ (by Bonferroni correction). The cells with counts above or below the expected count with statistical significance are shown in bold

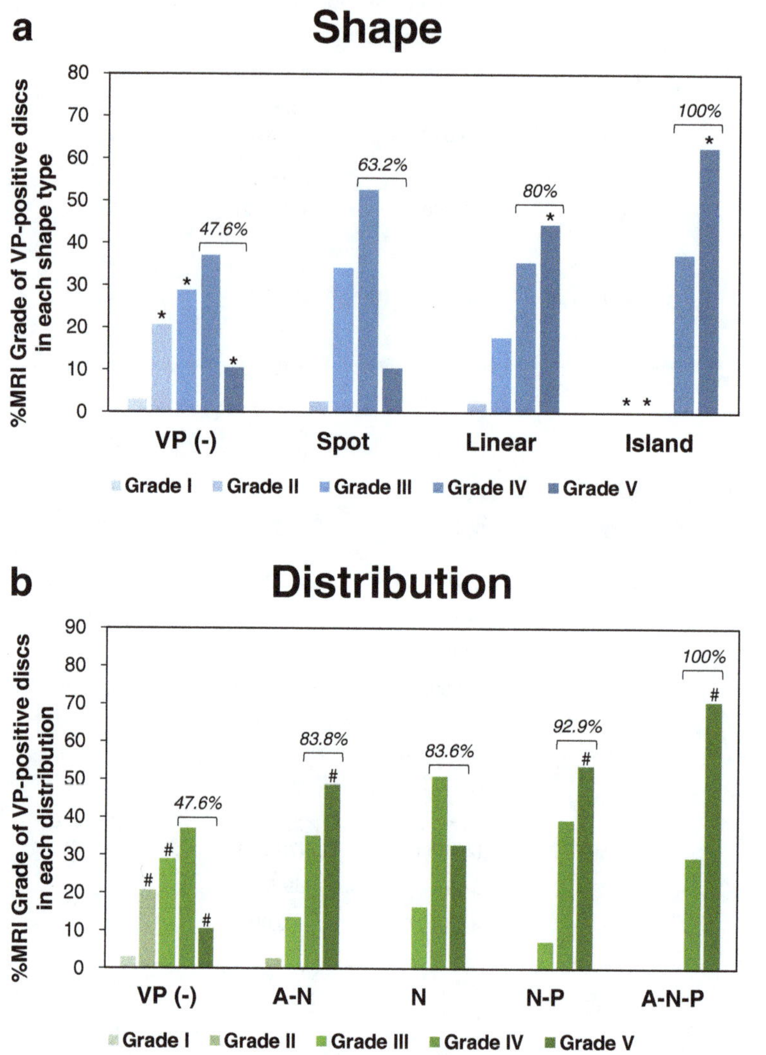

Fig. 8 Percentage of MRI grade of disc degeneration in vacuum phenomenon shape type and distribution analyses. The percentage of MRI grade (Pfirrmann's classification [10]) of disc degeneration in vacuum phenomenon (VP) shape type (**a**) and distribution (**b**) analyses. $^{*}P < 0.0025$, $^{\#}P < 0.002$ (by Bonferroni correction). The percentage of advanced degenerative stage discs (Pfirrmann grades IV and V) of each group is indicated by a bracket

Island type discs had a significantly lower proportion of discs with MRI grade 2 (0%) and grade 3 (0%), but significantly higher with MRI grade 5 (62.6%) ($P < 0.0001$, respectively) (Table 2A, Fig. 8a).

The distribution of intradiscal VPs was also significantly associated with MRI grade (Fisher's exact test, $P < 0.0001$) (Table 2B). The post-hoc test revealed that the discs with A-N, N-P and A-N-P distribution had the highest and significantly higher proportion of discs with MRI grade 5 (A-N: 48.6%, $P < 0.0001$; N-P: 53.6%, $P < 0.002$; A-N-P: 70.6%, $P < 0.0001$) than those with other MRI grades, respectively (Table 2B, Fig. 8b). Discs with N distribution were most frequently classified as MRI grade 4 (50.9%); however those discs showed no significant effect on the proportion of discs with different MRI grades (Table 2B, Fig. 8b).

Of all the discs analyzed by MRI (441 discs), 63.0% (278 discs) were in the advanced degenerative stage (Pfirrmann grades IV and V). In the VP shape type analysis, the percentage of discs with advanced stage of degeneration was highest in the island type (100%) followed by linear (80%) and spot (63.2%) types (Fig. 8a). In the VP distribution analysis, the discs with advanced stage of degeneration were most frequently distributed in the A-N-P (100%) area, followed by N-P (92.9%), A-N (83.8%) and N (83.6%) areas (Fig. 8b).

Association of VP type and distribution with lumbar spinal stenosis

The Fisher's exact test showed a significant association between VP shape type and MRI grade of canal stenosis ($P < 0.0001$) (Table 3A). VP (–) discs had a significantly

Table 3 Association between intradiscal vacuum phenomena (VPs) and lumbar spinal stenosis

A: Shape		MRI classification of lumbar spinal stenosis				Total
		A	B	C	D	
VP (−)	Count (% raw)	**171 *** **(81.8%)**	9 (4.3%)	22 (10.5%)	**7 *** **(3.3%)**	209
	Exp. Count	**147.5**	13.1	31.3	**17.1**	
	Corrected *P*-value	**< 0.0001**	0.07	0.006	**< 0.0001**	
Spot	Count (% raw)	21 (61.8%)	3 (8.8%)	7 (20.6%)	3 (8.8%)	34
	Exp. Count	24.0	2.1	5.1	2.8	
	Corrected *P*-value	0.23	0.51	0.34	0.89	
Linear	Count (% raw)	21 (55.3%)	4 (10.5%)	5 (13.2%)	**8 *** **(21.1%)**	38
	Exp. Count	26.8	2.4	5.7	**3.1**	
	Corrected *P*-value	0.03	0.35	0.74	**0.0022**	
Island	Count (% raw)	**46 *** **(53.5%)**	7 (8.1%)	21 (24.4%)	12 (14.0%)	86
	Exp. Count	**60.7**	5.4	12.9	7.0	
	Corrected *P*-value	**0.0001**	0.41	0.005	0.025	
B: Distribution		MRI classification of lumbar spinal stenosis				Total
		A	B	C	D	
VP (−)	Count (% raw)	**171 #** **(81.8%)**	9 (4.3%)	22 (10.5%)	**7 #** **(3.3%)**	209
	Exp. Count	**147.5**	13.1	31.3	**17.1**	
	Corrected *P*-value	**< 0.0001**	0.07	0.006	**< 0.0001**	
A-N	Count (% raw)	41 (63.1%)	5 (7.7%)	9 (13.8%)	10 (15.4%)	65
	Exp. Count	45.9	4.1	9.7	5.3	
	Corrected *P*-value	0.14	0.60	0.77	0.02	
N	Count (% raw)	26 (53.1%)	7 (14.3%)	9 (18.4%)	7 (14.3%)	49
	Exp. Count	34.6	3.1	7.3	4.0	
	Corrected *P*-value	0.0039	0.013	0.48	0.09	
N-P	Count (% raw)	**12 #** **(44.4%)**	2 (7.4%)	7 (25.9%)	6 (22.2%)	27
	Exp. Count	**19.1**	1.7	4.0	2.2	
	Corrected *P*-value	**0.0019**	0.07	0.005	0.0001	
A-N-P	Count (% raw)	9 (52.9%)	0 (0%)	**8 #** **(47.1%)**	0 (0%)	17
	Exp. Count	12.0	1.1	**2.5**	1.4	
	Corrected *P*-value	0.1	0.27	**0.00015**	0.21	

The results of a contingency-table test are presented. **A:** VP shape analysis. **B:** VP distribution analysis. Percentages of the raw marginal total (% raw) are in parentheses. Exp. Count: expected count; VP (−): non-ruptured group; Nucleus pulposus: N; anterior annulus fibrosus: A; and posterior annulus fibrosus: P. $^{*}P < 0.0025$, $^{\#}P < 0.002$ (by Bonferroni correction). The cells with counts above or below the expected count with statistical significance are shown in bold higher proportion of grade A stenosis (percentages of the raw marginal total: 81.8%), and significantly lower proportion of grade D stenosis (3.3%) at corresponding disc levels (Table 3A, Fig. 9a). Discs with a linear type VP had a significantly higher proportion of grade D stenosis (21.1%), and discs with an island type VP had a significantly lower proportion of grade A stenosis (53.5%) at corresponding disc levels (Table 3A, Fig. 9a).

The distribution of VPs also had a significant association with the MRI grade of canal stenosis (Fisher's exact test, $P < 0.0001$) (Table 3B). The discs with N-P distributions had a significantly lower proportion of MRI grade A canal stenosis (44.4%), and the discs with A-N-P distributions had a significantly higher proportion with MRI grade C canal stenosis (47.1%) at the corresponding disc levels (Table 3B, Fig. 9b). On the other hand, the discs with A-N and N distributions had no significant association with MRI grade of canal stenosis at corresponding disc levels (Table 3B, Fig. 9b).

The percentage of VP-positive discs with severe stenosis (grades C and D) at the corresponding disc level in all analyzed discs was 23.1%. The percentage of discs with severe stenosis in each shape type was highest in the island type (38.4%) followed by linear (34.2%) and spot (29.4%) types (Fig. 9a). The VP in discs with severe stenosis at the corresponding disc level was most frequently distributed to the N-P (48.1%) area, followed by A-N-P (47.1%), N (32.7%) and A-N (29.2%) areas (Fig. 9b).

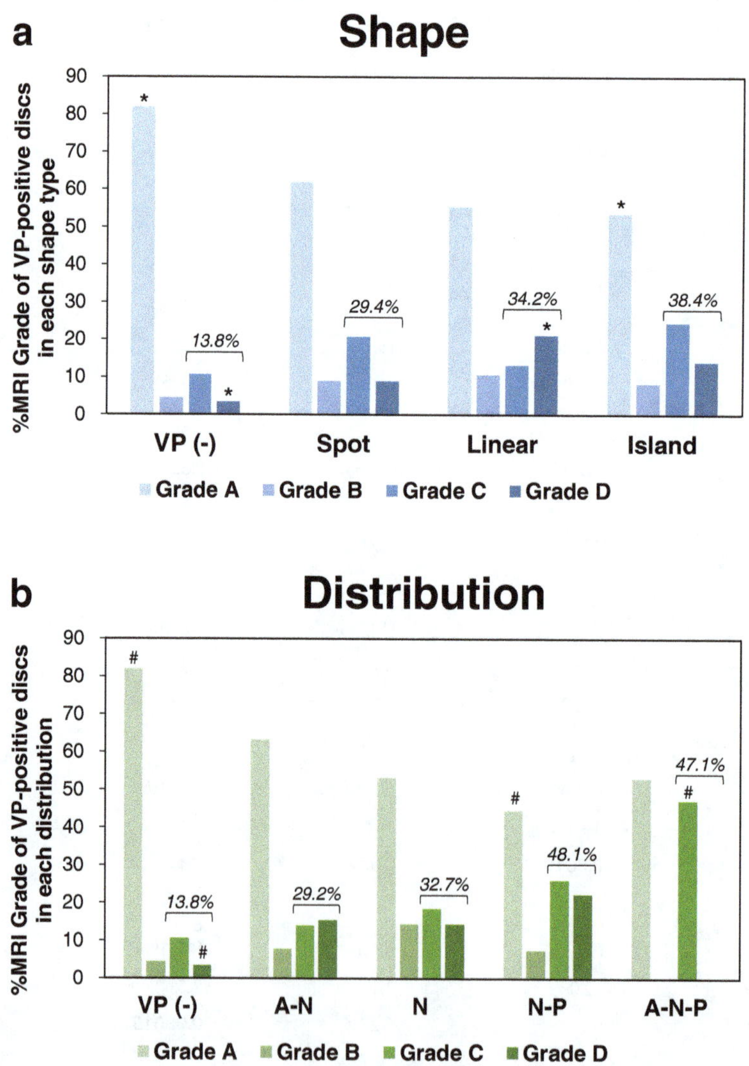

Fig. 9 Percentage of MRI grade of lumbar spinal stenosis in vacuum phenomenon shape type and distribution analyses. The percentage of MRI grade (Schizas's classification [11]) of lumbar spinal stenosis in vacuum phenomenon (VP) shape type (**a**) and distribution (**b**) analyses. $^{*}P < 0.0025$, $^{\#}P < 0.002$ (by Bonferroni correction). The percentage of VP-positive discs with severe stenosis (grades C and D) of each group is indicated by a bracket

Discussion

To evaluate the morphology of IVD ruptures in the lumbar spine, we performed a cross-sectional retrospective CT study to assess intradiscal VPs of consecutive patients who underwent spinal surgery. The results showed that VPs were found in 38.3% of the 587 discs analyzed, most prominently at the L4/5 level and highest in the seventy years-old population. The type and distribution of intradiscal VPs were significantly associated with severity of MRI grade of disc degeneration and disc height narrowing. The presence of VPs within the disc also had a significant effect on the lumbar spinal stenosis of corresponding IVDs.

Intradiscal VPs are most commonly seen in patients with disc degeneration, especially in the NP, where dehydration of the disc and enlarging clefts lead to the accumulation of gas [4, 16, 17]. VPs in IVDs were first described by Magnusson in 1937 [18] and are a common finding that can be observed in 1–3% of healthy adults on spinal radiographs [19–21], but can reach a prevalence of 20% in elderly patients [4, 22, 23]. Ford and colleagues reported that intradiscal VPs contain 90–92% nitrogen combined with oxygen, carbon dioxide and traces of other gases [24]. Because nitrogen gas is hard to metabolize within tissues in vivo, it can accumulate within the tissue organization.

With the progression of disc degeneration, the crevices extend peripherally, affecting first the inner fibers and later the outer fibers of the AF. At the same time, gas collections may become more prominent, extending from the interior to the exterior of the affected disc [4]. Therefore, the position and form of intradiscal VPs are considered to indicate the distribution and extent of ruptures within IVD tissues. Gas accumulation in the spinal canal or in disc herniation is reported to be associated with neurologic symptoms, although the clinical significance of intradiscal VPs has been controversial.

In this study, we first classified the morphology of intradiscal VPs, using CT images to evaluate the degree of disc rupture by shape (sagittal-plane) and distribution (axial–plane). Both intra- and inter-observer agreements of this two-part classification system are "substantial" by kappa statistics, and showed higher % agreements, suggesting that this classification system would be sufficient to distinguish between the different VP shapes and distributions.

The results of our study showed evidence that the presence of intradiscal VPs has a significant association with the degree of disc degeneration graded by MRI. In addition, the extent of disc ruptures evaluated by the types and distribution of intradiscal VPs also significantly affects the MRI grading of disc degeneration. Discs with linear and island shape VPs had a significantly higher proportion of MRI grade V discs, which indicated the collapse of discs with significant structural changes [10]. In the distribution analysis, except for the N distribution, all the discs with the VPs that extend from NP into anterior and/or posterior AF (A-N, N-P, A-N-P) had a significantly higher proportion of MRI grade V discs. These results suggested that intradiscal VPs extending from the N into AF area are associated with significant structural changes of IVDs.

The results of lumbar radiography also showed that there is a significant trend for disc height to decrease in accordance with the extent of disc rupture evaluated by the type of intradiscal VPs. Taking the distribution of VPs into account, disc height was significantly lower in discs that contained VPs in the area of the anterior AF. In the clinical setting, disc height narrowing is the commonly used radiographic finding indicating disc degeneration; however, according to Pfirrmann's classification [10], this change is recognized as a finding related to an advanced stage (more than grade IV) of disc degeneration with significant structural changes [9].

We also evaluated the association between intradiscal VPs and lumbar spinal stenosis. In this study, we also showed evidence that lumbar spinal stenosis was significantly associated with the presence of VPs at the corresponding IVD. Severe stenosis (grades C and D by MRI classification [11]) was most frequently identified in IVDs containing the island type VP, especially those including the posterior AF. Ligamentum flavum thickness, disc protrusion, and spondylolisthesis are major pathogeneses of lumbar spinal stenosis. Intradiscal VPs have been recognized as one of the signs of segmental instability [5, 25–27]. Therefore, the results of our study further support the possibility that the presence of intradiscal VPs would lead to segmental instability, which is responsible for the pathogenesis of lumbar spinal stenosis.

Clinical relevance: Recently, the effects of intradiscal VPs on the clinical (surgical) outcome of lumbar fusion surgery have been reported [5, 27, 28]. Liao et al. [5] reported that intradiscal VPs should be regarded as a sign of intervertebral instability. Hence, lumbar interbody fusion (LIF) surgery with intervertebral cage, but not posterolateral fusion only, should be performed for patients with degenerative lumbar spondylolisthesis containing intradiscal VPs. LIF surgery including lateral and posterior approaches with cages has been reported to be effective for restoration of disc height, lumbar lordosis and also for improving the bone fusion rate in lumbar spondylolisthesis patients with intradiscal VPs [5, 27, 28]. The results of this study also revealed that intradiscal VPs, especially those extending from the N into the AF region, were associated with structural destruction of IVD tissues, including disc height narrowing. Therefore, our morphological classification of

VPs might be advantageous in determining the surgical procedure used for treating degenerative lumbar diseases.

Limitations of this study were that most of the subjects were patients who had taken pre-operative CT images for elective spinal surgeries, and that an age-matched general population was not used as a control in this study. Therefore, the percentage of intradiscal VPs in our subjects would be much higher than that within an age-matched general population. This is the first study analyzing the shape type and distribution of intradiscal VPs using CT images to indicate that VPs were frequently distributed in the NP and anterior AF. However, it should be kept in mind that the anterior distribution of VPs would be more enhanced in a CT study using a supine position compared with the exact distribution of disc ruptures evaluated in cadaveric studies [1, 2]. Another limitation was that the morphological classification of intradiscal VPs was performed using sagittal and axial CT images analyzed separately with different classifications. A three-dimensional analysis of VPs may be needed for more precise evaluations of area, distribution and volume of intradiscal VPs.

Importantly, when the intradiscal VPs were evaluated by MRI T2-wighted images, approximately 10% of VP-positive discs showed high signal intensity, demonstrating MR imaging findings similar to those of infectious spondylodiscitis [7, 29, 30]. The presence of intradiscal VPs evaluated by CT images would aid in the exclusion diagnosis of infectious spondylodiscitis [31].

Conclusions

This study describes the assessment of IVD ruptures by the presence of intradiscal VPs using CT-imaging. This two-part classification can comprehensively present the shape and axial distribution of VPs within IVDs, with intra- and inter-observer reliability sufficient to classify different rupture shapes and distributions. This study also showed evidence that the presence of intradiscal VPs is associated with MRI-grading of disc degeneration and radiographic disc height narrowing. Therefore, the presence of intradiscal VPs represents one of the signs of disc ruptures with a significant structural change. This systematic analysis of intradiscal VPs also revealed that the shape and distribution of VPs were significantly associated with the MRI-grading of lumbar canal stenosis at the corresponding disc level. To further evaluate the clinical relevance of intradiscal VPs, it would be important in future studies to examine the association between segmental intervertebral instability and/or clinical symptoms using this CT-based analytical system.

Abbreviations

AF: annulus fibrosus; CT: computed tomography; DHI: disc height index; IVD: intervertebral disc; LSS: lumbar spinal stenosis; MDCT: multi-detector computed tomography; MRI: magnetic resonance imaging; NP: nucleus pulposus; VP: vacuum phenomenon

Authors' contributions

KMu performed data acquisition and statistical analysis and drafted the manuscript. KA helped to perform data acquisition and statistical analyses and drafted the manuscript, conceived of this study, and made substantial contributions to the study design. NT and KMa performed statistical analysis and revised the manuscript. KC performed data acquisition, and revised the manuscript. AS contributed to the study design and coordination, and revised the manuscript. All authors read and approved the final manuscript.

Competing interests

The authors declare that they have no competing interests.

Author details

[1]Department of Orthopaedic Surgery, Mie University Graduate School of Medicine, 2-174 Edobashi, Tsu City, Mie 514-8507, Japan. [2]Department of Orthopaedic Surgery, University of California, San Diego, 9500 Gilman Dr, La Jolla, CA 92093-0863, USA.

References

1. Osti OL, Vernon-Roberts B, Moore R, Fraser RD. Annular tears and disc degeneration in the lumbar spine. A post-mortem study of 135 discs. J Bone Joint Surg Br. 1992;74(5):678–82.
2. Vernon-Roberts B, Moore RJ, Fraser RD. The natural history of age-related disc degeneration: the pathology and sequelae of tears. Spine (Phila Pa 1976). 2007;32(25):2797–804. https://doi.org/10.1097/BRS.0b013e31815b64d2.
3. Videman T, Nurminen M. The occurrence of anular tears and their relation to lifetime back pain history: a cadaveric study using barium sulfate discography. Spine (Phila Pa 1976). 2004;29(23):2668–76.
4. Resnick D, Niwayama G, Guerra J Jr, Vint V, Usselman J. Spinal vacuum phenomena: anatomical study and review. Radiology. 1981;139(2):341–8. https://doi.org/10.1148/radiology.139.2.7220878.
5. Liao JC, Lu ML, Niu CC, Chen WJ, Chen LH. Surgical outcomes of degenerative lumbar spondylolisthesis with anterior vacuum disc: can the intervertebral cage overcome intradiscal vacuum phenomenon and enhance posterolateral fusion? J Orthop Sci. 2014;19(6):851–9. https://doi.org/10.1007/s00776-014-0618-z.
6. Kasai Y, Takegami K, Uchida A. Change of barometric pressure influences low back pain in patients with vacuum phenomenon within lumbar intervertebral disc. J Spinal Disord Tech. 2002;15(4):290–3.
7. Kumar Y, Gupta N, Chhabra A, Fukuda T, Soni N, Hayashi D. Magnetic resonance imaging of bacterial and tuberculous spondylodiscitis with associated complications and non-infectious spinal pathology mimicking infections: a pictorial review. BMC Musculoskelet Disord. 2017;18(1):244. https://doi.org/10.1186/s12891-017-1608-z.
8. Grenier N, Grossman RI, Schiebler ML, Yeager BA, Goldberg HI, Kressel HY. Degenerative lumbar disk disease: pitfalls and usefulness of MR imaging in detection of vacuum phenomenon. Radiology. 1987;164(3):861–5. https://doi.org/10.1148/radiology. 164.3.3615888.
9. Akeda K, Yamada T, Inoue N, Nishimura A, Sudo A. Risk factors for lumbar intervertebral disc height narrowing: a population-based longitudinal study in the elderly. BMC Musculoskelet Disord. 2015;16:344. https://doi.org/10.1186/s12891-015-0798-5.
10. Pfirrmann CW, Metzdorf A, Zanetti M, Hodler J, Boos N. Magnetic resonance classification of lumbar intervertebral disc degeneration. Spine (Phila Pa 1976). 2001;26(17):1873–8.
11. Schizas C, Theumann N, Burn A, Tansey R, Wardlaw D, Smith FW, et al. Qualitative grading of severity of lumbar spinal stenosis based on the morphology of the dural sac on magnetic resonance images. Spine (Phila Pa 1976). 2010;35(21):1919–24. https://doi.org/10.1097/BRS.0b013e3181d359bd.
12. Lombard M, Snyder-Duch J, Bracken CC. Content analysis in mass communication research: an assessment and reporting of intercoder reliability. Hum Commun Res. 2002;28:587–604.

13. Landis JR, Koch GG. The measurement of observer agreement for categorical data. Biometrics. 1977;33(1):159–74.
14. Beasley TM, Schumacker RE. Multiple regression approach to analyzing contingency tables: post hoc and planned comparison procedures. J Exp Educ. 1995;64(1):79–93.
15. GARCIA-PEREZ MA, NUNEZ-ANTON V. Cellwise residual analysis in two-way contingency tables. Educ Psychol Meas. 2003;63(5):825–39.
16. Fries JW, Abodeely DA, Vijungco JG, Yeager VL, Gaffey WR. Computed tomography of herniated and extruded nucleus pulposus. J Comput Assist Tomogr. 1982;6(5):874–87.
17. Knutsson F. The vacuum phenomenon in the intervertebral discs. Acta Radiologica [Old Series]. 1942;23(2):173–9. https://doi.org/10.3109/00016924209134912.
18. Magnusson W. Uber Die Bedingungen Des Hervortretens Der Wirklichen Gelenkspalte Auf Dem Rontgenbilde. Acta Radiol. 1937;18(5):733–41. https://doi.org/10.3109/00016923709132378.
19. Raines JR. Intervertebral disc fissures (vacuum intervertebral disc). Am J Roentgenol Radium Therapy, Nucl Med. 1953;70(6):964–6.
20. Marr JT. Gas in intervertebral discs. Am J Roentgenol Radium Therapy, Nucl Med. 1953;70(5):804–9.
21. Ford LT, Goodman FG. X-ray studies of the lumbosacral spine. South Med J. 1966;59(10):1123–8.
22. Pierpaolo L, Luciano M, Fabrizio P, Paolo M. Gas-containing lumbar disc herniation. A case report and review of the literature. Spine (Phila Pa 1976). 1993;18(16):2533–6.
23. Gershon-Cohen J, Schraer H, Sklaroff DM, Blumberg N. Dissolution of the intervertebral disk in the aged normal; the phantom nucleus pulposus. Radiology. 1954;62(3):383–7. https://doi.org/10.1148/62.3.383.
24. Ford LT, Gilula LA, Murphy WA, Gado M. Analysis of gas in vacuum lumbar disc. AJR Am J Roentgenol. 1977;128(6):1056–7. https://doi.org/10.2214/ajr.128.6.1056.
25. Iguchi T, Ozaki T, Chin T, Tsumura N, Kanemura A, Kasahara K, et al. Intimate relationship between instability and degenerative signs at L4/5 segment examined by flexion-extension radiography. Eur Spine J. 2011;20(8):1349–54. https://doi.org/10.1007/s00586-011-1793-7.
26. Hasegawa K, Shimoda H, Kitahara K, Sasaki K, Homma T. What are the reliable radiological indicators of lumbar segmental instability? J Bone Joint Surg Br. 2011;93(5):650–7. https://doi.org/10.1302/0301-620x.93b5.25520.
27. Lin TY, Liao JC, Tsai TT, Lu ML, Niu CC, Chen WJ, et al. The effects of anterior vacuum disc on surgical outcomes of degenerative versus spondylolytic spondylolisthesis: at a minimum two-year follow-up. BMC Musculoskelet Disord. 2014;15:329. https://doi.org/10.1186/1471-2474-15-329.
28. Yen CP, Beckman JM, Vivas AC, Bach K, Uribe JS. Effects of intradiscal vacuum phenomenon on surgical outcome of lateral interbody fusion for degenerative lumbar disease. J Neurosurg Spine. 2017;26(4):419–25. https://doi.org/10.3171/2016.8.SPINE16421.
29. Schweitzer ME. el-Noueam KI. Vacuum disc: frequency of high signal intensity on T2-weighted MR images. Skelet Radiol. 1998;27(2):83–6.
30. Wang HJ, Chen BB, Yu CW, Hsu CY, Shih TT. Alteration of disc vacuum contents during prolonged supine positioning: evaluation with MR image. Spine (Phila Pa 1976). 2007;32(23):2610–5. https://doi.org/10.1097/BRS.0b013e318158cb49.
31. Hong SH, Choi JY, Lee JW, Kim NR, Choi JA, Kang HS. MR imaging assessment of the spine: infection or an imitation? Radiographics. 2009;29(2):599–612. https://doi.org/10.1148/rg.292085137.

Short- and long-term reproducibility of diffusion-weighted magnetic resonance imaging of lower extremity musculature in asymptomatic individuals and a comparison to individuals with spinal cord injury

Jacob G. McPherson[1,2], Andrew C. Smith[2,3], Daniel A. Duben[1], Katie L. McMahon[4,5], Marie Wasielewski[2], Todd B. Parrish[6] and James M. Elliott[2,7,8*]

Abstract

Background: Diffusion-weighted magnetic resonance imaging (DW-MRI) of skeletal muscle has the potential to be a sensitive diagnostic and/or prognostic tool in complex, enigmatic neuromusculoskeletal conditions such as spinal cord injury and whiplash associated disorder. However, the reliability and reproducibility of clinically accessible DW-MRI parameters in skeletal muscle remains incompletely characterized – even in individuals without neuromusculoskeletal injury – and these parameters have yet to be characterized for many clinical populations. Here, we provide normative measures of the apparent diffusion coefficient (ADC) in healthy muscles of the lower limb; assess the rater-based reliability and short- and long-term reproducibility of the ADC in the same muscles; and quantify ADC of these muscles in individuals with motor incomplete spinal cord injury.

Methods: Twenty individuals without neuromusculoskeletal injury and 14 individuals with motor incomplete spinal cord injury (SCI) participated in this investigation. We acquired bilateral diffusion-weighted MRI of the lower limb musculature in all participants at 3 T using a multi-shot echo-planar imaging sequence with b-values of 0, 100, 300 and 500 s/mm^2 and diffusion-probing gradients applied in 3 orthogonal directions. Outcome measures included: (1) average ADC in the lateral and medial gastrocnemius, tibialis anterior, and soleus of individuals without neurological or musculoskeletal injury; (2) intra- and inter-rater reliability, as well as short and long-term reproducibility of the ADC; and (3) estimation of average muscle ADC in individuals with SCI.

Results: Intra- and inter-rater reliability of the ADC averaged 0.89 and 0.79, respectively, across muscles. Least significant change, a measure of temporal reproducibility, was 4.50 and 11.98% for short (same day) and long (9-month) inter-scan intervals, respectively. Average ADC was significantly elevated across muscles in individuals with SCI compared to individuals without neurological or musculoskeletal injury (1.655 vs. 1.615 mm^2/s, respectively).

(Continued on next page)

* Correspondence: jim.elliott@sydney.edu.au
[2]Department of Physical Therapy and Human Movement Sciences, Northwestern University Feinberg School of Medicine, Chicago, IL, USA
[7]School of Health and Rehabilitation Sciences, The University of Queensland, Brisbane, Australia
Full list of author information is available at the end of the article

(Continued from previous page)
Conclusions: These findings provide a foundation for future studies that track longitudinal changes in skeletal muscle ADC of the lower extremity and/or investigate the mechanisms underlying ADC changes in cases of known or suspected pathology.

Keywords: Magnetic resonance imaging, Skeletal muscle, Spinal cord injury, Diffusion-weighted imaging

Background

Diffusion-weighted magnetic resonance imaging (DW -MRI) provides a potential diagnostic and prognostic measure for the normal (and abnormal) movement of water through living soft-tissues. Skeletal muscle is an emerging application for DW-MRI [1], where it holds considerable potential in common, yet enigmatic, clinical conditions. For example, significant changes in DW-MRI metrics have been observed in individuals with rotator cuff tears [2], muscular dystrophy [3], myopathies [4, 5], radiculopathy [6, 7], and in animal models of denervation [7, 8]. In cases, diffusion-related changes may also precede findings on other diagnostic tests [7], opening a critical early window where diagnostic and prognostic data could better inform intervention. Additionally, DW-MRI could serve as a marker of muscle response to therapeutic exercise [9, 10]. Despite the increasing number of investigations utilizing DW-MRI in skeletal muscle – and in particular the use of skeletal muscle DW-MRI as a diagnostic or outcome measure – normative data remains sparse. Complicating matters further, the rater-based reliability and temporal reproducibility of DW-MRI-related parameters have also yet to be established for skeletal muscle.

Here, we investigate a clinically relevant DW-MRI parameter, the Apparent Diffusion Coefficient (ADC), in muscles of the lower limb. We estimate the rater-based reliability and the temporal reproducibility of ADC at both short- and long-inter-scan intervals, with the primary goal of providing an additional statistical reference for future investigations incorporating DW-MRI of skeletal muscle. We also quantify the ADC both in a cohort of individuals without neurological or musculoskeletal injury and in a cohort of individuals with motor incomplete spinal cord injury, a potential target for clinical use of DW-MRI. We hypothesize that ADC will be elevated in leg muscles innervated by spinal nerves below the level of lesion, given the previously documented elevations in ADC following denervation and/or trauma [2, 7].

Methods

Study participants

In total, 20 individuals without known neurological or musculoskeletal injury ("control cohort"; 11 males, 9 females; age: 31 ± 10 yrs) and 14 individuals with motor incomplete spinal cord injury ("SCI cohort"; 13 males, 1 female; age: 43 ± 12 yrs.; Table 1; see also [11]) participated in this investigation. All individuals provided informed, written consent to participate, and the protocol was approved by the Institutional Review Board of Northwestern University in accordance with the guidelines established by the Declaration of Helsinki for research involving human participants.

Participants with any of the following were excluded from participation: previous diagnosis of cervical or lumbar radiculopathy; history of neurological disorders (e.g. Multiple Sclerosis, previous stroke, myelopathy), inflammatory diseases (e.g. Hepatitis, Systemic Lupus Erythematosus, Rheumatoid Arthritis or Osteoarthritis, Alzheimers, Ankylosing Spondylitis, Chron's Disease, Fibromyalgia) or metabolic disorders (e.g. Diabetes, hyper- and hypo-thyroidism); previous spinal fracture or spinal surgery and/or history of one or more motor vehicle collisions (neither criteria applied to participants in the SCI cohort); and standard/institutional contraindications to MRI, including claustrophobia, metallic implants, pacemaker and pregnancy or thought to be pregnant in the absence of contraception since the last normal menstrual period.

Average ADC per muscle was estimated in all participants (control: $N = 20$; SCI: $N = 14$). For the control cohort, we also quantified the rater-based reliability, short-term reproducibility, and long-term reproducibility of the ADC in subsets of these individuals: intra- and inter-rater reliability were estimated from 6 individuals (3 male, 3 female), short-term reproducibility was estimated in 3 of these 6 (2 male, 1 female), and long-term reproducibility was estimated in a separate subset of 12 individuals (8 males, 4 females). Reliability metrics were not computed for the SCI cohort because it would not have been feasible to decouple ADC changes related to evolution of the post-SCI recovery/impairment sequelae from variability inherent to the DW-MRI technique itself at this early, foundational stage of investigation.

DW-MRI acquisition and analysis

MRI scans were performed on a Siemens 3 T TRIO MRI scanner (Siemens; Erlangen, Germany). A 16-channel body array coil positioned anteriorly over the lower legs. Segments 3 and 4 of the spine matrix coil were also turned on to improve signal posteriorly. The legs were comfortably stabilized (to minimize movement) using sandbags. Axial diffusion-weighted images (DWI) were acquired bilaterally using a multi-shot echo-planar imaging sequence

Table 1 Spinal cord injury cohort demographic and clinical data

Participant	Gender	Age	Time since injury (years)	Level of injury	ASIA Impairment Scale	Primary ambulation
1	M	53	6	C5	C	Wheelchair
2	M	57	8	C3	D	Walk with A.D.
3	F	52	0.5	C6	D	Walk with A.D.
4	M	31	4	C5	D	Walk with A.D.
5	M	28	3	C5	D	Walk
6	M	50	2	C6	D	Walk
7	M	30	4	C6	C	Wheelchair
8	M	27	4	C5	C	Wheelchair
9	M	32	5	C7	D	Walk
10	M	45	3.5	C3	D	Walk with A.D.
11	M	36	1.5	C6	C	Wheelchair
12	M	50	5	C4	D	Wheelchair
13	M	64	4	C5	D	Wheelchair
14	M	52	31	C5	D	Wheelchair

Cx cervical spinal segment number, *A.D.* assistive device

(readout segmentation of long variable echo-trains; RESOLVE [12]) with the following parameters: repetition time: 2500 ms; echo time 1: 67 ms; echo time 2: 113 ms; matrix: 224 × 224; field of view: 320 mm; echo spacing: 0.34 ms; bandwidth: 531 Hz/Px; number of averages: 1; slice thickness: 5 mm with a gap spacing of 5 mm; total scan time: 4:39 mins. Fat suppression was used to eliminate signal from subcutaneous fat. Diffusion-probing gradients were applied in 3 orthogonal directions (*x, y,* and *z)* at the following levels of diffusion weighting (b-values): 0, 100, 300 and 500 s/mm^2, where b_0 reflects no diffusion weighting (i.e., a T2-weighted image). Isotropic DWI's were calculated automatically at each b-value as part of the image reconstruction (Siemens VB17A software).

Ten equidistant image slices were acquired between the proximal tibial epiphysis and the distal tibial epiphysis at each b-value. In each slice, regions of interest (ROI) were defined bilaterally using the native axial T1 image as a guide, then transferred to the corresponding isotropic DWI at each successive b value. Blinded, novice raters with ≤1-year experience manually produced all ROI's. ROIs delineated the tibialis anterior (TA), soleus (SOL), and lateral and medial gastrocnemius (LG, MG, respectively). ROI were identified using Analyze 11.0 (Biomedical Imaging Resource, Mayo Clinic, Rochester, MN) and OsiriX 7.5.1 (Pixmeo SARL, Bernex, Switzerland), with the perimeter of each ROI defined as the fascial plane of each muscle at a given proximal-distal location (Fig. 1a).

For a given ROI and b-value, we extracted the mean pixel intensity per DWI and averaged across slices to arrive at the grand mean throughout the muscle's proximal-distal extent. This resulted in 4 discrete estimates of signal intensity per muscle (i.e., one for each b-value), as seen in Fig. 1a-d. From these values, we computed the apparent diffusion coefficient (ADC) for each muscle, using regression analysis to fit pixel intensity and b-value to the standard mono-exponential diffusion equation: $SI_b = SI_0 \times e^{(-b^*ADC)}$ (Fig. 1e). In this equation, SI_b is signal intensity at a particular non-zero b-value and SI_0 is signal intensity at b = 0 s/mm^2. Figure 1f shows a pixel-wise ADC map for a single representative participant without known neurological or musculoskeletal injury; Fig. 1g, h depict ADC maps for the right and left legs of a participant with spinal cord injury. All statistical calculations described below are based upon whole muscle ADC estimates.

To estimate short-term reproducibility, we acquired two DW-MRI scans approximately 30 min apart. Between scans, participants fully exited the MRI scanner environment and waited in a temperature-controlled room (72.6 ° F); activity level and fluid intake were kept to a minimum during this interval. To estimate long-term reproducibility, we acquired two DW-MRI scans approximately 9 months apart. We did not control for activity level, hydration, or time of day between long-term reliability scans.

Statistical analyses

We used both relative and absolute estimates of measurement error to quantify the reliability and reproducibility of skeletal muscle ADC. Relative estimates of measurement error were based on intra-class correlation coefficients ($ICC_{2,1}$; two-way random, absolute agreement), and were used to compute intra- and inter-rater reliability of single scans, as well as short- and long-term ADC reproducibility. For inter-rater reliability, 4 raters independently defined each ROI. Two of these raters also performed duplicate ratings on the same images,

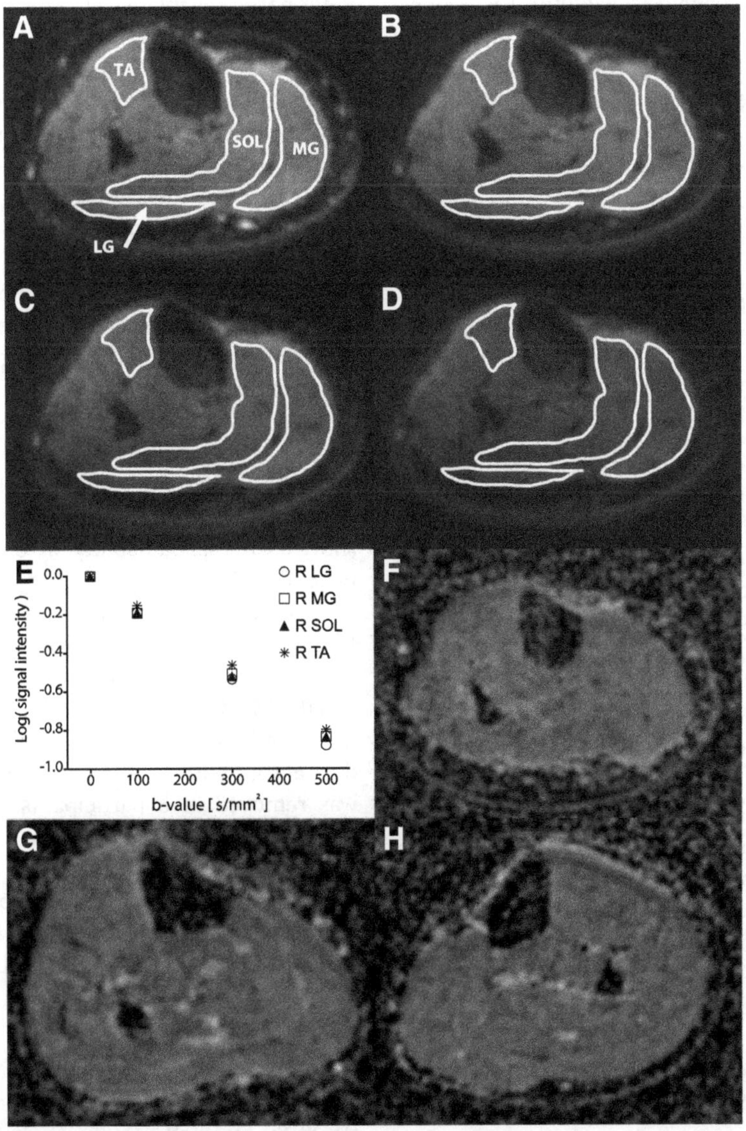

Fig. 1 Representative DW-MRI images. All images acquired at the same proximal-distal level, approximately halfway between the proximal and distal tibial epiphyses, in the right leg of a single, representative participant. **a-d** Diffusion-weighted images acquired at progressively increasing diffusion-probing gradient strength: (**a**) b = 0 s/mm^2, (**b**) b = 100 s/mm^2, (**c**) b = 300 s/mm^2, and (**d**) b = 500 s/mm^2. **e** logarithm of signal intensity is plotted as a function of diffusion-probing gradient strength in a single participant. **f** ADC map for the same participant at (**a-e**). **g**, **h** ADC maps for the right and left legs of a representative participant with spinal cord injury. Abbreviations: TA, Tibialis Anterior; SOL, Soleus; LG, Lateral Gastrocnemius; MG, Medial Gastrocnemius

and these data were used to compute intra-rater reliability. Two additional raters defined all ROI used to compute estimates of short- and long-term reproducibility.

Absolute measures of reliability and reproducibility, also known as precision statistics, included root-mean-square standard deviation (RMS-SD), root-mean-square coefficient of variation (RMS-CV), and least significant change (LSC), expressed at the 95% confidence level. For reference, LSC is based upon the Repeatability Coefficient originally defined by Bland and Altman [13]. The formula for RMS-SD is as follows,

$$RMS\text{-}SD\left(\times 10e^{-3}\ \frac{mm^2}{s}\right) = \sqrt{\frac{\Sigma_{i=1}^{N}\left(\Sigma_{r=1}^{R}\frac{\left(\widehat{ADC}_r - \overline{ADC}\right)^2}{R}\right)}{N}}$$

where r is an individual rating of a given image (for intra-rater reliability) or a single rater (for inter-rater reliability), R is the total number of individual ratings of a given image (for intra-rater reliability) or the total number of raters (for inter-rater reliability), i is a single image of a given muscle, and N is the total number of images rated across all study participants in a given comparison (i.e., number of images i multiplied by the number of participants). The formulae for RMS-CV and LSC follow from RMS-SD, and are:

$$RMS\text{-}CV\ (\%) = \left(\frac{RMS\text{-}SD}{grand\ mean\ (ADC)}\right) \times 100$$

$$LSC\ (\%) = (RMS\text{-}CV) \times 2.77$$

Absolute measures of error were computed for rater-based reliability as well as short- and long-term reproducibility.

We used a linear mixed model to assess potential differences in ADC between individuals without neuromuscular injury and individuals with SCI. The model tested the main fixed effects of cohort (i.e., control vs. SCI) and muscle on average ADC, as well as the cohort-by-muscle interaction and the effect of ambulation type (i.e., walking vs. wheelchair) within the SCI cohort. Participant was included in the model as a correlated random effect. Nominal sample size was determined a priori to be 13 individuals per cohort. Sample size estimates were based on the following model parameters: a small standardized effect size (0.2), α error probability of 0.05, power (1-β error probability) of 0.85, 2 groups (control and SCI), 4 repeated measures (i.e., 4 muscles), and a moderate correlation among repeated measures (0.7). All statistical comparisons were considered significant at the $\alpha = 0.05$ level. All statistical analyses were performed with IBM SPSS Statistics software (Version 19; SPSS Inc., Armonk, NY, USA).

Results

ADC by muscle

Table 2 summarizes the average ADC per muscle across the control and SCI cohorts. For the SCI cohort, we also computed the average ADC per muscle when the legs were grouped by residual strength rather than left/right.

Rater-based reliability

Rater-based reliability statistics of the first time-point can be seen in Table 3. Data are presented as the mean of left and right legs, and excluded images are the same as those described above. ICC-based estimates are presented per muscle, and absolute measures of error are presented as averages across muscles. The LG and SOL were the most inconsistently defined muscles. For LG, errors appeared to stem from an inability to reliably distinguish the border between the LG and MG on the DW-MRI image; for SOL, errors appeared to stem from an inability to reliability distinguish the interior perimeter of the SOL from deeper muscles such as the flexor digitorum longus, flexor hallucis longus, and the tibialis posterior.

Short- and long-term reproducibility

Given the high rater-based reliability, we estimated short-term reproducibility in only one leg per participant. For these analyses, no data required removal due to artifacts. Short-term reproducibility, assessed by $ICC_{2,1}$, was 0.94. Short-term RMS-SD averaged 0.03×10^{-3} mm^2/s across muscles and participants, with a mean RMS-CV of 1.63% and an LSC of 4.50%. For estimates of long-term reproducibility, we used all available data across both legs of the 11 participants (the left LG was removed in 8 participants due to artifacts, as was the left SOL in 1 participant and the MG bilaterally in 2 participants). With a 9-month inter-scan interval, we found an ICC-based reproducibility of 0.34. RMS-SD averaged 0.07×10^{-3} mm^2/s over this interval, with a mean RMS-CV of 4.33% and an LSC of 11.98%.

ADC in chronic SCI

We found a significant main effect of participant cohort on average ADC per muscle ($F = 5.94$; $P = 0.016$), reflective of an elevated average ADC across muscles in individuals with SCI compared to individuals without neuromuscular injury (Table 2). We also found a significant effect of ambulation type on average ADC within the SCI cohort, driven by a higher average ADC across muscles in community walkers than wheelchair users ($F = 19.06$; $P < 0.001$; Fig. 2). Neither the main effect of muscle ($F = 1.77$, $P = 0.095$) nor the muscle-by-cohort interaction ($F = 1.47$, $P = 0.18$) were significant at the α

Table 2 Mean ADC by muscle ($\times 10^{-3}$ mm^2/s)

	Control L	Control R	SCI L	SCI R	SCI more impaired	SCI less impaired
MG	1.62 ± 0.08	1.63 ± 0.13	1.66 ± 0.12	1.65 ± 0.10	1.65 ± 0.11	1.67 ± 0.12
LG	1.62 ± 0.12	1.60 ± 0.17	1.69 ± 0.14	1.70 ± 0.08	1.67 ± 0.08	1.72 ± 0.13
TA	1.61 ± 0.08	1.59 ± 0.10	1.61 ± 0.11	1.58 ± 0.09	1.59 ± 0.09	1.59 ± 0.10
SOL	1.63 ± 0.09	1.63 ± 0.09	1.69 ± 0.12	1.66 ± 0.10	1.66 ± 0.10	1.69 ± 0.12
Average	1.62 ± 0.09	1.61 ± 0.13	1.66 ± 0.04	1.65 ± 0.05	1.64 ± 0.10	1.67 ± 0.12

Data presented as mean ± standard deviation

Table 3 Relative and absolute rater-based reliability

	MG (ICC)	LG (ICC)	TA (ICC)	SOL (ICC)	RMS-SD ($\times 10^{-3}$ mm²/s)	RMS-CV (%)	LSC (%)
Intra-rater (R1)	1.00	0.90	0.91	0.60	0.06	3.53	9.77
Intra-rater (R2)	0.99	0.79	0.97	0.99	0.04	2.58	7.16
Inter-rater	0.81	0.72	0.87	0.76			

Abbreviations ICC intra-class correlation coefficient, *RMS-SD* root-mean-square standard deviation, *RMS-CV* root-mean-square coefficient of variation, *LSC* least significant change

= 0.05 level. Qualitatively, the non-significant main effect of muscle appeared to be driven primarily by low ADC values for the TA muscle in the SCI cohort. We confirmed this observation by conducting a separate one-way repeated measures ANOVA on the SCI cohort alone; a within-subject factor of muscle and an independent variable of average ADC revealed a significant main effect of muscle on average ADC ($F = 6.25$; $P = 0.002$). Post-hoc analyses (after Bonferroni correction) confirmed that the effect of muscle was due to significantly lower average ADC in the TA compared to the MG, LG, and SOL ($P = 0.004$ and $P = 0.0005$ for L and R TA, respectively).

Discussion

The objectives of this investigation were to provide normative ADC values in healthy skeletal muscle at 3 T, to further establish the rater-based reliability and temporal reproducibility of DW-MRI in muscle, and to estimate ADC in a cohort of individuals with motor incomplete spinal cord injury. Although previous reports of mean ADC for healthy skeletal muscles exhibit considerable variability, our estimates are generally consistent with the available data. In the earliest results, obtained at 0.5 T, Morvan et al. reported mean ADC of resting muscle at 1.82×10^{-3} mm²/s [14]. ADC estimates obtained at 1.5 T have generally been lower than our results, ranging from 1.26×10^{-3} mm²/s to 1.51×10^{-3} mm²/s [7, 15, 16], although more recently, values of 1.8×10^{-3} mm²/s have again been reported (albeit at the shoulder) [2]. ADC estimates of leg muscles obtained at 3 T appear to be more closely aligned with our findings, ranging from 1.51–1.85×10^{-3} mm²/s [3–5].

Overall, we found excellent absolute rater-based reliability and short-term reproducibility for ADC in skeletal muscle. Our average rater-based LSC was less than 10% across muscles, and our average LSC for short-term reproducibility was 4.5% for scans acquired on the same day. Both findings are consistent with the available literature [17, 18]. Based upon standard reporting conventions for relative reliability metrics [19], our ICC estimates for rater-based reliability and short-term reproducibility were also excellent. We caution against direct comparisons of our ICC values to other studies however, given that ICC estimates are highly sensitive to sample size and across -participant variability not attributable to the instrument itself. For example, while Heemskerk et al. [18] report much lower ICCs of 0.7 and 0.17 for rater-based reliability and short-term reproducibility, their repeatability coefficients (i.e., LSC) for the same data were closely aligned with our results, at 6 and 12%, respectively.

Experimental and/or physiological factors likely contributed to our lower long-term ICC estimates. For example, our study implicitly assumed that ADC values

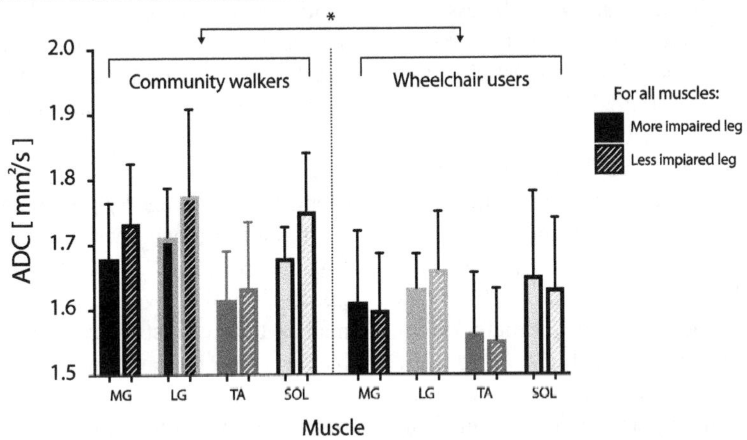

Fig. 2 Average ADC is elevated in community walkers compared to wheelchair users post-SCI. Average ADC is shown per muscle for the SCI cohort, parsed by ambulation type (community walkers vs. wheelchair users) and grouped by overall impairment of each leg. Solid tone columns: more impaired leg; cross-hatched columns: less impaired leg. MG: medial gastrocnemius; LG: lateral gastrocnemius; TA, Tibialis Anterior; SOL, Soleus

in healthy skeletal muscle are stable over time in the absence of trauma, disease, etc. This is a clear oversimplification, as changes in temperature, activity level, and hydration are all capable of influencing the ADC of skeletal muscles [9, 10, 15, 20]. Because we did not explicitly control for these factors, our slightly lower long-term performance is presumably related, at least in part, to true changes in muscle physiology that were unaccounted for by our experimental design. Nevertheless, our estimate of absolute long-term reproducibility is consistent with those reported in the literature, which range from repeatability coefficients of 7–15% with scans acquired 1–2 weeks apart [18, 21].

We found a modest but statistically significant increase in average ADC across muscles in individuals with motor incomplete SCI compared to individuals without neurological or musculoskeletal injury. These increases were confined to the plantarflexor muscles (MG, LG, and SOL), with the TA showing no clear differences between cohorts. Given that elevations of muscle ADC, not reductions, are most commonly associated with pathology, it was somewhat surprising that average ADC was higher in individuals with SCI for whom walking is the primary means of ambulation compared to wheelchair users. It should be reiterated however that neural drive to leg muscles was not altogether absent in our wheelchair user cohort; these participants could perform standing transfers and engage in some therapist assisted walking. Nevertheless, changes in ADC both within the SCI cohort and between the SCI and control cohorts presumably reflect a combination of direct, SCI-induced alterations in neural drive to muscles and indirect effects associated with reduced motor output. Indeed, denervation, atrophy, and changes in physical activity level are all known to influence skeletal muscle ADC [7, 8, 10, 22].

Because our study was not intended to correlate ADC with motor function, the relevance of elevated ADC to impairment – if any – remains unclear. Nevertheless, it is interesting to note that plantarflexor spasms represent one of the most common presentations of spasticity after SCI [23], and we observed preferential elevation of ADC in these muscles. Future work that explores the mechanisms of ADC elevation post-SCI and their potential relevance to motor function, as well as normative estimates of ADC in motor complete SCI, is clearly warranted.

Our study has important limitations. Unlike previous investigations, our ROI definition was performed by raters with minimal imaging experience yet an intimate knowledge of the relevant anatomical structures (Doctor of Physical Therapy students). Although this choice was motivated by a desire to estimate a potential lower bound on rater-based reliability, it also complicates the interpretation of our findings by making it harder to decouple the sources of experimental, physiological, and rater-induced variability. Another limitation is that we used the same MRI scanner for all imaging sessions. As a result, our ADC values, as well as our reliability estimates, should be interpreted only in this context. In purest terms, our results may over-estimate rater-based reliability and/or reproducibility and thus be much different if compared to results from multi-site investigations incorporating different community imaging centers. Finally, we did not control leg temperature in the cohort of individuals with SCI. Thus, it is possible that subtle temperature differences existed between the SCI and control cohorts and/or between the more and less impaired legs of individuals with SCI. Reduced temperature in the extremities, as has been reported in SCI [24], could change our estimates of ADC independently of SCI-induced alterations of muscle physiology [15, 20]. It seems unlikely that changes in temperature could explain the differences in ADC we found between individuals with and without SCI, however. Specifically, leg temperature in individuals with SCI is generally lower than that of individuals without SCI [24], suggesting that ADC should be lower in SCI than controls [20]. However, we found a significantly *elevated* ADC across muscles in the SCI cohort compared to the control cohort, indicating that temperature was not the primary factor driving the observed ADC differences. We also found no significant differences in ADC between legs within the SCI cohort for any muscle (Fig. 2). This finding also suggests that the influence of leg temperature on our results was likely minimal (although it was presumably a source of overall variability in our estimates of ADC). Nevertheless, future work investigating skeletal muscle ADC in individuals with SCI (or other neurological injuries) should systematically monitor and control extremity temperature to avoid undue experimental confounds.

Conclusions

Despite the promise of DW-MRI in skeletal muscle as an additional tool for clinical evaluation and basic scientific investigation, its utility has remained limited at least in part due to a lack of normative data and an incomplete assessment of its precision and reliability. Our results demonstrate that its reproducibility is excellent over short time scales, reinforcing the available literature. We also extend these findings by providing insights into the stability of the approach over the longest inter-scan interval available to date (9 months). Although performance was expectedly lower over this time scale, ADC changes as small as 12% were still discernable. Considering that ADC changes of ~ 24% have been reported in radiculopathy [7], ~ 35% following rotator cuff tear [2], and ~ 20% immediately following vigorous contraction of the same muscles included in this investigation [10], we conclude that controlled experiments using DW-MRI of skeletal muscle are sufficiently reproducible for longitudinal analyses. With evolving scanner and sequence technologies, DW-MRI may prove to be a highly sensitive measure of physiological changes to peripheral muscles after neurological injury and in any number of common, yet enigmatic, neuro-musculoskeletal conditions (e.g., low back pain, whiplash). Such knowledge could help to improve clinical decision making at a time when therapeutic intervention may have its largest effect.

Abbreviations

3T: 3-Tesla; ADC: Apparent diffusion coefficient; DW-MRI: Diffusion-weighted magnetic resonance imaging; ICC: Intra-class correlation coefficient; LG: Lateral gastrocnemius; LSC: Least significant change; MG: Medial gastrocnemius; MRI: Magnetic resonance imaging; RMS-CV: Root-mean-square coefficient of variation; RMS-SD: Root-mean-square standard deviation; ROI: Region of interest; SCI: Spinal cord injury; SOL: Soleus; TA: Tibialis anterior

Acknowledgements

The authors thank Nicholas Fendt, D.P.T., Samuel Gallardo, D.P.T., Brian Greenfield, D.P.T., Bethany Locicero, D.P.T., Joshua Ostrom, D.P.T., and Andrew Wayda, D.P.T. for assistance with participant recruitment, data collection, and definition of regions of interest.

Funding

This work was supported by National Institutes of Health Grant: R01 HD079076-01A1. The funder played no role in the design, collection, analysis, or interpretation of the data associated with this study, nor did it contribute to the writing of the associated manuscript.

Authors' contributions

JGM, ACS, TBP, and JME designed the experiments; JGM, ACS, MW, and TBP collected data; KLM, TBP, and JME determined MRI sequence parameters; JGM, ACS, DAD analyzed data; all authors contributed to the interpretation of data and writing of the manuscript. All authors read and approved the final version of the manuscript.

Consent for publication

Not applicable.

Competing interests

The authors declare that they have no competing interests.

Author details

[1]Department of Biomedical Engineering, Florida International University, Miami, FL, USA. [2]Department of Physical Therapy and Human Movement Sciences, Northwestern University Feinberg School of Medicine, Chicago, IL, USA. [3]School of Physical Therapy, Regis University, Denver, CO, USA. [4]Herston Imaging Research Facility, University of Queensland Centre for Clinical Research, Herston, QLD, Australia. [5]School of Clinical Sciences, Institute of Health and Biosciences Innovation, Queensland University of Technology, Brisbane, Australia. [6]Department of Radiology, Northwestern University, Chicago, IL, USA. [7]School of Health and Rehabilitation Sciences, The University of Queensland, Brisbane, Australia. [8]Faculty of Health Sciences, The University of Sydney, Northern Sydney Local Health District, St Leonards, NSW, Australia.

References

1. Oudeman J, Nederveen AJ, Strijkers GJ, Maas M, Luijten PR, Froeling M. Techniques and applications of skeletal muscle diffusion tensor imaging: a review. J Magn Reson Imaging. 2016;43(4):773–88.
2. Lo HC, Hung ST, Kuo DP, Chen YL, Lee HM. Quantitative diffusion-weighted magnetic resonance imaging for the diagnosis of partial-thickness rotator cuff tears . J Shoulder Elb Surg. 2016;25(9):1433-41.
3. Hooijmans MT, Damon BM, Froeling M, Versluis MJ, Burakiewicz J, Verschuuren JJ, Niks EH, Webb AG, Kan HE. Evaluation of skeletal muscle DTI in patients with duchenne muscular dystrophy. NMR Biomed. 2015;28(11):1589–97.
4. Ai T, Yu K, Gao L, Zhang P, Goerner F, Runge VM, Li X. Diffusion tensor imaging in evaluation of thigh muscles in patients with polymyositis and dermatomyositis. Br J Radiol. 2014;87(1043):20140261.
5. Ran J, Liu Y, Sun D, Morelli J, Zhang P, Wu G, Sheng Y, Xie R, Zhang X, Li X. The diagnostic value of biexponential apparent diffusion coefficients in myopathy. J Neurol. 2016;263(7):1296–302.
6. Cohen-Adad J, Buchbinder B, Oaklander AL. Cervical spinal cord injection of epidural corticosteroids: comprehensive longitudinal study including multiparametric magnetic resonance imaging. Pain. 2012;153(11):2292–9.
7. Holl N, Echaniz-Laguna A, Bierry G, Mohr M, Loeffler JP, Moser T, Dietemann JL, Kremer S. Diffusion-weighted MRI of denervated muscle: a clinical and experimental study. Skelet Radiol. 2008;37(12):1111–7.
8. Goyault G, Bierry G, Holl N, Lhermitte B, Dietemann JL, Beregi JP, Kremer S. Diffusion-weighted MRI, dynamic susceptibility contrast MRI and ultrasound perfusion quantification of denervated muscle in rabbits. Skelet Radiol. 2012;41(1):33–40.
9. Yanagisawa O, Shimao D, Maruyama K, Nielsen M. Evaluation of exercised or cooled skeletal muscle on the basis of diffusion-weighted magnetic resonance imaging. Eur J Appl Physiol. 2009;105(5):723–9.
10. Yanagisawa O, Kurihara T. Intramuscular water movement during and after isometric muscle contraction: evaluation at different exercise intensities. Clin Physiol Funct Imaging. 2016;36(5):368–75.
11. Smith AC, Weber KA, Parrish TB, Hornby TG, Tysseling VM, McPherson JG, Wasielewski M, Elliott JM. Ambulatory function in motor incomplete spinal cord injury: a magnetic resonance imaging study of spinal cord edema and lower extremity muscle morphometry. Spinal Cord. 2017;55(7):672–8.
12. Porter DA, Heidemann RM. High resolution diffusion-weighted imaging using readout-segmented echo-planar imaging, parallel imaging and a two-dimensional navigator-based reacquisition. Magn Reson Med. 2009;62(2):468–75.
13. Bland JM, Altman DG. Statistical methods for assessing agreement between two methods of clinical measurement. Lancet. 1986;1(8476):307–10.
14. Morvan D. In vivo measurement of diffusion and pseudo-diffusion in skeletal muscle at rest and after exercise. Magn Reson Imaging. 1995;13(2):193–9.
15. Yanagisawa O, Fukubayashi T. Diffusion-weighted magnetic resonance imaging reveals the effects of different cooling temperatures on the diffusion of water molecules and perfusion within human skeletal muscle. Clin Radiol. 2010;65(11):874–80.
16. Yanagisawa O, Shimao D, Maruyama K, Nielsen M, Irie T, Niitsu M. Diffusion-weighted magnetic resonance imaging of human skeletal muscles: gender-, age- and muscle-related differences in apparent diffusion coefficient. Magn Reson Imaging. 2009;27(1):69–78.
17. Elliott J, Pedler A, Beattie P, McMahon K. Diffusion-weighted magnetic resonance imaging for the healthy cervical multifidus: a potential method for studying neck muscle physiology following spinal trauma. J Orthop Sports Phys Ther. 2010;40(11):722–8.
18. Heemskerk AM, Sinha TK, Wilson KJ, Ding Z, Damon BM. Repeatability of DTI-based skeletal muscle fiber tracking. NMR Biomed. 2010;23(3):294–303.
19. Cicchetti DV, Sparrow SA. Developing criteria for establishing interrater reliability of specific items: applications to assessment of adaptive behavior. Am J Ment Defic. 1981;86(2):127–37.
20. Morvan D, Leroy-Willig A, Malgouyres A, Cuenod CA, Jehenson P, Syrota A. Simultaneous temperature and regional blood volume measurements in human muscle using an MRI fast diffusion technique. Magn Reson Med. 1993;29(3):371–7.
21. Froeling M, Oudeman J, van den Berg S, Nicolay K, Maas M, Strijkers GJ, Drost MR, Nederveen AJ. Reproducibility of diffusion tensor imaging in human forearm muscles at 3.0 T in a clinical setting. Magn Reson Med. 2010;64(4):1182–90.

24

Simultaneous multi-slice MR imaging of the hip at 3 T to reduce acquisition times and maintain image quality

Mayuko Haraikawa*, Masashi Suzuki, Kaiji Inoue, Eito Kozawa, Junji Tanaka and Mamoru Niitsu

Abstract

Background: Newly developed simultaneous multi-slice (SMS) scans are now being introduced as a clinical application in neuroimaging. We examined the feasibility of SMS scans for joint imaging. The purpose of the present study was to prospectively compare the resolution and specific absorption rate (SAR) obtained using SMS to those of conventional methods in hip joint magnetic resonance imaging (MRI) and establish whether imaging times may be reduced using SMS in 3 T MRI and if image quality is affected.

Methods: Twenty-one patients (4 men and 17 women, average age, 51.5 years, range: 22 to 76 years) with hip pain underwent MR examinations of the unilateral hip joint. Three board-certified radiologists independently and blindly evaluated the images obtained with and without SMS using window and level settings and magnification according to personal preferences. Individual SAR values were measured for each protocol. A Wilcoxon signed-rank test and a *t*-statistic test were used for statistical analyses. Signal-to-noise ratio (SNR) was also compared using a phantom.

Results: SMS imaging maintained equivalent image quality to conventional imaging for evaluating the morphology of the hip joint, and also reduced imaging times by approximately 40%. SMS images had significantly higher SAR values than conventional images. The rate of difference (SMS/conventional) in SNR ranged between 80 and 111%.

Conclusions: Based on its significantly lower acquisition times and the maintenance of similar image quality to conventional imaging, SMS may be applied to morphological evaluations of hip joint disorders without significantly increasing SAR.

Keywords: Simultaneous multi-slice, Turbo spin echo, Magnetic resonance imaging, Hip joint, Fast imaging, Musculoskeletal disorders

Background

Magnetic resonance imaging (MRI) with high tissue contrast is essential for diagnostic imaging of the hip joint [1]. In order to facilitate initial treatments, cartilage, labrum, ligament, and tendon diseases need to be precisely diagnosed in the early stages using MRI [2]. MRI plays an important role in decision making for surgical treatments, the alleviation of symptoms, and improved prognoses [3, 4].

MRI with a high magnetic field strength and phased array coil provides a higher signal-to-noise-ratio (SNR) and enables thin-sliced images to be obtained while maintaining high spatial resolution. In 2D multi-slice imaging, each slice excitation and signal reception are conducted sequentially, with the shortest repetition time (TR) becoming longer with increases in the number of slices. Therefore, imaging times are prolonged. Prolonged scanning duration may inconvenience patients and result in unwarranted movements, leading to blurred images due to motion artifact. Furthermore, patients with hip joint pain move more. Decreases in image acquisition times improved patient satisfaction and cost effectiveness by reducing scan times.

Simultaneous multi-slice (SMS) imaging is a method that reduces the scan time of 2D imaging by simultaneously exciting several slices [5, 6]. Since the information obtained on simultaneously excited slices is superimposed in the MR signal received, it is divided into each

* Correspondence: hmayuko@saitama-med.ac.jp
Department of Radiology, Saitama Medical University, 38 Morohongo, Moroyama-machi, Iruma-gun, Saitama 350-0495, Japan

slice with slice-GRAPPA (Generalized Auto Calibrating Partially Parallel Acquisitions) reconstruction. SMS is now mainly applied to echo planar imaging sequences, and has been used for diffusion and functional MRI [7–9]. If SMS becomes applicable to turbo spin echo (TSE) sequences, which are commonly used, it will be more useful [10]. The scan parameters that need to be changed in order to reduce the scan time in SMS include TR, the turbo factor, and concatenations. These parameters are related to image contrast. Moreover, care is needed in order to avoid exceeding the regulatory limits of the specific absorption rate (SAR).

The objective of the present study was to prospectively compare the resolution and SAR obtained using SMS to those of conventional methods in hip joint MRI and establish whether imaging times may be reduced using SMS in 3 T MRI and if image quality is affected.

Methods

Patients

The study design is outlined in Fig. 1. Twenty-one patients (4 men and 17 women, average age: 51.5 years, age range: 22 to 76 years) with hip pain and a presumed acetabular labral tear underwent MR examinations of the unilateral hip joint. All patients presented at the hip surgery clinic of the orthopedic department of our institution. This prospective study was performed between November 2016 and March 2017, was approved by the local Ethics Committee, and written informed consent was obtained from all patients prior to MR examinations.

MRI

All examinations were performed on a 3.0 T whole-body scanner (MAGNETOM Skyra; Siemens Healthcare GmbH, Erlangen, Germany) and a 18-channel body array coil. In addition to our routine protocols using TSE sequences, including oblique coronal proton-density weighted (PDW), oblique axial T1-weighted (T1W), and oblique coronal fat-saturated T2-weighted (FS-T2W) imaging, SMS protocols using a prototype sequence were also acquired in an identical geometry. All SMS images were acquired in the latter half of examinations.

Fixed sequence parameters in all protocols were as follows: number of slices: 30; slice thickness: 2.5 mm; slice gap: 0.25 mm; field-of-view (FOV): 160 × 160 mm^2. Other individual parameters of conventional and SMS imaging are shown in Table 1.

Image evaluation and analysis

We initially excluded some MR examinations with poor image quality from the analysis. Three board-certified radiologists (with 31, 26, and 19 years of experience in musculoskeletal MRI) evaluated pairs of images with and without SMS. Delineative imaging quality was assessed in the delineation of the following structures: the acetabular labrum (labrum), articular cartilage (cartilage), and bony trabecula of the femoral neck (trabecula) (Figs. 2, 3 and 4). The evaluation incorporated the recognition of normal structures as well as pathologies, including labral tears, cartilage defects, and trabecular irregularities. The evaluation also included image blurring, edge sharpness, contrast, and flow/motion artifacts. The labrum and cartilage were evaluated on PDW, T1W, and FS-T2W, while the trabecula was assessed on PDW and T1W. The reviewers independently and blindly evaluated images using window and level settings and magnification according to personal preferences.

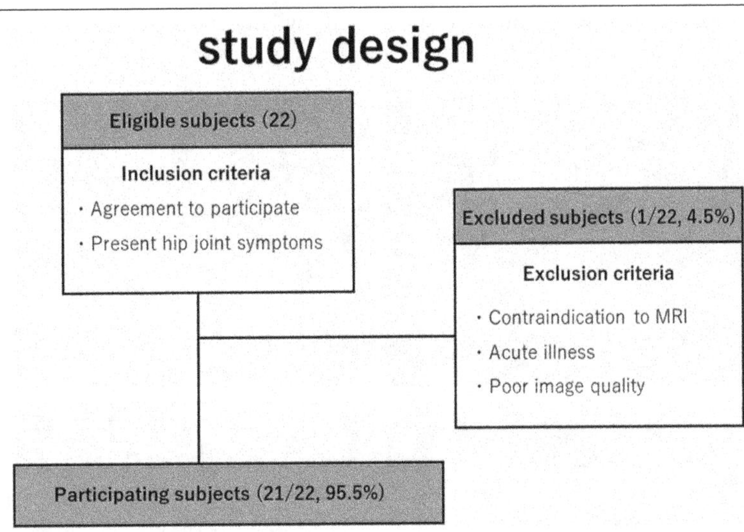

Fig. 1 Study design

Table 1 Scan parameters of conventional and SMS scans

	Conventional			SMS		
	PDW	T1W	FS-T2W	PDW	T1W	FS-T2W
AT	4:36	3:42	3:58	2:22	2:17	2:56
Total AT	12:16			7:35		
TR (ms)	2000	712	3500	2000	650	3500
TE (ms)	20	27	61	21	14	62
Averages	1	2	2	1	1	2
Concatenations	2	3	2	1	2	1
Flip angle (deg)	150	120	150	150	120	150
Fat suppression	none	none	CHESS	none	none	CHESS
Base resolution	320	384	320	320	384	320
Phase resolution (%)	100	75	70	100	75	70
Parallel imaging	none	GRAPPA	GRAPPA	CAIPIRINHA	CAIPIRINHA	CAIPIRINHA
Acceleration factor phase	–	2	2	1	1	1
Acceleration factor slice	–	–	–	2	2	2
FOV shift factor	–	–	–	2	2	2
Bandwidth (Hz/Px)	240	250	220	240	250	279

PDW proton-density weighted, *T1W* T1-weighted, *FS-T2W* fat-saturated T2-weighted, *SMS* simultaneous multi-slice, *AT* acquisition time, *TR* repetition-time, *TE* echo time, *GRAPPA* generalized auto calibrating partially parallel acquisitions, *CAIPIRINHA* controlled aliasing in parallel imaging results in higher acceleration, *CHESS* chemical shift selective, *FOV* field-of-view

Delineative quality was rated using a five-point scale: Conventional (CNV) + 2: the conventional image is superior to SMS, CNV + 1: the conventional image is better than SMS, 0: the conventional image is equal (EQUAL) to SMS, SMS + 1: SMS is better than the conventional image, SMS + 2: SMS is superior to the conventional image.

The five-point evaluation scale was scored as follows: + 2 (CNV + 2), + 1 (CNV + 1), 0 (EQUAL), – 1 (SMS + 1), and – 2 (SMS + 2). A score for each sequence represented the difference between the two groups being compared. A Wilcoxon signed-rank test was used for the statistical analysis. Data analyses were performed with the software JMP® 12 (SAS Institute Inc., Cary, NC, USA), and $p < 0.05$ was considered to be significant.

SAR

Individual SAR values predicted by the scanner system before the scan (0–100%) were recorded. The average and standard deviation (SD) were calculated in every sequence for all patients. Values with and without SMS were compared through the *t*-statistic test. A data analysis was performed with the software JMP® 12 (SAS Institute Inc., Cary, NC, USA). $p < 0.05$ was considered to be significant. Although parameters had to be changed when the predicted SAR value exceeded the

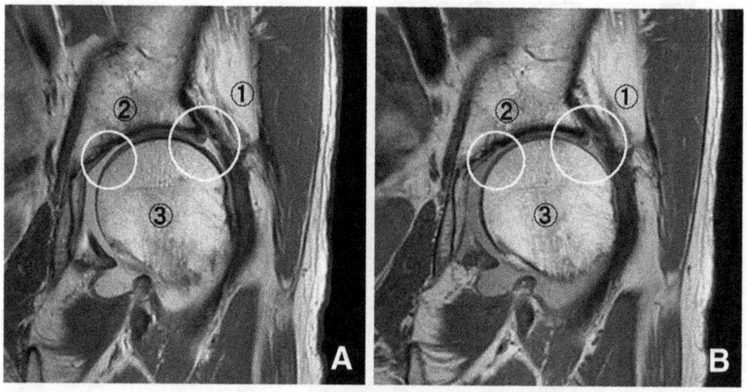

Fig. 2 A 76-year-old woman with left hip pain. Oblique coronal proton density-weighted images with conventional (**a**) and simultaneous multi-slice (SMS) sequences (**b**). Circles indicate areas for image evaluations: ① acetabular labrum, ② articular cartilage, ③ bony trabecula. Joint fluid in the conventional image appears brighter than that in SMS in this patient

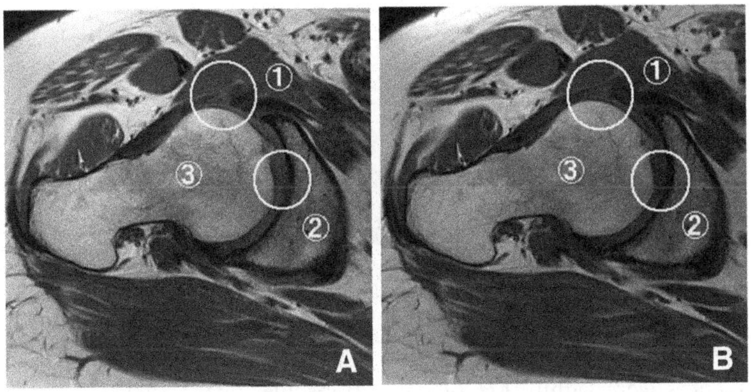

Fig. 3 A 50-year-old woman with right hip pain. Oblique axial T1-weighted images with conventional (**a**) and simultaneous multi-slice sequences (**b**). Circles indicate areas for image evaluations: ① acetabular labrum, ② articular cartilage, ③ bony trabecula

regulated level, we used the values obtained before changes for the evaluation.

SNR measurements using a phantom

Phantom SNRs were measured by the consecutive method to evaluate the intrinsic SNR of each protocol [11]. A polypropylene cylinder with a length of 200 mm and diameter of 120 mm filled with polyvinyl alcohol was used as a phantom (Fig. 5a). By using an identical MR scanner and the coil (Fig. 5b), scan parameters were identical to those of the patient scan. Axial PDW, T1W, and FS-T2W images were consecutively scanned 50 times each. In a series of 50 images, the signal intensity (SI) of each pixel was measured and then averaged SI and SD were also calculated. The SNR of each pixel was calculated as the SI value divided by the SD value, and SNR maps were created (Fig. 5c). In the center slice of the SNR map, the average SNR value was measured in the region of interest enclosing 75% of the area of the phantom (Fig. 5c). ImageJ software (National Institutes of Health, Bethesda, MD, USA) was used for this procedure.

Results

The imaging times of each conventional sequence were as follows: PDW 4 min 36 s, T1W 3 min 42 s, and FS-T2W 3 min 58 s. The following imaging times were obtained with SMS: PDW 2 min 22 s, T1W 2 min 17 s, and FS-T2W 2 min 56 s (Table 1). SMS reduced the total acquisition time of the three sequences from 12 min 16 s to 7 min 35 s.

In image evaluations, no significant differences were observed in image quality for labrum PDW and cartilage T1W and FS-T2W between conventional and SMS images. Conventional image qualities for labrum T1W ($p = 0.0072$), labrum FS-T2W ($p = 0.0007$), and cartilage PDW ($p = 0.0042$) were significantly superior to those by SMS. However, SMS image qualities for trabecula PDW ($p = 0.0083$) and T1W ($p = 0.0179$) were significantly superior to those by conventional images (Figs. 6, 7 and 8).

SMS images had significantly higher SAR values than conventional images ($p < 0.001$ for all sequences). The

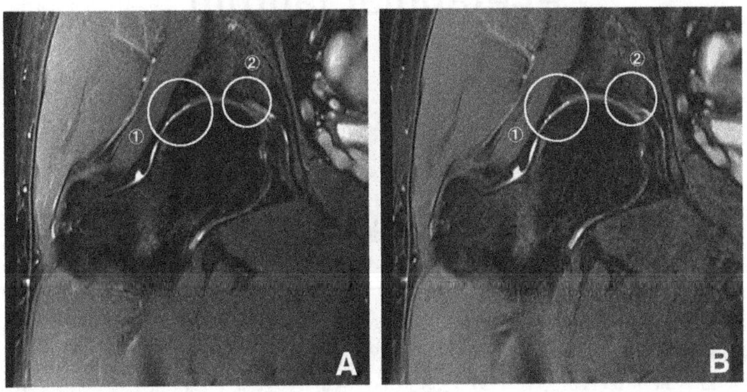

Fig. 4 A 22-year-old man with right hip pain. Oblique coronal fat-saturated T2-weighted images with conventional (**a**) and simultaneous multi-slice sequences (**b**). Circles indicate areas for image evaluations: ① acetabular labrum, ② articular cartilage

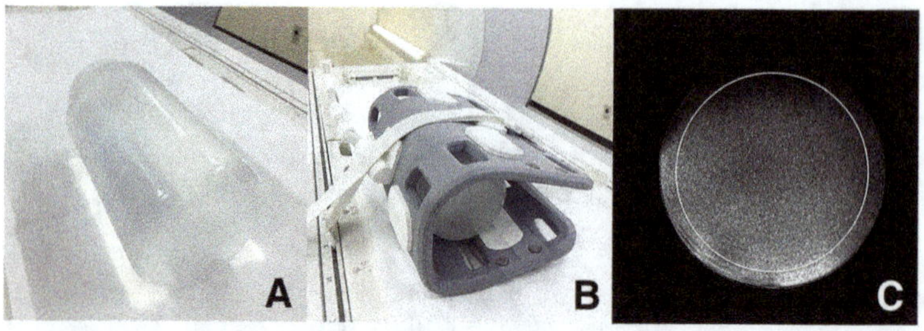

Fig. 5 (**a**) A phantom for SNR measurements: A polypropylene cylinder filled with polyvinyl alcohol. **b** An 18-channel body array coil. **c** An SNR map and the 75% region of interest (circle)

mean values of SMS sequences were within 90% of the simulated limit (Fig. 9).

Table 2 summarizes the SNR of sequences. The rates of difference (SMS/conventional) in each sequence were PDW 86%, T1W 80%, and FS-T2W 111%.

Discussion

The present results showed that the quality of SMS images was similar to that of conventional images and also that imaging times were reduced by 40%. None of the protocols for conventional images enabled the acquisition of all slices needed during 1TR; thus, concatenations were set to 2–3. The application of SMS resulted in fewer concatenations for all protocols and reduced imaging times.

Regarding visual assessments, conventional methods are better than SMS for bone/cartilage and soft tissues; however, no marked differences were observed on a 5-point scale basis. This result indicates the absence of any marked differences between the image qualities of SMS and conventional methods in terms of how the labrum and cartilage are shown. Regarding the bone trabecula, SMS was superior to conventional methods. Although the reason for this currently remains unclear, it is conceivable that in the evaluation of the bone trabecula, image evaluations placed more emphasis on contrast rather than shape, and image reconstruction may have reduced noise. It is advantageous for joint MRI, which requires high spatial and contrast resolution, that SMS reduced imaging times while producing similar resolution to conventional methods. Due to reductions in imaging times, it will be possible to increase the number of additions for higher resolution images and obtain more images for another section. At the hip joint, MRI is often performed on both sides of patients being treated with steroid medication [12, 13]. This reduced imaging time with SMS will be beneficial for acquiring high resolution images of both hip joints.

Image reconstruction by SMS was performed using the slice GRAPPA method, and overlapped signals were divided into each individual slice [14]. The GRAPPA kernel for SMS was calculated from the gradient echo signal acquired before the SMS scan. The arithmetic precision of this GRAPPA kernel has a prominent influence on the quality of reconstructed images. Inferior quality indicates the appearance of an artifact and decrease in SNR. In SMS, each slice was excited in order to have a different FOV shift toward the phase-encoding direction [15].With CAIPIRINHA (Controlled aliasing in parallel imaging results in higher acceleration),

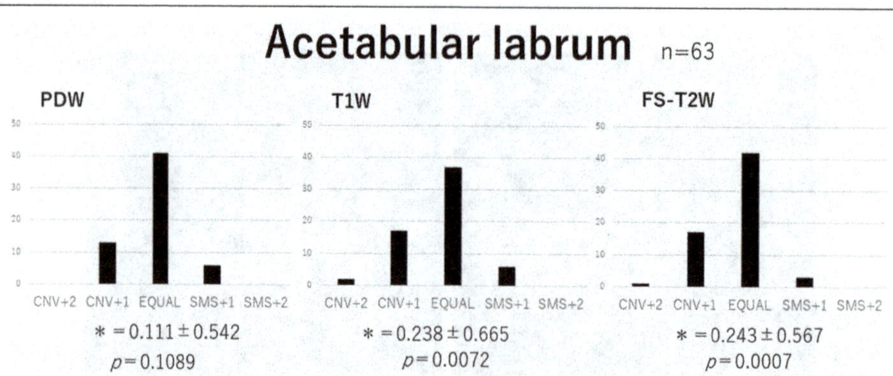

Fig. 6 Visual image evaluation of the acetabular labrum. Bar chart of the total score obtained from three readers. Wilcoxon signed-rank test values (MEAN ± SD:*) were as follows: PDW 0.111 ± 0.542, T1W 0.238 ± 0.665, and FS-T2W 0.248 ± 0.567. No significant differences were observed in PDW, whereas T1W and FS-T2W of the labrum by conventional methods were significantly superior to those of SMS. PDW: proton density-weighted; T1W: T1-weighted; FS-T2W: fat-saturated T2-weighted; SMS: Simultaneous multi-slice; CNV: Conventional; EQUAL: equal

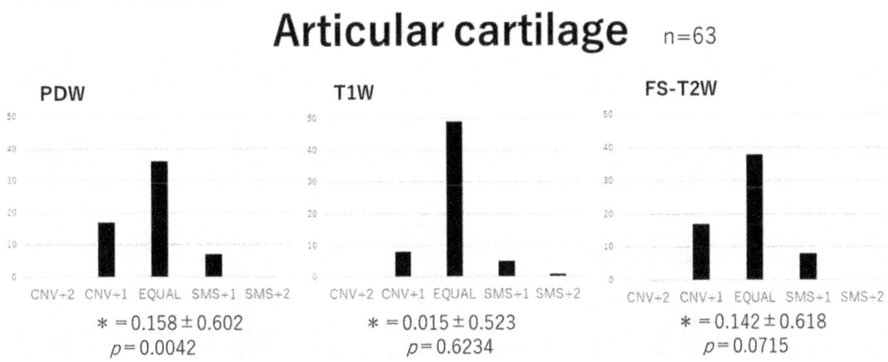

Fig. 7 Visual image evaluation for articular cartilage. Bar chart of the total score obtained from the three readers. Wilcoxon signed-rank test values (MEAN ± SD:*) were as follows: PDW 0.158 ± 0.601, T1W 0.015 ± 0.523, and FS-T2W 0.142 ± 0.618. PDW for articular cartilage by conventional methods was significantly superior to that by SMS. No significant differences were noted in T1W and FS-T2W. PDW: proton density-weighted; T1W: T1-weighted; FS-T2W: fat-saturated T2-weighted; SMS: Simultaneous multi-slice; CNV: Conventional; EQUAL: equal

separation performance is significantly improved [16]. In the present study, although we set the shift amount to 1/2 FOV for slice GRAPPA factor = 2 in all protocols, the effect on a reconstructed image was expected to depend not only on these values, but also on the distance between overlapped slices, number of coils used, and slice geometry to coil configuration. Regarding the results of the phantom measurement, the SNR change was less than 20% at the maximum. Although there is a difference based on positions, no marked difference was observed from that without SMS. Slice GRAPPA may be used in conjunction with in-plane GRAPPA, but will result in a decrease in image quality due to the total acceleration factor. Although we performed a test a priori and decreased the in-plane GRAPPA factor for some protocols, we adjusted the parameters to reduce the overall imaging time.

Some points need to be emphasized for SMS: an increase in peak voltage due to a change in the radio frequency (RF) pulse shape and increase in SAR [6]. Regarding peak voltage, since it is not possible to exceed the limiting values of the hardware, methods such as prolonging the RF time and decreasing the peak voltage by shifting the peak position of each slice have been suggested [17, 18].

The SAR limitation is important for clinical use. Imaging parameters need to be changed when the SAR value exceeds its peak. Therefore, the reduced imaging time is prolonged again. Based on the measurements of SAR values for each protocol, SMS achieved high values. We need to consider patient conditions that may be more strongly affected by high SAR, such as pregnant or pediatric patients. However, the average values for all protocols were less than 100% against the limiting values, and there were only a few cases that required a change in imaging parameters during the study.

This study has several limitations. The number of subjects was small, but sufficient for a technical feasibility

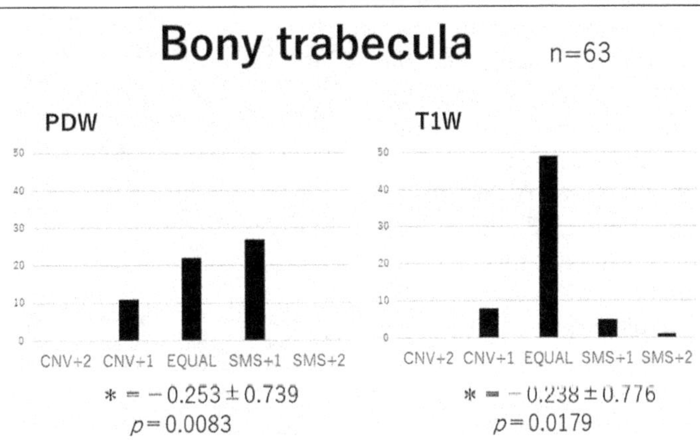

Fig. 8 Visual image evaluation for the bony trabecula. Bar chart of the total score obtained from three readers. Wilcoxon signed-rank test values (MEAN ± SD:*) were as follows: PDW -0.253 ± 0.739 and T1W -0.238 ± 0.776. PDW and T1W for the bony trabecula by SMS were significantly superior to those by conventional methods. PDW: proton-density weighted; T1W: T1-weighted; SMS: simultaneous multi-slice; CNV: conventional; EQUAL: equal

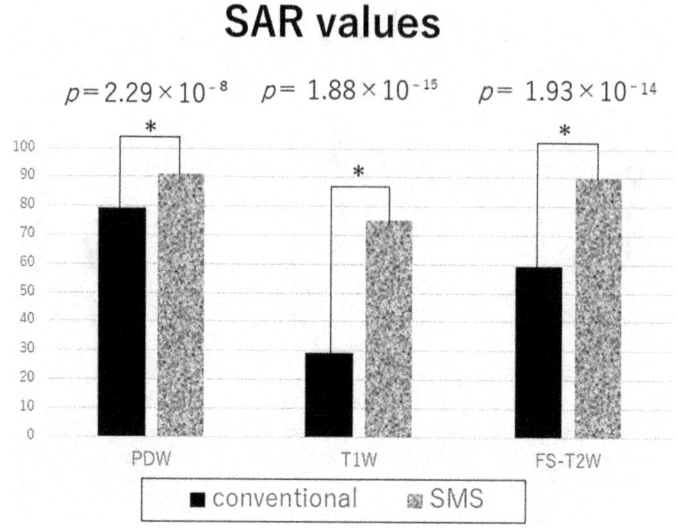

Fig. 9 SAR values of each sequence. In all sequences, the SAR of SMS significantly increased. SAR: specific absorption rate; SMS: simultaneous multi-slice; PDW: proton density-weighted; T1W: T1-weighted; FS-T2W: fat-saturated T2-weighted

study. The qualitative analysis focused on the reader's ability to evaluate intact anatomical structures. The three radiologists in our study were experienced radiologists. The addition of a relatively inexperienced reader may have increased the validity of the present study. Echo time (TE), TR, and other imaging parameters are not completely equivalent, and the resultant image contrast was greater between joint fluid and articular cartilage on the conventional scan than on the SMS scan. This contrast change may lead to the superior delineation of cartilage on PDW of a conventional scan. Furthermore, a difference exists in the magnetization transfer effect due to the simultaneous application of RF pulses with different frequencies, which may affect image contrast. In the present study, SMS imaging was performed sequentially after all conventional methods had been completed. A body motion artifact is more likely to appear due to a prolonged examination time in the magnet. In the present study, the image quality of SMS was evaluated under unfavorable conditions; however, no definite artifact was observed in the visual assessment.

The present results indicate the potential of SMS to significantly reduce imaging times and maintained equivalent image quality to conventional imaging. Images with high spatial resolution are mandatory for the evaluation of subtle morphologies in cartilage, the labrum, and trabecula. Therefore, reduced imaging times are useful for improving spatial resolution. This study approach has not been previously tested in musculoskeletal applications. Our results appear to support the replacement of conventional techniques with this imaging technique, particularly for the evaluation of musculoskeletal diseases, and applications to more advanced techniques. Therefore, the study of other joints, such as the shoulder and knee, is needed. Before actual clinical application of the new protocol, the diagnostic accuracy of the proposed image acquisition will need to be tested for chondrolabral pathology in a future study.

Table 2 Signal-to-noise ratio of each sequence

PDW		T1W		FS-T2W	
CNV	SMS	CNV	SMS	CNV	SMS
113	98	25	20	159	178

PDW proton-density weighted, *T1W* T1-weighted, *FS-T2W* fat-saturated T2-weighted, *CNV* Conventional, *SMS* Simultaneous multi-slice

Conclusions

In conclusion, the present results indicate that due to significantly shorter acquisition times and similar quality to conventional imaging, SMS may be applied to morphological evaluations of hip joint disorders without significantly increasing SAR.

Abbreviations

CAIPIRINHA: Controlled aliasing in parallel imaging results in higher acceleration; CNV: conventional; FOV: field-of-view; FS-T2W: fat-saturated T2-weighted; GRAPPA: Generalized Auto Calibrating Partially Parallel Acquisitions; PDW: proton-density weighted; RF: radio frequency; SAR: specific absorption rate; SI: signal intensity; SMS: simultaneous multi-slice; SNR: Signal-to-noise ratio; T1W: T1-weighted; TE: echo time; TR: repetition time; TSE: turbo spin echo

Acknowledgments

The authors would like to thank Dingxin Wang (Siemens Medical Solutions, USA) for providing the prototype sequence that he developed. We would also like to thank Hiroshi Imai (Siemens Healthcare K.K.) for providing thorough technical assistance with the experiments.

Funding
Not applicable.

Authors' contributions
Substantial contributions to study conception and design: MH, MS, MN. Substantial contributions to the acquisition of data: MH, MS, MN. Substantial contributions to the analysis and interpretation of data: MH, MS KI, EK, JT, MN. Drafting the article or revising it critically for important intellectual content: MH, MS, MN. All authors read and approved the final manuscript. Final approval of the version of the article to be published: MH, MS, MN.

Consent for publication
Not applicable.

Competing interests
The authors declare that they have no competing interests.

References
1. Aguilar HN, Battie MC, Jaremko JL. MRI-based hip cartilage measures in osteoarthritic and non-osteoarthritic individuals: a systematic review. RMD Open. 2017;3(1):e000358.
2. Crema MD, Watts GJ, Guermazi A, Kim YJ, Kijowski R, Roemer FW. A narrative overview of the current status of MRI of the hip and its relevance for osteoarthritis research - what we know, what has changed and where are we going? Osteoarthr Cartil. 2017;25(1):1–13.
3. Naraghi A, White LM. MRI of labral and chondral lesions of the hip. AJR Am J Roentgenol. 2015;205(3):479–90.
4. Ragab Y, Nabih M, Aly I, Kamal A, Abd-Allah MA, El-Refai R, Emad Y, El-Naggar A, El-Shaarawy N, Rasker JJ. Magnetic resonance imaging features of hip disorders in an Egyptian pediatric population. Reumatismo. 2015;67(2): 68–77.
5. Barth M, Breuer F, Koopmans PJ, Norris DG, Poser BA. Simultaneous multislice (SMS) imaging techniques. Magn Reson Med. 2016;75(1):63–81.
6. Hamilton J, Franson D, Seiberlich N. Recent advances in parallel imaging for MRI. Prog Nucl Magn Reson Spectrosc. 2017;101:71–95.
7. Kenkel D, Wurnig MC, Filli L, Ulbrich EJ, Runge VM, Beck T, Boss A. Whole-body diffusion imaging applying simultaneous multi-slice excitation. Rofo. 2016;188(4):381–8.
8. Setsompop K, Cohen-Adad J, Gagoski BA, Raij T, Yendiki A, Keil B, Wedeen VJ, Wald LL. Improving diffusion MRI using simultaneous multi-slice echo planar imaging. NeuroImage. 2012;63(1):569–80.
9. Zahneisen B, Poser BA, Ernst T, Stenger AV. Simultaneous Multi-Slice fMRI using spiral trajectories. NeuroImage. 2014;92:8–18.
10. Fritz J, Fritz B, Zhang J, Thawait GK, Joshi DH, Pan L, Wang D. Simultaneous multislice accelerated Turbo spin Echo magnetic resonance imaging: comparison and combination with in-plane parallel imaging acceleration for high-resolution magnetic resonance imaging of the knee. Investig Radiol. 2017;52(9):529–37.
11. Imai H, Miyati T, Ogura A, Doi T, Tsuchihashi T, Machida Y, Kobayashi M, Shimizu K, Kitou Y. Signal-to-noise ratio measurement in parallel MRI with subtraction mapping and consecutive methods. Nihon Hoshasen Gijutsu Gakkai Zasshi. 2008;64(8):930–6.
12. Zhao FC, Hu HX, Zheng X, Cang DW, Liu X, Zhang JZ, Guo KJ. Clinical analysis of 23 cases of steroid-associated osteonecrosis of the femoral head with normal initial magnetic resonance imaging presentation. Medicine (Baltimore). 2017;96(49):e8834.
13. Nagasawa K, Tada Y, Koarada S, Horiuchi T, Tsukamoto H, Murai K, Ueda A, Yoshizawa S, Ohta A. Very early development of steroid-associated osteonecrosis of femoral head in systemic lupus erythematosus: prospective study by MRI. Lupus. 2005;14(5):385–90.
14. Runge VM, Richter JK, Heverhagen JT. Speed in clinical magnetic resonance. Investig Radiol. 2017;52(1):1–17.
15. Setsompop K, Gagoski BA, Polimeni JR, Witzel T, Wedeen VJ, Wald LL. Blipped-controlled aliasing in parallel imaging for simultaneous multislice echo planar imaging with reduced g-factor penalty. Magn Reson Med. 2012;67(5):1210 24.
16. Yokota H, Sakai K, Tazoe J, Goto M, Imai H, Teramukai S, Yamada K. Clinical feasibility of simultaneous multi-slice imaging with blipped-CAIPI for diffusion-weighted imaging and diffusion-tensor imaging of the brain. Acta Radiol. 2017;58(12):1500–10.
17. Auerbach EJ, Xu J, Yacoub E, Moeller S, Ugurbil K. Multiband accelerated spin-echo echo planar imaging with reduced peak RF power using time-shifted RF pulses. Magn Reson Med. 2013;69(5):1261–7.
18. Zaitsev M, Schultz G, Hennig J, Gruetter R, Gallichan D. Parallel imaging with phase scrambling. Magn Reson Med. 2015;73(4):1407–19.

25

MRI findings of low-grade fibromyxoid sarcoma

Yali Yue[1], Yongkang Liu[1], Lina Song[1], Xiao Chen[1], Yaohui Wang[2] and Zhongqiu Wang[1*]

Abstract

Background: Low-grade fibromyxoid sarcoma (LGFMS) is a distinctive slow growing soft tissue neoplasm, mostly affecting young individuals with no gender difference. It usually arises in deep soft tissue of the lower limbs and trunk, but few cases of LGFMS located in pelvis have been reported.

Case presentation: We describe the magnetic resonance imaging(MRI) features of LGFMS located in the anterior pelvic wall of a 21-year-old female and correlate them with clinicopathological features. The tumor was completely resected and there is no recidivism during the follow-up one year.

Conclusions: We report on the radiological findings of LGFMS with histological correlation. Awareness of the imaging features may be useful for the diagnosis of LGFMS and helpful to distinguish among mimics.

Keywords: Magnetic resonance imaging, Anterior pelvic wall, Low-grade fibromyxoid sarcoma

Background

Low-grade fibromyxoid sarcoma (LGFMS) is a slow growing sarcoma that originally described by Evans [1]. LGFMS is defined by the World Health Organization (WHO) as a malignant fibroblastic/myofibroblastic tumor usually arise from deep soft tissue with potential for recurrence and late metastatic spread [2, 3]. The incidence is estimated 0.18 per million, accounting for 0.6% of all soft tissue sarcomas [4]. Due to the relative rarity, it is difficult to distinguish LGFMS from other mesenchymal tumors and make accurate diagnosis for the radiologists. To make a deep understanding of this kind of disease, we describe MRI findings of a 21-year-old woman LGFMS patient and review relevant literature. This study may be conducive to future diagnosis and differential diagnosis of LGFMS for radiologists.

Case presentation

A 21-year-old female with a palpable painless mass in her lower abdomen which was gradually increasing in size was admitted to our institution. Physical examination demonstrated a firm, non-tender and non-movable mass measuring 8 × 9 cm in size protruding through the anterior pelvic wall. The index of hemotology and biochemistry were all in the normal scope. The patient has no history of injury or surgery, and no family history was identified.

The nosocomial MRI revealed a well-defined, 12 × 10 × 9 cm-sized, lobulated mass within the mid-pelvis. The mass exhibited isointensity relative to muscle in fat-supressed T1-weighted MR image (Fig. 1a) and heterogeneous relatively hyperintensity with a little stip and patchy hypointensity inside on fat-suppression T2-weighted MR image (Fig. 1b). Meanwhile, circinate low signal intensity can be found around the tumor, indicating that there was a capsule or pseudocapsule. Sagittal T2WI showed that the rectus abdominis was open with umbrella shape (Fig. 1c). The tumor showed restricted diffusion on diffusion weighted imaging (DWI) (Fig. 1d) and apparent diffusion coefficient (ADC) map (Fig. 1e), which presented as heterogeneous hyperintensity and hypointensity, respectively. It also showed heterogeneous enhancement on fat-suppression T1WI after the contrast agent injected (Fig. 1f-1h). The area of higher signal intensity exhibited more obvious enhancement compared with lower signal intensity area on T2WI. At surgery, the mass was located at the symphysis ossium pubis, invading the lower right rectus abdominis and the bottom of the bladder. It was well circumscribed, firm and lobulated

* Correspondence: zhq2001us@163.com
[1]Department of Radiology, Affiliated Hospital of Nanjing University of Chinese Medicine, 155 Hanzhong Road, Nanjing, Jiangsu 210029, People's Republic of China
Full list of author information is available at the end of the article

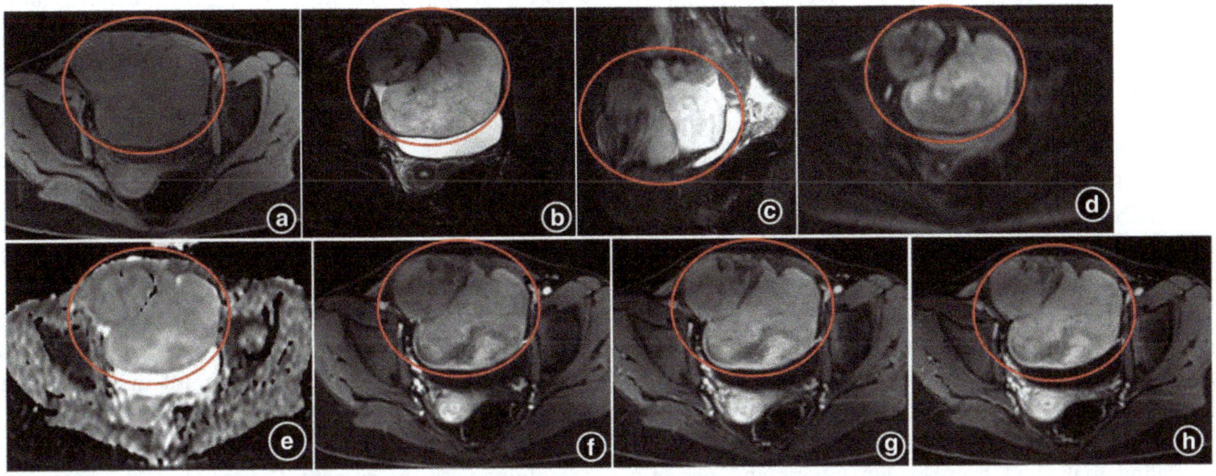

Fig. 1 The magnetic resonance imaging findings of low grade fibromyxoid sarcoma. **a**: T1-weighted MR images; **b**: T2-weighted MR images; **c**: Sagittal T2WI showed that the rectus abdominis was open with umbrella shape; **d**: The tumor showed high signal intensity on diffusion weighted imaging; **e**: The tumor showed low signal intensity on apparent diffusion coefficient (ADC) map; **f-h**: On Gadolinium-enhanced T1-weighted MR images with fat suppression at arterial (**f**), portal (**g**) and delayed phases (**h**), the tumor showed heterogeneous enhancement

appearance. The cut surface of the lesion was pale white and glistening with neither necrosis nor hemorrhage. Microscopic examination identified alternating fibrous and myxoid stroma areas inside the tumor, the tumor cells arranging in a whorled growth pattern with curvilinear capillaries (Fig. 2a). Immunohistochemically, the tumor cells were positive for smooth muscle actin (SMA) (Fig. 2b). MRI findings combined with histopathological analysis made a final diagnosis of LGFMS. The patient was discharged from hospital 10 days after the operation. During one year of follow-up, the patient was in a good status without evidence of recurrence.

Discussion and conclusions

LGFMS was first depicted by Evans in 1987 [1], who subsequently reported the clinicopathologic features of these tumors in subsequent studies [5]. It has been shown that LGFMS seem to occur mainly in young adults without difference in gender (median age 34 years old) [6]. LGFMS usually occur in deep soft tissue, manifestating as a slow-growing, non-tender and solid tumor [5, 6]. It usually presents as a well circumscribed soft tissue mass, without hemorrhage, nodularity or infiltrative border, and is usually favor of a benign lesion. The microscopic appearance of LGFMS is composed of alternative fibrous and myxoid zones and spindle cells arranging in a swirling pattern with no obvious atypia [7, 8].

Radiological examination plays a crucial part in both diagnosis and treatment of this kind of disease. CT and MRI can visually characterize lesions' morphological features, textural features, and relationships with adjacent structures. On CT or MRI, LGFMS is solitary and well circumscribed, which is similar to the lesion in our study, although it may present as multiple infiltrating masses at recurrence [9]. Several previous case reports have described CT and MRI observations of LGFMS. On plain CT scan, the fibrous component has been depicted as isodense while the myxoid component has been depicted as hypodense [6]. Conventional and advanced MR techniques can be more helpful than CT in the assessment of various muscle

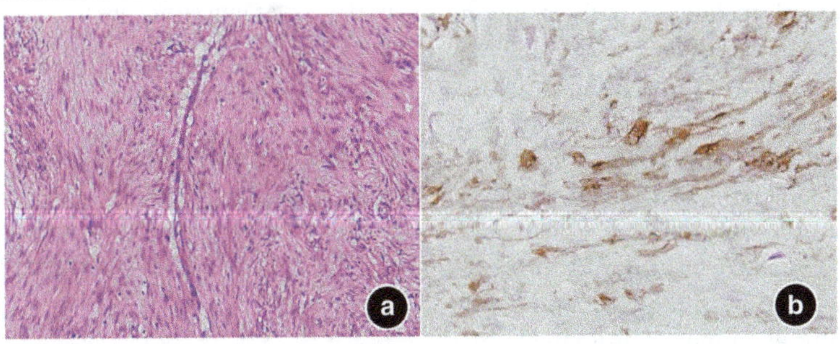

Fig. 2 Microscopic findings of low grade fibromyxoid sarcoma. **a**: Hematoxylin-eosin staining (magnification, × 100); **b**: immunochemical staining for smooth muscle actin (SMA) (magnification, × 400)

disorders for its further subtle multi-sequence imaging [10]. MRI performances of LGFMS have previously been reported [11, 12]. On MRI, LGFMS is inhomogeneous, owing to its two distinct internal zones: myxoid and fibrous. Generally, the low T1/T2 signal intensity and slight enhancement correspond to fibrous components [13, 14]. The low T1 signal intensity, high T2 signal intensity and variable enhancement after gadolinium injection correspond to the myxoid components [6, 15]. In our case, the tumor had an inhomogeneous appearance on T1WI and T2WI. The internal components were hypointense to muscle on T2WI. The relative higher signal intensity zone showed more intense enhancement compared with lower signal intensity on T2WI, as formerly reported [11]. Additionly, DWI also plays an important part in differentiating malignant from benign lesions and necrotic tumors from infections [16, 17]. DWI is a noninvasive method used to measure the motion of water molecules and can be quantified as ADC. Both soft tissue tumors and infectious diseases may present hyperintense signal on DWI and hypointense signal on the ADC map. However, hyperintensity relative to skeletal muscle is more frequent in malignant than benign tumors on DWI, ADCs of malignant tumors are remarkably lower than benign tumors. Most necrotic tumors show higher ADC values and low-to-intermediate signal intensity on DWI, whereas abscesses has lower ADC values and higher signal intensity on DWI in contrast.

Although MRI and CT can detect the fibrous and myxoid components of the tumor, sometimes, it is very difficult to distinguish theses lesions from LGFMS only depending on imageological examinations. The definite diagnosis depends on histopathological examination. Immunohistochemical staining showed positive expression of vimentin in the tumor cells, but SMA, β-catenin, desmin, S100, cytokeratin, CD34 and CD56 were negative [18]. In the present case, the LGFMS was negative for vimentin and positive for SMA.

Various similar benign or malignant soft tissue lesions should be considered in the differential diagnosis of LGFMS, of which has the significant potential for recurrence and late metastatic spread. Low-grade myxofibrosarcoma is the most important malignant entities among various mimics. It is usually confused with LGFMS, partially due to similar nomenclature. LGFMS commonly locate in the deep soft tissue which tend to occur in young adults, while low-grade myxofibrosarcoma primarily locate in subcutaneous layer of the extremities of elderly individuals. Most myxofibrosarcoma cases histologic expressions include: homogeneous myxoid zone, lack of alternative fibrous zones, pleomorphic cells, and hyperchromatic nuclei [19]. Intra-abdominal fibromatosis may have myxoid areas and pluricellular areas with a fascicular pattern of growth just mimic LGFMS [20]. However, unlike LGFMS, fibromatosis is a poorly-defined tumor with infiltrative borders and exhibits myofibroblastic differentiation morphologically and immunohistochemically [21]. Nodular fasciitis can also have variably myxoid and fibrous zones with well circumscribed boundary [20]. However, histological features including a loose storiform pattern of growth, myxoid degeneration and extravasation of lymphocytes and erythrocytes, which are characteristics of nodular fasciitis, are absent in LGFMS. LGFMS should also be differentiated from Morel-Lavallee Lesions, which is a post-traumatic soft tissue degloving injury. The appropriateclinical history and a fluid collection in a typical location are useful in determining the diagnosis of Morel-Lavallee Lesions [22].

In conclusion, we reviewed previously publications combining with the current 21-year-old female case, and some relative characteristics of LGFMS can be summarized as following. LGFMS is an uncommon soft tissue tumor that usually arise from deep soft tissue of young individuals and has high risk of recurrence and late metastatic spread. Fibrous component areas show low T1/T2 signal intensity. Myxoid component areas show low T1 signal intensity, high T2 signal intensity and variable enhancement. Awareness of the above may be useful for the diagnosis of LGFMS.

Abbreviations

ADC: Apparent diffusion coefficient; DWI: Diffusion weighted imaging; LGFMS: Low-grade fibromyxoid sarcoma; MRI: Magnetic resonance imaging; SMA: Smooth muscle actin; WHO: World health organization

Acknowledgements

Not applicable.

Funding

This report was funded by national natural science foundation of China (81471705).

Authors' contributions

YLY wrote the initial draft of this manuscript and subsequent revisions. YKL and LNS assisted with drafting the manuscript and data collection. YHW analyzed the pathological features. XC and ZQW are responsible for the oversight of the report and editing the manuscript. All authors read and approved the final manuscript.

Consent for publication

The authors have obtained the patient's written informed consent for print and electronic publication of this case report.

Competing interests

The authors declare that they have no financial or other conflicts of interest in relation to this research and its publication.

Author details
[1]Department of Radiology, Affiliated Hospital of Nanjing University of Chinese Medicine, 155 Hanzhong Road, Nanjing, Jiangsu 210029, People's Republic of China. [2]Department of Pathology, Affiliated Hospital of Nanjing University of Chinese Medicine, Nanjing, Jiangsu 210029, China.

References

1. Evans HL. Low-grade fibromyxoid sarcoma. A report of two metastasizing neoplasms having a deceptively benign appearance. Am J Clin Pathol. 1987;88(5):615–9.
2. Kurisakiarakawa A, Suehara Y, Arakawa A, Takagi T, Takahashi M, Mitani K, Kaneko K, Yao T, Saito T. Deeply located low-grade fibromyxoid sarcoma with FUS-CREB3L2 gene fusion in a 5-year-old boy with review of literature. Diagn Pathol. 2014;9(1):1–8.
3. Doyle LA, Möller E, Dal CP, Fletcher CD, Mertens F, Hornick JL. MUC4 is a highly sensitive and specific marker for low-grade fibromyxoid sarcoma. Am J Surg Pathol. 2011;35(5):733–41.
4. Marettynielsen K, Baerentzen S, Keller J, Dyrop HB, Safwat A. Low-Grade Fibromyxoid Sarcoma: Incidence, Treatment Strategy of Metastases, and Clinical Significance of the FUS Gene. Sarcoma. 2013,(2013-5-30) 2013; 2013(2013):256280.
5. Evans HL. Low-grade fibromyxoid sarcoma. A report of 12 cases. American. J Surg Pathol. 1993;17(6):595–600.
6. Miyake M, Tateishi U, Maeda T, Arai Y, Seki K, Hasegawa T, Sugimura K. CT and MRI features of low-grade fibromyxoid sarcoma in the shoulder of a pediatric patient. Radiat Med. 2006;24(7):511–4.
7. Evans HL. Low-grade fibromyxoid sarcoma: a clinicopathologic study of 33 cases with long-term follow-up. Am J Surg Pathol. 2011;35(10):1450.
8. Kim SY, Kim MY, Hwang YJ, Han YH, Seo JW, Kim YH, Cha SJ, Hur G. Low-grade fibromyxoid sarcoma: CT, sonography, and MR findings in 3 cases. J Thorac Imaging. 2005;20(4):294.
9. Hwang S, Kelliher E, Hameed M. Imaging features of low-grade fibromyxoid sarcoma (Evans tumor). Skelet Radiol. 2012;41(10):1263–72.
10. Kumar Y, Wadhwa V, Phillips L, Pezeshk P, Chhabra A. MR imaging of skeletal muscle signal alterations: systematic approach to evaluation. Eur J Radiol. 2016;85(5):922.
11. Kim SK, Jee WH, Lee AW, Chung YG. Haemorrhagic low-grade fibromyxoid sarcoma: MR findings in two young women. Br J Radiol. 2011;84(1003):146–50.
12. Sargar K, Kao SC, Spunt SL, Hawkins D, Parham DM, Coffin C, Mccarville MB. MR and CT imaging of low grade Fibromyxoid sarcoma in children: a report from Children's oncology group study ARST0332. AJR Am J Roentgenol. 2015;205(2):414.
13. Arnaoutoglou C, Lykissas MG, Gelalis ID, Batistatou A, Goussia A, Doukas M, Xenakis TA. Low grade fibromyxoid sarcoma: a case report and review of the literature. Journal of Orthopaedic Surgery & Research. 2010;5(1):49.
14. Lee BJ, Park WS, Jin JM, Ha CW, Lee SH. Low grade fibromyxoid sarcoma in thigh. Clinics in Orthopedic Surgery. 2009;1(4):240.
15. Bajpai J, Shukla S, Jah M, Singh AK, Goel M, Mourya A, Sachdeva N. Low-grade fibromyxoid sarcoma around the knee involving the proximal end of the tibia and patella: a rare case report. Oncol Lett. 2014;7(4):1308.
16. Kumar Y, Khaleel M, Boothe E, Awdeh H, Wadhwa V, Chhabra A. Role of diffusion weighted imaging in musculoskeletal infections: current perspectives. Eur Radiol. 2016;27(1):1–10.
17. Lee SY, Jee WH, Jung JY, Park MY, Kim SK, Jung CK, Chung YG. Differentiation of malignant from benign soft tissue tumours: use of additive qualitative and quantitative diffusion-weighted MR imaging to standard MR imaging at 3.0 T. Eur Radiol. 2016;26(3):743–54.
18. Mastoraki A, Strigkos T, Tatakis FP, Christophi A, Smyrniotis V. Recurrent low-grade Fibromyxoid sarcoma of the neck: report of a case and review of the literature. Indian Journal of Surgical Oncology. 2015;6(3):296.
19. Oda Y, Takahira T, Kawaguchi K, Yamamoto H, Tamiya S, Matsuda S, Tanaka K, Iwamoto Y, Tsuneyoshi M. Low-grade fibromyxoid sarcoma versus low-grade myxofibrosarcoma in the extremities and trunk. A comparison of clinicopathological and immunohistochemical features. Histopathology. 2004;45(1):29–38.
20. Billings SD, Giblen G, Fanburgsmith JC. Superficial low-grade fibromyxoid sarcoma (Evans tumor): a clinicopathologic analysis of 19 cases with a unique observation in the pediatric population. Am J Surg Pathol. 2005;29(2):204.
21. Fisher C, Thway K. Aggressive fibromatosis. Pathology. 2014;46(2):135–40.
22. Diviti S, Gupta N, Hooda K, Sharma K, Lo L. Morel-Lavallee lesions-review of pathophysiology, clinical findings, imaging findings and management. J Clin Diagn Res. 2017;11(4):TE01–4.

Grade of retraction and tendon thickness correlates with MR-spectroscopically measured amount of fatty degeneration in full thickness supraspinatus tears

F. Gilbert[1*], R. H. Meffert[1], J. Schmalzl[2], A. M. Weng[3], H. Köstler[3] and L. Eden[1]

Abstract

Background: The amount of fatty degeneration (FD) has major impact on the clinical result and cuff integrity after rotator cuff repair. A quantitative analysis with magnet resonance imaging (MRI) spectroscopy was employed to analyze possible correlation of FD with tendon retraction, tendon thickness and patients' characteristics in full thickness supraspinatus tears.

Methods: Forty-two patients with full-thickness supraspinatus tears underwent shoulder MRI including an experimental spectroscopic sequence allowing quantification of the fat fraction in the supraspinatus muscle belly. The amount of fatty degeneration was correlated with tendon retraction, tendon thickness, patients' age, gender, smoker status, symptom duration and body mass index (BMI). Patients were divided in to three groups of retraction (A) 0-10 mm (*n*=), (B) 11-20 mm (*n*=) and (C) < 21 mm (*n*=) and the means of FD for each group were calculated.

Results: Tendon retraction ($R = 0.6$) and symptom duration ($R = 0.6$) correlated positively, whereas tendon thickness correlated negatively ($R = -0.6$) with the amount of FD. The fat fraction increased significantly with tendon retraction: Group (A) showed a mean fat mount of 3.7% (±4%), group (B) of 16.7% (±8.2%) and group (C) of 37.5% (±19%). BMI, age and smoker-status only showed weak to moderate correlation with the amount of FD in this cohort.

Conclusion: MRI spectroscopy revealed significantly higher amount of fat with increasing grade of retraction, symptom duration and decreased tendon thickness. Thus, these parameters may indirectly be associated with the severity of tendon disease.

Keywords: Rotator cuff, MRI, Spectroscopy, Muscle degeneration

Background

Fatty degeneration (FD) of the rotator cuff (RC) muscles is a major influencing factor for the anatomical and the clinical result after RC repair, with significant FD leading to inferior clinical results and showing higher failure rates of RC repair [1, 2]. Investigation of FD is thus essential in preoperative planning of RC repair [3–6]. The clinically widely used Goutallier scale represents a five-point semi-quantitative grading of the amount of FD and shows only low to moderate inter-observer reliability and low correlation compared to quantitative analyses [7–11]. As FD is irreversible even after successful RC repair, the surgeon has to rely on early detection and a reliable quantification of the fat fraction [12, 13]. Semi-quantitative studies using the Goutallier scale indicate a correlation between tear size, age, retraction and number of tendons involved. Several efforts to quantify the fat fraction, as single voxel spectroscopy, MR spectroscopy and chemical shift-based water-fat separation have been made. These methods have demonstrated a strong correlation of tear size and amount of FD in heterogeneous cohorts [14–16]. Nevertheless quantitative methods are lacking methodical standardization and may be difficult to apply in a clinical

* Correspondence: gilbert_f@ukw.de
[1]Department of Trauma, Hand, Plastic and Reconstructive Surgery, Julius-Maximilians-University of Würzburg, Oberdürrbacherstr. 6, D-97080 Würzburg, Germany
Full list of author information is available at the end of the article

setting, thus these techniques inevitably remain experimental and the semi-quantitative Goutallier-scale is still regarded as the "gold standard". MR Spectroscopy has been shown to enable accurate and reliable quantification of fat tissue in the RC and has been tested with other quantitative methods [8, 15, 17, 18]. The possible integration into a clinical MR scanner and the relatively easy post-processing make it attractive for clinical investigations regarding fat quantification and may add value and accuracy to evaluate the context of FD in RC tears [17].

The SPLASH technique (spectroscopic fast low angle shot) as an MR based spectroscopy allows quantification of the emitted tissue-specific spectrum in a 2nd MRI layer, its reproducibility and reliability has been reported previously [8, 15, 17]. This study investigates whether the amount of FD correlates with tendon retraction and tendon thickness and patient's baseline characteristics as age, sex, BMI, smoker status and symptom duration when MR spectroscopy is used for quantification in full thickness supraspinatus tears.

Methods

Forty-Two Patients with full thickness supraspinatus tears were included in the study. A regular MRI shoulder image was performed, which included a spectroscopy using the SPLASH (spectroscopic fast low angle shot) technique. The exact technical background, post processing and calculation of the fat fraction have been previously described by our workgroup [8, 17]. MR-Spectroscopy allows quantification in a random region of interest; for all scans a 3 Tesla MRI (Skyra, Siemens, Germany) was used. MRI parameters for the t1-weighted images were: TR = 653 ms, TE = 12 ms, FOV 180 mm and for the SPLASH Sequence: TR = 35 ms, TE = 5-25 ms, FOV 278 mm (TR = repetition time, TE = echo time, FOV = field of view). Slices were 5 mm for the spectroscopy (SPLASH technique) and 3 mm for the standard MRI. For spectroscopic analysis, the muscular borders of the supraspinatus were delineated manually, and the quantitative evaluation of the spectra was obtained using a home-built reconstruction program (MATLAB 2014b, The MathWorks, Inc., Natick, Massachusetts, United States) and the time domain fit program AMARES implemented in jMRUI) (Fig. 1).

Patient's demographic data as sex, age, smoker status, BMI and the onset of symptoms were collected from our clinical database.

One shoulder specialist resident measured the grade of retraction in mm between the lateral border of the tear and a tangent to the lateral border humeral head footprint in a coronary-t2-weighted image. Tendon thickness was measured at the thinnest portion of the tendon (Fig. 2). Patients were divided into three groups of tendon retraction (A) 0-10 mm, (B) 11-20 mm, and (C) > 20 mm. For tendon thickness 2 groups with (A) > 4 mm and (B) < 4 mm were distinguished.

Patients were divided into 2 groups for BMI: (A) < 25 (normal weight) and (B) < 25 (over weight).

For all groups the mean fat fraction and standard deviation were calculated. Parameters were tested for normal distribution using student's T Test. Level of significance was calculated using the independent samples Mann-Whitney U-test and the Kruskal-Wallis test. For correlation between fat fraction and different parameters Pearson's R was calculated. All statistical analyses were performed using SPPS version 14 (IBM, Armonk NY, USA). Differences were considered as statistically significant, when $p < 0.05$. Written informed consent of every patient and institutional ethic committee approval were obtained.

Results

Twenty-nine of the patients were male and 13 were female. The mean age was 62 years (± 7.7; minimum: 43; maximum: 79 years). The mean fat fraction for all individuals was 19% (± 18). For males the mean fat fraction

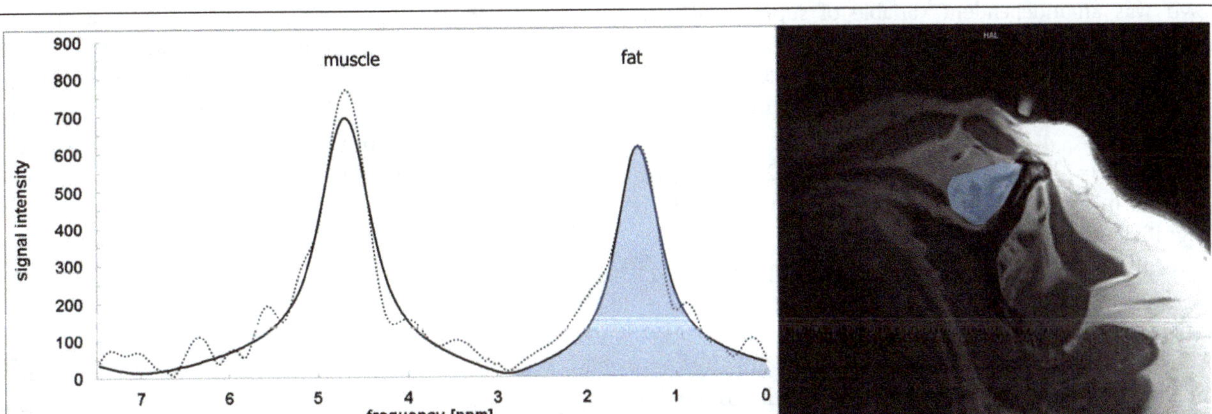

Fig. 1 MRI Spectroscopy and para sagittal MRI of the Fossa supraspinata: MRI spectroscopy revealed a fat fraction of 44%. The amount of fat is represented as the area under the curve from the second peak in the spectrogram, the first peak represents water respectively muscle

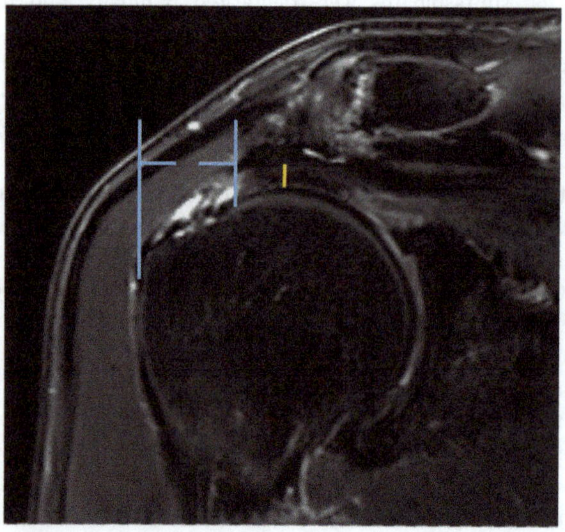

Fig. 2 Tendon retraction and thickness were measured in the coronar plane of a t2-weighted MRI slice. Tendon retraction was measured between the lateral margin of the ruptured tendon and the lateral border of the supraspinatus foot print. Tendon thickness was measured at the thinnest portion of the tendon (yellow line)

was 16.2% and for females 25.1% ($p = 0.23$) However, the differences did not reach the level of significance.

Subdivision of tendon retraction into three groups revealed a significant increase of the fat fraction with growing tendon retraction. The mean retraction for all individuals was 15 mm (±14). Individuals with tendons retracted between 0 and 10 mm had a mean fat fraction of 3.7% between 11 and 20 mm 16.7% and greater 20 mm had a mean fat fraction of 37% ($p = 0.0008$).

Tendons thinner than 4 mm had significant higher fat fraction (31.5%) than tendons thicker than 4 mm (9.6%). Duration of symptoms showed significant differences as patients with symptoms longer than 12 months had a mean fat amount of 32.5 and patients with symptoms lesser than 12 months of 8.9% ($p < 0.0001$).

BMI was an independent variable of supraspinatus fat fraction as patients with a BMI < 25 had a mean fat fraction of 15.9% and patients with a BMI > 25 of 17.8% ($p = 0.78$).

Correlation between age and amount of FD was $R = 0.21$ (p0.18).

Smokers (n=) had a mean fat fraction of 25.5% regarding 17.5% in non-smokers (n) without reaching the level of significance ($p = 0.64$). The patients' demographic data and results are shown in Tables 1 and 2 (Fig. 3).

Discussion

Spectroscopic analysis of the fat fraction in full thickness supraspinatus tears revealed positive correlation of tendon retraction and duration of symptoms with the amount of fat in the supraspinatus muscle belly and negative correlation with tendon thickness. Whereas BMI, smoker status and gender seemed to be independent from the intramuscular fat fraction.

Numerous studies reported the impact of these parameters previously, but the majority of these studies relied on the Goutallier scale [5, 19, 20]. Reliability and accuracy of this scale is debatable, as quantitative comparisons revealed a lack of accuracy especially when high amounts of fat occur, as the division between grade 3 and 4 becomes imprecise [8, 16]. The exact pathophysiologic mechanisms of FD are not completely understood and distinction between fatty atrophy and infiltration and vice versa remains imprecise. Scientifically differentiation between these two entities may not be prudent, both may be merged under the term fatty degeneration.

Table 1 Amount of fat fraction in the supraspinatus muscle belly in the different subgroups

Tendon Retraction [mm]	n	Fat fraction [%]	SD [%]
0–10	15×	3.7	4.2
11–20	13×	16.7	8.2
20	14×	37.5	19.7
Tendon Thickness [mm]			
Larger than 4	24×	9.6	12
Thinner than 4	18×	31.5	19.3
Duration [months]			
1–12	20×	8.9	8.7
> 12	22×	32.5	21.3
Age [years]			
43–55	11×	12.9	15.9
56–65	17×	22.1	20.3
> 65	14×	20	18.4
BMI			
< 25	16×	15.9	19.6
> 25	26×	17.8	18.3
Sex			
Male	11×	16.2	18.2
Female	31×	25.1	19.24
Smoker Status			
Smoker	7×	25,50	18,2
Non-smoker	35×	17,50	18,85

Table 2 Patients characteristics

Patients' features	
Total No. of patients	42
Sex, female: male	29:13
Age [years]	62 (±7.7)
Duration of symptoms [months]	12.3 (±7)
BMI [kg/m^2]	29 (±4.4)
Tendon retraction [mm]	15.6 (13.7)

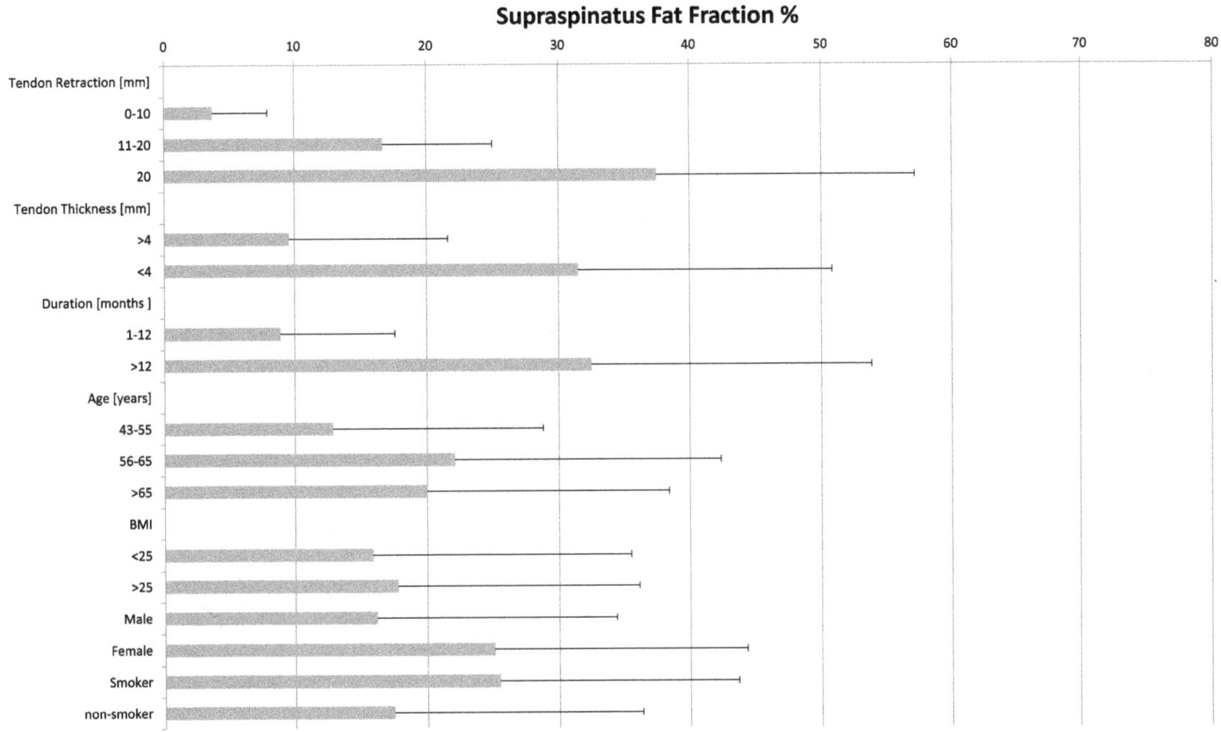

Fig. 3 Diagram of mean fat fraction and standard deviation in the supraspinatus muscle belly in different subgroups

This study found high correlation of tendon retraction with the supraspinatus fat fraction. Tendon retraction is known to strongly correlate with the amount of FD, as it leads to ultrastructural changes in muscle fiber orientation and accumulation of fat cells in the disorientated myofibrillar structure [21, 22]. Different clinical and experimental study designs using the Goutallier method and quantitative methods have revealed that retraction and the amount of fat fraction show high correlation, which has been recently supported by a quantitative study by Lee et al. who found a linear relationship between those variables [14, 16, 21]. Another MRI investigation by Fukuta et al. showed reduction of the cross sectional area of the infraspinatus muscle with progressing retraction [23]. This study furthermore supports these findings, with only very few studies using quantitative methods to this date.

Histological analysis showed that tendon degeneration increases with the progress of tendon disease [24]. Tendon thickness has not been assessed yet in correlation with FD. This study could clearly demonstrate that decrease of tendon thickness correlates with increasing fat fraction.

Symptom duration was also a strong predictor of fatty degeneration in this cohort. This supports the findings of Lee et al., who found a nearly linear relationship in a cohort of 187 patients between symptom duration and the RC fat fraction using a chemical shift MRI [16].

The role of gender to the muscular fat fraction remains controversial, as Barry et al. found that older women with substantial defects more likely develop high fat fractions. Our data indicate higher amount of fat in the female cohort without reaching the level of significance. As only 11 women were included in our study these results may not be representative. Yet, the surgeon should be aware of accelerated development of FD in women.

BMI was independent from intramuscular fat fraction in our cohort. In contrast to our findings Lee et al. found a linear relation between BMI and fat fraction. As increasing BMI has been described to correlate with the fat fraction in the paravertebral muscles its impact to shoulder girdle has not been investigated yet [25]. The difference of the studies remains unclear, but as this study focuses on individuals with full thickness tears, the study of Lee et al. involved healthy and younger individuals. So, the effect of BMI might be attenuated by the other factors with higher impact to the development of FD.

Smokers in this cohort showed higher fat fractions without reaching the level of significance, if smoking has a direct effect to the muscle structure ore promotes FD is not known, but it may represent a less active life style which is related to development of sarcopenia [26].

While this study is an analysis of FD and correlating findings, it may be concluded decreasing tendon diameter as well as increasing retraction may indicate the severity of FD. Although a clinical algorithm cannot be established yet, quantitative analyzation might be able to help identify irreparable RC tears and predict postoperative results after RC repair.

Conclusion

Detailed understanding of tendon disease needs quantitative methods as the widely used semi-quantitative scales are imprecise and implicate a high amount of guessing. Prospective quantitative assessment of the fat fraction may be a valuable tool to understand the dynamic of fatty degeneration in tendon disease and the effect of RC-repair to its development. The long-distance goal would be identification of a fat fraction threshold when RC repair might be no more beneficial.

Abbreviations

BMI: Body mass index; FD: Fatty degeneration.; mm: Millimeter.; MRI: Magnet resonance imaging.; RC: Rotator cuff.; SPLASH: Spectroscopic fast low angle shot.

Funding

This publication was funded by the German Research Foundation (DFG) and the University of Würzburg in the funding program Open Access Publishing.

Authors' contributions

FG: made substantial contribution in design and conception of the study, wrote the manuscript, RM: made substantial contribution in design and conception of the study, revisited the manuscript critically, JS: made substantial contribution in design and conception of the study, revisited the manuscript critically, AW: performed acquisition of data and interpretation of data (spectroscopy), revisited the manuscript critically, HK: performed acquisition of data and interpretation of data (spectroscopy), revisited the manuscript critically, LE: made substantial contribution in design and conception of the study, revisited the manuscript.

All authors approved the final version of the manuscript.

Competing interests

The authors declare that they have no competing interests.

Author details

[1]Department of Trauma, Hand, Plastic and Reconstructive Surgery, Julius-Maximilians-University of Würzburg, Oberdürrbacherstr. 6, D-97080 Würzburg, Germany. [2]Department of Traumatology and Hand Surgery, St. Vincentius Klinik, ViDia Kliniken, Suedendstraße 32, D-76137 Karlsruhe, Germany. [3]Department of Radiology, Julius-Maximilians-University of Würzburg, Oberdürrbacherstr. 6, D-97080 Würzburg, Germany.

References

1. Gerber C, Schneeberger AG, Hoppeler H, Meyer DC. Correlation of atrophy and fatty infiltration on strength and integrity of rotator cuff repairs: a study in thirteen patients. J Shoulder Elb Surg. 2007;16:691–6.
2. Yamaguchi H, Suenaga N, Oizumi N, Hosokawa Y, Kanaya F. Will preoperative atrophy and fatty degeneration of the shoulder muscles improve after rotator cuff repair in patients with massive rotator cuff tears? Adv Orthop. 2012;2012:195876.
3. Gladstone JN, Bishop JY, Lo IKY, Flatow EL. Fatty infiltration and atrophy of the rotator cuff do not improve after rotator cuff repair and correlate with poor functional outcome. Am J Sports Med. 2007;35:719–28.
4. Goutallier D, Postel JM, Lavau L, Bernageau J. Impact of fatty degeneration of the suparspinatus and infraspinatus msucles on the prognosis of surgical repair of the rotator cuff. Rev Chir Orthop Reparatrice Appar Mot. 1999;85:668–76.
5. Oh JH, et al. Prognostic factors affecting anatomic outcome of rotator cuff repair and correlation with functional outcome. Arthrosc -J Arthrosc Relat Surg. 2009;25:30–9.
6. Ohzono H, et al. Effect of preoperative fatty degeneration of the rotator cuff muscles on the clinical outcome of patients with intact tendons after arthroscopic rotator cuff repair of large/massive cuff tears. Am J Sports Med. 2017;45:2975–81.
7. Battaglia PJ, Maeda Y, Welk A, Hough B, Kettner N. Reliability of the Goutallier classification in quantifying muscle fatty degeneration in the lumbar multifidus using magnetic resonance imaging. J Manip Physiol Ther. 2014;37(3):190–7. https://doi.org/10.1016/j.jmpt.2013.12.010.
8. Gilbert F, Böhm D, Eden L, Schmalzl J, Meffert RH, Köstler H, Ziegler D.Comparing the MRI-based Goutallier Classification to an experimental quantitative MR spectroscopic fat measurement of the supraspinatus muscle. BMC Musculoskelet Disord. 2016;17(1). https://doi.org/10.1186/s12891-016-1216-3.
9. Lippe J, et al. Inter-rater agreement of the Goutallier, Patte, and Warner classification scores using preoperative magnetic resonance imaging in patients with rotator cuff tears. Arthroscopy. 2012;28:154–9.
10. Oh JH, Kim SH, Choi J-A, Kim Y, Oh CH. Reliability of the grading system for fatty degeneration of rotator cuff muscles. Clin Orthop Relat Res. 2010;468:1558–64.
11. Slabaugh Ma, et al. Interobserver and Intraobserver reliability of the Goutallier classification using magnetic resonance imaging: proposal of a simplified classification system to increase reliability. Am J Sports Med. 2012;40:1728–34.
12. Burkhart SS, Barth JRH, Richards DP, Zlatkin MB, Larsen M. Arthroscopic repair of massive rotator cuff tears with stage 3 and 4 fatty degeneration. Arthroscopy. 2007;23:347–54.
13. Oh JH, Kim SH, Kang JY, Oh CH, Gong HS. Effect of age on functional and structural outcome after rotator cuff repair. Am J Sports Med. 2010;38:672–8.
14. Pfirrmann CWA, et al. Assessment of fat content in supraspinatus muscle with proton MR spectroscopy in asymptomatic volunteers and patients with supraspinatus tendon lesions. Radiology. 2004;232:709–15.
15. Kenn W, et al. 2D SPLASH: a new method to determine the fatty infiltration of the rotator cuff muscles. Eur Radiol. 2004;14:2331–6.
16. Lee S, et al. Magnetic resonance rotator cuff fat fraction and its relationship with tendon tear severity and subject characteristics. J Shoulder Elb Surg. 2015;24:1442–51.
17. Köstler H, Kenn W, Hümmer C, Böhm D, Hahn D. 2D-SPLASH spectroscopy to determine the fat/water ratio in the muscle of the rotator cuff. Rofo. 2002;174:991–5.
18. Gilbert F, Klein D, Weng AM, Köstler H, Schmitz B, Schmalzl J, Böhm D. Supraspinatus muscle elasticity measured with real time shear wave ultrasound elastography correlates with MRI spectroscopic measured amount of fatty degeneration. BMC Musculoskelet Disord. 2017;18(1). https://doi.org/10.1186/s12891-017-1911-8.
19. Shen PH, et al. Long-term functional outcomes after repair of rotator cuff tears correlated with atrophy of the supraspinatus muscles on magnetic resonance images. J Shoulder Elb Surg. 2008;17(1 Suppl):1S-7S.
20. Mellado JM, et al. Surgically repaired massive rotator cuff tears: MRI of tendon integrity, muscle fatty degeneration, and muscle atrophy correlated with intraoperative and clinical findings. AJR Am J Roentgenol. 2005;184:1456–63.
21. Gerber C, Meyer DC, Schneeberger AG, Hoppeler H, von Rechenberg B. Effect of tendon release and delayed repair on the structure of the muscles of the rotator cuff: an experimental study in sheep. J Bone Joint Surg Am. 2004;86–A:1973–82.
22. Meyer DC, Hoppeler H, von Rechenberg B, Gerber C. A pathomechanical concept explains muscle loss and fatty muscular changes following surgical tendon release. J Orthop Res. 2004;22:1004–7.

Permissions

All chapters in this book were first published in MD, by BioMed Central; hereby published with permission under the Creative Commons Attribution License or equivalent. Every chapter published in this book has been scrutinized by our experts. Their significance has been extensively debated. The topics covered herein carry significant findings which will fuel the growth of the discipline. They may even be implemented as practical applications or may be referred to as a beginning point for another development.

The contributors of this book come from diverse backgrounds, making this book a truly international effort. This book will bring forth new frontiers with its revolutionizing research information and detailed analysis of the nascent developments around the world.

We would like to thank all the contributing authors for lending their expertise to make the book truly unique. They have played a crucial role in the development of this book. Without their invaluable contributions this book wouldn't have been possible. They have made vital efforts to compile up to date information on the varied aspects of this subject to make this book a valuable addition to the collection of many professionals and students.

This book was conceptualized with the vision of imparting up-to-date information and advanced data in this field. To ensure the same, a matchless editorial board was set up. Every individual on the board went through rigorous rounds of assessment to prove their worth. After which they invested a large part of their time researching and compiling the most relevant data for our readers.

The editorial board has been involved in producing this book since its inception. They have spent rigorous hours researching and exploring the diverse topics which have resulted in the successful publishing of this book. They have passed on their knowledge of decades through this book. To expedite this challenging task, the publisher supported the team at every step. A small team of assistant editors was also appointed to further simplify the editing procedure and attain best results for the readers.

Apart from the editorial board, the designing team has also invested a significant amount of their time in understanding the subject and creating the most relevant covers. They scrutinized every image to scout for the most suitable representation of the subject and create an appropriate cover for the book.

The publishing team has been an ardent support to the editorial, designing and production team. Their endless efforts to recruit the best for this project, has resulted in the accomplishment of this book. They are a veteran in the field of academics and their pool of knowledge is as vast as their experience in printing. Their expertise and guidance has proved useful at every step. Their uncompromising quality standards have made this book an exceptional effort. Their encouragement from time to time has been an inspiration for everyone.

The publisher and the editorial board hope that this book will prove to be a valuable piece of knowledge for researchers, students, practitioners and scholars across the globe.

List of Contributors

Rebecca J. Crawford
Institute for Health Sciences, Zurich University of Applied Sciences, Technikumstrasse 81, Postfach, CH-8401 Winterthur, Switzerland
Faculty of Health Professions, Curtin University, Perth, Australia

Jon Cornwall
Institute for Health Sciences, Zurich University of Applied Sciences, Technikumstrasse 81, Postfach, CH-8401 Winterthur, Switzerland
Graduate School of Nursing, Midwifery and Health, Victoria University of Wellington, Wellington, New Zealand

Rebecca Abbott
Department of Physical Therapy and Human Movement Sciences, Feinberg School of Medicine, Northwestern University, Chicago, USA

James M. Elliott
Institute for Health Sciences, Zurich University of Applied Sciences, Technikumstrasse 81, Postfach, CH-8401 Winterthur, Switzerland
Department of Physical Therapy and Human Movement Sciences, Feinberg School of Medicine, Northwestern University, Chicago, USA
School of Health and Rehabilitation Sciences, University of Queensland, Brisbane, Australia

Okihiro Onishi, Kazuya Ikoma, Masamitsu Kido, Yukichi Kabuto, Keiichiro Ueshima and Toshikazu Kubo
Department of Orthopaedics, Graduate School of Medical Science, Kyoto Prefectural University of Medicine, 602-8566 465, Kajiicho, Kamigyo-ku Kyoto-shi, Kyoto, Japan

Ken-ichi Matsuda and Masaki Tanaka
Department of Anatomy and Neurobiology, Graduate School of Medical Science, Kyoto Prefectural University of Medicine, Kyoto, Japan

Judith E. Gold
Centre for Musculoskeletal Research, Department of Occupational and Public Health Sciences, University of Gävle, Gävle, Sweden
Gold Standard Research Consulting, 830 Montgomery Ave, Bryn Mawr, PA, USA

David M. Hallman, Fredrik Hellström, Albert G. Crenshaw and Svend Erik Mathiassen
Centre for Musculoskeletal Research, Department of Occupational and Public Health Sciences, University of Gävle, Gävle, Sweden

Martin Björklund
Centre for Musculoskeletal Research, Department of Occupational and Public Health Sciences, University of Gävle, Gävle, Sweden
Department of Community Medicine and Rehabilitation, Physiotherapy, Umeå University, Umeå, Sweden

Mary F. Barbe
Department of Anatomy and Cell Biology, Temple University Medical School, Philadelphia, PA, USA

Sayed Ali
Department of Radiology, Temple University Medical School, Philadelphia, PA, USA

Tae Hyung Kim, Sung Gyu Moon and Na Ra Kim
Department of Radiology, Konkuk University Medical Center, Konkuk University School of Medicine, 120-1 Neungdong-ro, Gwangjin-gu, Seoul 05030, South Korea

Hong-Geun Jung
Department of Orthopedic Surgery, Konkuk University Medical Center, Konkuk University School of Medicine, Seoul, South Korea

L. Torén and H. Hebelka
Department of Radiology, Sahlgrenska University Hospital, Gothenburg, Sweden
Institute of Clinical Sciences, Sahlgrenska Academy, University of Gothenburg, Gothenburg, Sweden

I. Kasperska
Department of Radiology, Sahlgrenska University Hospital, Gothenburg, Sweden

H. Brisby
Department of Orthopaedics, Sahlgrenska University Hospital, Gothenburg, Sweden
Institute of Clinical Sciences, Sahlgrenska Academy, University of Gothenburg, Gothenburg, Sweden

K. Lagerstrand
Department of Medical Physics and Techniques, Sahlgrenska University Hospital, Gothenburg, Sweden
Institute of Clinical Sciences, Sahlgrenska Academy, University of Gothenburg, Gothenburg, Sweden

Vikas V. Patel
The Spine Center, University of Colorado Hospital, Denver, CO, USA

Gunnar B. J. Andersson
Midwest Orthopaedics, RUSH University Medical Center, Chicago, IL, USA

Steven R. Garfin
Department of Orthopaedic Surgery, University of California, San Diego, CA, USA

Donald L. Resnick
Department of Radiology, University of California, San Diego, CA, USA

Jon E. Block
2210 Jackson Street, Ste. 401, San Francisco, CA 94115, USA

Takashi Nawata, Makoto Kubo, Keiji Oishi, Tadayoshi Ikegami, Shigeki Kobayashi and Masafumi Yano
Department of Medicine and Clinical Science, Yamaguchi University Graduate School of Medicine, 1-1-1 Minamikogushi, Ube, Yamaguchi 755-8505, Japan

Takafumi Nomura and Munemasa Okada
Department of Radiology, Yamaguchi University Graduate School of Medicine, 1-1-1 Minamikogushi, Ube 755-8505, Japan

Kosaku Shiragami
Department of Internal Medicine, Saiseikai Yamaguchi General Hospital, 2-11, Midorimachi, Yamaguchi 753-8517, Japan

Jonas Pogorzelski, Knut Beitzel, Francesco Ranuccio, Andreas B. Imhoff and Sepp Braun
Department of Orthopaedic Sports Medicine, Hospital Rechts der Isar, University of Munich, Ismaninger Street 22, 81675 Munich, Germany

Klaus Wörtler
Department of Radiology, Hospital Rechts der Isar, University of Munich, Munich, Germany

Peter J. Millett
Orthopaedic Surgery, The Steadman Clinic, Vail, CO, USA

David B. Berry
Department of Bioengineering, University of California San Diego, La Jolla, CA, USA

Jennifer Padwal
Department of Medicine, University of California San Diego, La Jolla, CA, USA

Seth Johnson and Callan L. Parra
Department of Orthopaedic Surgery, University of California San Diego, 9500 Gilman Drive (MS 0863), La Jolla, CA 92093, USA

Samuel R. Ward
Department of Bioengineering, University of California San Diego, La Jolla, CA, USA
Department of Orthopaedic Surgery, University of California San Diego, 9500 Gilman Drive (MS 0863), La Jolla, CA 92093, USA
Department of Radiology, University of California San Diego, 9500 Gilman Drive (MS 0863), La Jolla, CA 92093, USA

Bahar Shahidi
Department of Orthopaedic Surgery, University of California San Diego, 9500 Gilman Drive (MS 0863), La Jolla, CA 92093, USA
Department of Radiology, University of California San Diego, 9500 Gilman Drive (MS 0863), La Jolla, CA 92093, USA

Anne Heizelmann, Sümeyra Tasdemir, Julian Schmidberger and Wolfgang Kratzer
Department of Internal Medicine I, Ulm University Hospital, Albert-Einstein-Allee, 23 89081 Ulm, Germany

Tilmann Gräter
Department of Diagnostic and Interventional Radiology, Ulm University Hospital, Albert-Einstein-Allee 23, Ulm 89081, Germany

Beate Grüner
Department of Internal Medicine III, Ulm University Hospital, Albert-Einstein-Allee 23, Ulm 89081, Germany

Yeon Ho Kim, Jin Woo Park and Kahyun Kim
Department of Orthopedic Surgery, Seoul National University Bundang Hospital, Seongnam, South Korea

Hyun Sik Gong
Department of Orthopedic Surgery, Seoul National University Bundang Hospital, Seongnam, South Korea
Department of Orthopedic Surgery, Seoul National University Bundang Hospital, Seoul National University College of Medicine, 300 Gumi-dong, Bundang-gu, Seongnam-si, Gyeonggi-do 463-707, South Korea

Hyun Kyung Yang
Department of Radiology, Seoul National University Bundang Hospital, Seongnam, South Korea

Goo Hyun Baek
Department of Orthopedic Surgery, Seoul National University Hospital, Seoul, South Korea

Marina Katsu, Tetsuro Ohba, Shigeto Ebata and Hirotaka Haro
Department of Orthopaedic Surgery, University of Yamanashi, 1110, Shimokato, Chuo, Yamanashi 409-3898, Japan

C. Sifuentes-Cantú, I. Contreras-Yáñez and V. Pascual-Ramos
Department of Immunology and Rheumatology. Instituto Nacional de Ciencias Médicas y Nutrición Salvador Zubirán, Vasco de Quiroga 15, colonia sección XVI, Tlalpan, 14000 México City, Mexico

L. Saldarriaga, A. C. Lozada and M. Gutiérrez
Division of Musculoskeletal Ultrasound. Instituto Nacional de Rehabilitación y Ortopedia, Calzada México-Xochimilco 289, Arenal de Guadalupe, 14389 México City, Mexico

Joel Glenn Buikstra
Austin Health, Austin Hospital, Heidelberg, VIC 3084, Australia

Camdon Fary and Phong Tran
Orthopaedic Surgery, Western Health, Footscray, VIC, Australia

F. Gilbert, T. M. Heintel, M. G. Jakubietz, C. Sebald and R. H. Meffert
Department of Trauma, Hand, Plastic and Reconstructive Surgery, Julius-Maximilians-University of Würzburg, Oberdürrbacherstr. 6, D-97080 Würzburg, Germany

H. Köstler and A. M. Weng
Department of Radiology Julius-Maximilians-University of Würzburg, Oberdürrbacherstr. 6, D-97080 Würzburg, Germany

Yogesh Kumar
Department of Radiology, Yale New Haven Health System at Bridgeport Hospital, 267 Grant Street, Bridgeport 06610, CT, USA

Nishant Gupta
Department of Radiology, St. Vincent's Medical Center, 2800 Main Street, Bridgeport 06606, CT, USA

Avneesh Chhabra
Department of Radiology, University of Texas Southwestern Medical Center, 5323 Harry Hines Blvd, Dallas 75390, TX, USA

Takeshi Fukuda
Department of Radiology, The Jikei University School of Medicine, 3-25-8 Nishi-shimbashi, Minato-ku, Tokyo 105-8461, Japan

Neetu Soni
Department of Neuroradiology, Sanjay Gandhi Postgraduate Institute of Medical Sciences, Lucknow, U.P, India

Daichi Hayashi
Department of Radiology, Yale New Haven Health System at Bridgeport Hospital, 267 Grant Street, Bridgeport 06610, CT, USA
Department of Radiology, Boston University School of Medicine, 820 Harrison Avenue, FGH Building 3rd Floor, Boston 02118, MA, USA

Jingyu Jia, Qiangqiang Wei and Xigao Cheng
Department of Orthopaedics, The Second Affiliated Hospital of Nanchang University, Nanchang City 330006, Jiangxi Province, China

Tianlong Wu and Dingwen He
Department of Orthopaedics, The Second Affiliated Hospital of Nanchang University, Nanchang City, Jiangxi Province, China

Kazuhiro Hasegawa, Masashi Okamoto and Shun Hatsushikano
Niigata Spine Surgery Center, 2-5-22 Nishi-machi, Niigata City 950-0165, Japan

Gabriel Caseiro
EOS imaging, Paris, France

Kei Watanabe
Department of Orthopaedic Surgery, Niigata University Medical and Dental Hospital, Niigata, Japan

Kyra De Coninck, Karen Hambly, John W. Dickinson and Louis Passfield
School of Sport and Exercise Sciences, University of Kent, Medway Building, Chatham Maritime, Chatham, Kent ME4 4AG, UK

Akihiko Hiyama, Hiroyuki Katoh, Daisuke Sakai, Masato Sato, Masahiro Tanaka and Masahiko Watanabe
Department of Orthopaedic Surgery, Tokai University School of Medicine, 143 Shimokasuya, Isehara, Kanagawa 259-1193, Japan

Xiaohui Zhang, Yuanjun Teng, Xinxin Yang, Rui Li, Chongwen Ma, Hong Wang, Hua Han, Bin Geng and Yayi Xia
Department of Orthopaedics, Lanzhou University Second Hospital, Lanzhou University, No. 82 Cuiyingmen, Chengguan District, Lanzhou City, Gansu Province 730030, People's Republic of China
Orthopedics Key Laboratory of Gansu Province, Lanzhou University Second Hospital, Lanzhou University, No. 82 Cuiyingmen, Chengguan District, Lanzhou City, Gansu Province 730030, People's Republic of China

Koichiro Murata, Koji Akeda, Norihiko Takegami and Akihiro Sudo
Department of Orthopaedic Surgery, Mie University Graduate School of Medicine, 2-174 Edobashi, Tsu City, Mie 514-8507, Japan

Kevin Cheng and Koichi Masuda
Department of Orthopaedic Surgery, University of California, San Diego, 9500 Gilman Dr, La Jolla, CA 92093-0863, USA

Jacob G. McPherson
Department of Biomedical Engineering, Florida International University, Miami, FL, USA
Department of Physical Therapy and Human Movement Sciences, Northwestern University Feinberg School of Medicine, Chicago, IL, USA

Andrew C. Smith
Department of Physical Therapy and Human Movement Sciences, Northwestern University Feinberg School of Medicine, Chicago, IL, USA
School of Physical Therapy, Regis University, Denver, CO, USA

Daniel A. Duben
Department of Biomedical Engineering, Florida International University, Miami, FL, USA

Katie L. McMahon
Herston Imaging Research Facility, University of Queensland Centre for Clinical Research, Herston, QLD, Australia
School of Clinical Sciences, Institute of Health and Biosciences Innovation, Queensland University of Technology, Brisbane, Australia

Marie Wasielewski
Department of Physical Therapy and Human Movement Sciences, Northwestern University Feinberg School of Medicine, Chicago, IL, USA

Todd B. Parrish
Department of Radiology, Northwestern University, Chicago, IL, USA

James M. Elliott
Department of Physical Therapy and Human Movement Sciences, Northwestern University Feinberg School of Medicine, Chicago, IL, USA
School of Health and Rehabilitation Sciences, The University of Queensland, Brisbane, Australia
Faculty of Health Sciences, The University of Sydney, Northern Sydney Local Health District, St Leonards, NSW, Australia

Mayuko Haraikawa, Masashi Suzuki, Kaiji Inoue, Eito Kozawa, Junji Tanaka and Mamoru Niitsu
Department of Radiology, Saitama Medical University, 38 Morohongo, Moroyama-machi, Iruma-gun, Saitama 350-0495, Japan

Yali Yue, Yongkang Liu, Lina Song, Xiao Chen and Zhongqiu Wang
Department of Radiology, Affiliated Hospital of Nanjing University of Chinese Medicine, 155 Hanzhong Road, Nanjing, Jiangsu 210029, People's Republic of China

Yaohui Wang
Department of Pathology, Affiliated Hospital of Nanjing University of Chinese Medicine, Nanjing, Jiangsu 210029, China
Department of Trauma, Hand, Plastic and Reconstructive Surgery, Julius-Maximilians-University of Würzburg, Oberdürrbacherstr. 6, D-97080 Würzburg, Germany

J. Schmalzl
Department of Traumatology and Hand Surgery, St. Vincentius Klinik, ViDia Kliniken, Suedendstraße 32, D-76137 Karlsruhe, Germany

A. M. Weng and H. Köstler
Department of Radiology, Julius-Maximilians-University of Würzburg, Oberdürrbacherstr. 6, D-97080 Würzburg, Germany

Index

R

S

T

U

Z